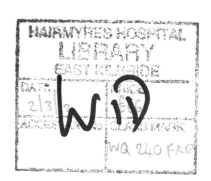

# Early Pregnancy

Edited by

**Roy G. Farquharson**
Liverpool Women's Hospital

**Mary D. Stephenson**
University of Chicago

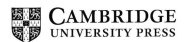

CAMBRIDGE UNIVERSITY PRESS
Cambridge, New York, Melbourne, Madrid, Cape Town, Singapore, São Paulo, Delhi, Dubai, Tokyo, Mexico City

Cambridge University Press
The Edinburgh Building, Cambridge CB2 8RU, UK

Published in the United States of America by Cambridge University Press, New York

www.cambridge.org
Information on this title: www.cambridge.org/9780521517089

First published 2010

Printed in the United Kingdom at the University Press, Cambridge

*A catalogue record for this publication is available from the British Library*

*Library of Congress Cataloguing in Publication data*
Early pregnancy / edited by Roy G. Farquharson and Mary D. Stephenson.
    p. ; cm.
Includes bibliographical references and index.
ISBN 978-0-521-51708-9 (hardback)
1. Pregnancy – Complications.   I. Farquharson, Roy G.   II. Stephenson, Mary D.
[DNLM:   1. Pregnancy Complications – diagnosis.   2.  Pregnancy Trimester, First.   3.  Early Diagnosis.
4.  Pregnancy Complications – therapy.   WQ 240 E12   2010]   I. Title.
RG571.E27   2010
618.2–dc22

2010002817

ISBN 978-0-521-51708-9 Hardback

Cambridge University Press has no responsibility for the persistence or
accuracy of URLs for external or third-party internet websites referred to in
this publication, and does not guarantee that any content on such
websites is, or will remain, accurate or appropriate.

# Contents

# Contributors

**Willem M. Ankum**
Department of Obstetrics
and Gynecology
Academic Medical Centre
Amsterdam
The Netherlands

**Ruth Bender Atik**
The Miscarriage Association
Wakefield
West Yorkshire
UK

**Carolien M. Boomsma**
Infertility and Periconceptual Medicine
Department of Reproductive Medicine
University Medical Centre Utrecht
Utrecht
The Netherlands

**Tom H. Bourne**
Department of Obstetrics and Gynaecology
Queen Charlotte's & Chelsea Hospital
London
UK

**Larry W. Chamley**
Department of Obstetrics
and Gynecology
University of Auckland
Auckland
New Zealand

**Ole B. Christiansen**
Fertility Clinic
Righospitalet
Cophenhagen
Denmark

**Fatima Crispi**
Department of Maternal Fetal Medicine
Institute's Clinic of Gynaecology, Obstetrics
and Neonatology

Hospital Clinic
Universitat de Barcelona
Barcelona
Spain

**Feroza Dawood**
University Department
Liverpool Women's Hospital
Liverpool
UK

**Pat Doyle**
London School of Hygiene and Tropical Medicine
London
UK

**Niek Exalto**
Erasmus MC
University Medical Centre
Rotterdam
The Netherlands

**Roy G. Farquharson**
Liverpool Women's Hospital
Liverpool
UK

**M. Goddijn**
Centre for Reproductive Medicine
Department of Obstetrics and Gynecology
Academic Medical Centre
University of Amsterdam
The Netherlands

**Eduard Gratacos**
Department of Maternal Fetal Medicine
Institute's Clinic of Gynaecology, Obstetrics
and Neonatology
Hospital Clinic
Universitat de Barcelona
Barcelona
Spain

**Mike Greaves**
School of Medicine and Dentistry
University of Aberdeen
Division of Applied Medicine
Aberdeen
UK

**Aisha Hameed**
Department of Obstetrics
and Gynaecology
Imperial College London
London
UK

**Barbara E. Hepworth-Jones**
The Miscarriage Association
Wakefield
West Yorkshire
UK

**Kristin Holoch**
Department of Obstetrics and
Gynecology
Greenville Hospital System
Greenville
USA

**José A. Horcajadas**
Instituto Valenciano de Infertilidad
Valencia
Spain

**Eric R. M. Jauniaux**
Academic Department of Obstetrics
and Gynaecology
Institute for Women's Health
University College London
London
UK

**Jemma Johns**
Academic Department of Obstetrics
and Gynaecology
Early Pregnancy Unit
King's College Hospital
London
UK

**Davor Jurkovic**
Department of Obstetrics and Gynaecology
University College Hospital
London
UK

**Anne Kennedy**
Department of Radiology
University Hospital
Salt Lake City
USA

**Emma Kirk**
Department of Obstetrics and Gynaecology
Whittington Hospital
London
UK

**Ruth Bunker Lathi**
Department of Obstetrics and Gynecology
Stanford University School of Medicine
Stanford
USA

**Nico J. Leschot**
Department of Clinical Genetics
Academic Medical Centre
University of Amsterdam
The Netherlands

**Bruce A. Lessey**
Department of Obstetrics and Gynecology
Greenville Hospital System
Greenville
USA

**Nick S. Macklon**
Department of Obstetrics and Gynaecology
University of Southampton
Southampton
UK

**Dimitrios Mavrelos**
Department of Obstetrics and Gynaecology
University College Hospital
London
UK

**Saskia Middeldorp**
Leiden University Medical Center
Department of Clinical Epidemiology and
Department of General Internal Medicine
Leiden
The Netherlands

**Gillian Norrie**
School of Medicine and Dentistry
University of Aberdeen
Division of Applied Medicine

Aberdeen
UK

**Errol R. Norwitz**
Department of Obstetrics and Gynecology
Tufts Medical Center
Boston
USA

**Thomas Philipp**
Danube Hospital Vienna
Vienna
Austria

**Anja Pinborg**
Fertility Clinic
Copenhagen University Hospital
Righospitalet
Copenhagen
Denmark

**Siobhan Quenby**
Liverpool Women's Hospital
Liverpool
UK

**Lesley Regan**
Department of Obstetrics
and Gynaecology
Imperial College London
London
UK

**Dominique Royère**
Department of Gynecology and Obstetrics
Hospital Bretonneau
Cedex
France

**Isaac E. Sasson**
Division of Maternal-Fetal Medicine
Department of Obstetric, Gynecological and
Reproductive Science

Yale-New Haven Hospital
New Haven
USA

**Sony Sierra**
Division of Reproductive Endocrinology
and Infertility
Department of Obstetrics and Gynecology
University of Toronto
Ontario
Canada

**Mary D. Stephenson**
Department of Obstetrics and Gynecology
University of Chicago
Chicago
USA

**Peter R. Stone**
Department of Obstetrics and Gynaecology
School of Medicine
Faculty of Medical and Health
University of Auckland
Auckland
New Zealand

**Ai-Wei Tang**
Liverpool Women's Hospital
Liverpool
UK

**Etienne Van den Abbeel**
Centre for Reproductive Medicine
AZVUB
Brussels

**Nicole S. Winkler**
Department of Radiology
University Hospital
Salt Lake City
USA

# Preface

The clear enthusiasm of clinicians and scientists engaged in early pregnancy care and research has been the springboard for the launch of this first book on early pregnancy. Authors from international organizations such as The European Society for Human Reproduction and Embryology (ESHRE), The American Society for Reproductive Medicine (ASRM) and the Royal College of Obstetrics and Gynaecology (RCOG) have been brought together through several fascinating and engaging meetings as the burgeoning area of early pregnancy research has "come of age" and matured into sentinel areas of basic science research and evidence-based practice.

In professional terms, early pregnancy sits between fertility practice and obstetrics. Early pregnancy has become an expanding area of research for embryologists, geneticists, endocrinologists and ultrasound experts plus many related core specialist areas. It truly requires a multidisciplinary team, both at the bench and at the bedside, who can work together to translate the exciting new developments in the field into clinical practice.

The editors are indebted to all of the authors for their contributions in the field of early pregnancy and for writing chapters on their unique expertise. Their enthusiasm has made the production of this book much easier than anticipated.

Roy G. Farquharson
Liverpool
Mary D. Stephenson
Chicago

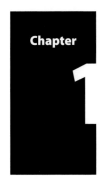

**Chapter**

**1**

# Early pregnancy – models of healthcare

Roy G. Farquharson and Niek Exalto

## Introduction

Early pregnancy problems form a major part of all gynecological emergencies. In the past, patients were admitted to the emergency receiving ward and waited for a considerable length of time before undergoing ultrasound scan and clinical assessment. With the appearance of early pregnancy assessment units (EPU), an increasing number of women are being assessed and managed as outpatient or office attenders. The advent of high-resolution transvaginal ultrasound coupled with the improved access to hCG measurements has allowed the development of models of care and improved delivery of care.

Within the UK the growth of EPU numbers has increased to the extent that over 200 active units are registered with the Association of Early Pregnancy Units (AEPU). The AEPU has set out, since it's inception in 2001, to improve the standards of early pregnancy care and to provide a clearer pathway for the patient's journey (earlypregnancy.org.uk).

In recent years ultrasound diagnosis and improved understanding of problems related to early pregnancy have led to the introduction of medical and expectant management of miscarriage and selected cases of ectopic pregnancy. Randomized controlled trials have provided evidence-based practice (rcog.org.uk/guidelines). Patient choice has emerged as a powerful selector for treatment. The mission statement from the Association of Early Pregnancy Units has the patient at the center of all activity and the multidisciplinary care structure reflects the multitasking approach of care providers.

> All women with early pregnancy problems will have prompt access to a dedicated Early Pregnancy Assessment Unit (EPU) that provides efficient evidence based care with access to appropriate information and counseling. At all times women will be supported in making informed choices about their care and management.

## Evolution

Early pregnancy loss before 12 weeks' gestation is a common event that causes a great deal of distress to women and their partners alike. Approximately 1 in 5 pregnancies will end in pregnancy loss which represents a considerable burden on individuals as well as the health-care providers.

As miscarriage causes such strong emotional reaction it is apparent that the great majority of sufferers clearly remember the event process leading up to the pregnancy loss. Most early pregnancy complications will have undergone ultrasound scan assessment. Many women recall precise details of ultrasound findings before or at the time of diagnosis. As a consequence there is a need to improve our description of early pregnancy events so that care providers and patients understand each other and use the same language to describe these findings. Upon this basis and using a pragmatic ultrasound-based approach, an attempt to replace old and misunderstood terms like blighted ovum has been made.

The nomenclature used to describe clinical events in early pregnancy has been criticized for lack of clarity and promoting confusion. There is no agreed glossary of terms or consensus regarding important gestational milestones. In particular there are old and poorly descriptive terms such as missed abortion or blighted ovum which have persisted since their introduction many years ago [1] and have not undergone revision despite the widespread application of ultrasound for accurate clinical assessment and diagnosis.

The authors are aware of these shortcomings in terminology and are keen to provide an updated glossary. The attached summary hopes to facilitate the introduction of a revised terminology in an attempt to provide clarity and to enhance uptake and use in the literature, especially patient information leaflets, as well as clinical assessment and documentation (Table 1.1).

## Recognizing the event

The commonest early pregnancy complication of spontaneous miscarriage occurs in approximately 15–20% of all pregnancies, as recorded by hospital episode statistics. The actual figure, from community-based assessment, may be up to 30%, as many cases remain unreported to hospital [2]. The great majority occurs early before 12 weeks gestational age and less than 5% occur after identification of fetal heart activity [3]. Second trimester loss, between 12 and 24 weeks, occurs less frequently and constitutes <4% of pregnancy outcomes [4]. The clinical assessment of every pregnancy loss history requires clarification of pregnancy loss type and accurate classification, whenever possible [5].

The traditional grouping of all pregnancy losses prior to 24 weeks as "abortion" may have had pragmatic origins, but it is poor in terms of definition and makes little sense. The term abortion is also confusing for the patient and its use should be abandoned. She may not realize that (spontaneous) abortion is not a termination of pregnancy because the terms medical abortion or legal abortion are used in the same way.

Increasing knowledge about early pregnancy development, with the more widespread availability of serum beta hCG measurement, the advent of high-resolution transvaginal ultrasound (TVU) and a clearer description of gestational age at pregnancy loss make for a more sophisticated assessment of previous miscarriage history. The advent of these important information milestones has not been fully realized nor incorporated into clinical event description for article publication.

The emergence of early pregnancy units (EPU) in many hospitals has addressed the need for a dedicated clinical area for the diagnosis of miscarriage and patient support at a distressing time (Box 1.1) [6,7]. With the establishment of an EPU network, it becomes more important that a standardized diagnostic classification system be employed for accurate and reproducible reporting of ultrasound findings and clinical outcomes so that direct comparisons between units can be readily understandable for both research and audit purposes.

The most recent Confidential Enquiry into Maternal Deaths (2007) conclusively demonstrates that mortality from ectopic pregnancy has not declined and is still on the increase on rates described 10 years ago [8]. As the EPU represents the most likely point of ectopic pregnancy diagnosis, the importance of standardized reporting of very early pregnancy changes requires a robust approach following recent recommendations [9].

## Length of pregnancy

Just as postnatal age begins at birth, prenatal age begins at fertilization. The embryonic period occupies the first 8 postfertilization weeks, during which organogenesis takes place. Thereafter, the fetal period is characterized by growth. Embryologists prefer the term embryonic age and assess this by using 23 internationally recognized morphological stages [10]. Clinicians, however, conventionally calculate from the first day of the last normal menstrual period (LMP). Confusion about the definition of pregnancy duration derives from use of terms such as postovulatory age, conceptual age or even misnomers like menstrual age within the published literature.

Clinicians do have to acknowledge that a woman does not become pregnant during the LMP, or during ovulation but exclusively after conception. Gestation is the condition of being carried in the womb during the interval between conception and birth. The term "gestational age" (GA) is therefore confusing, although generally accepted, and its widespread use can only be legitimized using a clear definition. The appropriate way to overcome this confusion is to choose GA based on a theoretical ovulation plus 2 weeks. As early ultrasound (US) measurements of the fetus (crown–rump length, CRL) are reproducible [11] and more accurate than the use of the LMP there is a need in publications to define GA as based on LMP and/or US. The continuing refinement of early pregnancy dating and growth studies will clearly help the patient's experience and clarify uncertainty in the clinician's mind [12].

## Ultrasound criteria

With the introduction of transvaginal ultrasound, longitudinal assessment of early pregnancy development can be made, in terms of viability and growth. Ultrasound plays a major role in maternal reassurance, where fetal cardiac activity is seen and is pivotal in the assessment of early pregnancy complications, such as vaginal bleeding [13]. However, there are limits to ultrasound resolution of normal early pregnancy development. Recent advice concludes that a

**Table 1.1** Revised nomenclature 2005 [5].

| Avoid | Prefer | Ultrasound findings |
|---|---|---|
| 1. Egg | Oocyte | |
| 2. Embryo | Fetus | Ultrasound-based definition to include fetal heart activity and/or crown–rump length >10 mm |
| 3. Embryonic age<br>Postovulatory age<br>Conceptual age<br>Menstrual age | Gestational age based on last menstrual period and/or ultrasound fetal measurement | |
| 4. Threatened abortion | Threatened miscarriage | |
| 5. Spontaneous abortion | Spontaneous miscarriage | |
| 6. Medical abortion<br>Legal abortion | Termination of pregnancy | |
| 7. Recurrent abortion<br>Habitual abortion | Recurrent miscarriage consisting of 3 early consecutive losses or 2 late pregnancy losses | |
| 8. Pregnancy test | Serum/urine level of human chorionic gonadotrophin (hCG) | |
| 9. Pre-clinical embryo loss | Biochemical pregnancy loss with description of falling low positive serum/urinary hCG | No definition of pregnancy location |
| 10. Trophoblast regression | Biochemical pregnancy loss | |
| 11. Menstrual abortion<br>Pre-clinical abortion | Biochemical pregnancy loss | Pregnancy not located on scan |
| 12. Early embryonic demise<br>Anembryonic pregnancy | Empty sac | Gestation sac with absent structures or minimal embryonic debris without heart rate activity |
| 13. Embryonic death | Fetal loss | Previous identification of crown–rump length and fetal heart activity followed by loss of heart activity |
| 14. Early abortion | Early pregnancy loss | Ultrasound definition of intrauterine pregnancy with reproducible evidence of lost fetal heart activity and/or failure of increased crown–rump length over one week, or persisting presence of empty sac, at less than 12 weeks' gestation |
| 15. Missed abortion | Delayed miscarriage | Same as for early pregnancy loss (vide supra) |
| 16. Late abortion | Late pregnancy loss | After 12 weeks gestational age where fetal measurement was followed by loss of fetal heart activity |
| 17. Hydatidiform mole<br>Partial mole<br>Molar pregnancy | Gestational trophoblastic disease (complete or partial) | |
| 18. Heterotopic pregnancy | Intrauterine plus ectopic pregnancy (e.g. tubal, cervical, ovarian, abdominal) | |
| 19. | Pregnancy of unknown location (PUL) | No identifiable pregnancy on ultrasound with positive blood/urine hCG |

**Box 1.1**  Standards in early pregnancy care

| Standard | Core | Aspirational |
|---|---|---|
| Patient information | Designated reception area. Universal use of clear, understandable terminology by all staff. | Dedicated staff constantly at reception desk to provide greeting, obtain patient details and explain structure and triage function of EPU. |
| Patient choice of management | Education of patient relevant to diagnosis and management. Open explanation of expectant, medical and surgical options. | Dedicated phone line for patient queries and electronic access to protocols from outside unit. |
| Dedicated quiet room | Room for breaking bad news away from work area. | Single-use room only with soft furnishing and absence of medical equipment. |
| Availability of service | 5 day opening during office hours. | 7/24 opening and service provision with full staffing and daily scan support. |
| Competence of scanning | Recognized ultrasound training and RCOG/BMUS preceptor assessment and validation. Register of staff competent at scanning. | Lead clinician. Presence of RCOG/BMUS trainer in EPU. Annual assessment of audited activity. |
| Blood hCG level measurement | Laboratory access to blood hCG measurement and result within 48 hours of sampling. | Same-day sampling and result with electronic result link to laboratory. |
| Written information leaflets | Visible open access to written information leaflets in EPU. | Online external access to PIL. |
| Acknowledgment of privacy and dignity | To provide individualized patient support and acknowledge confidentiality. | Place one to one care as best practice at all times. |
| Bereavement counseling | All staff trained in emotional aspects of early pregnancy loss. To enable access to counseling and provide immediate support. | To provide all emotional and psychological counseling requirements within EPU and supported by dedicated staff and related agencies. |
| Site of EPU | Geographically separate from all maternity areas. | Own EPU entrance/exit. |

diagnosis of an empty sac (previously named: anembryonic pregnancy, early embryonic demise or embryo loss) should not be made if the visible crown–rump length is less than 6 mm, as only 65% of normal embryos will display cardiac activity [14]. Repeat transvaginal ultrasound examination after at least a week showing identical features and/or the presence of fetal bradycardia is strongly suggestive of impending miscarriage [15]. The possibility of incorrect dates should always be remembered by the alert clinician. In addition, it should be remembered that when the fetus has clearly developed and the fetal heart is absent, the term "missed abortion" should be replaced by "delayed miscarriage" [16].

Gynecologists and ultrasonographers acknowledge the "embryonic" period by speaking about fetal heart action and fetal activity before the end of organogenesis. This evidence of heart action is vital to the patient who sees clear signs of life. Embryologists, by contrast, may debate the meaning of embryo in early pregnancy but embryo is more synonymous with cells and gametes in an IVF laboratory than as the pre-clinical scientific description of anatomic organogenesis. Although a clear distinction between embryonic and fetal periods is significant in teratology, we have to accept that modern terminology should reflect daily clinical practice whose description has changed in the last two decades and is more patient-centered. The term fetus receives an ultrasound definition to include fetal heart activity and/or a crown–rump length >10 mm.

## Classification of events

There has been a plea to classify pregnancy losses according to the gestational age at which they occur

**Table 1.2** Commonest pregnancy loss types based on ultrasound features.

| | | **Pregnancy loss classification** | | |
|---|---|---|---|---|
| **Type of loss** | **Typical gestation (range in weeks)** | **Fetal heart activity** | **Principal ultrasound finding** | **Beta hCG level** |
| Biochemical loss | **<6** (0–6) | Never | Pregnancy not located on ultrasound | Low then fall |
| **Early** Pregnancy loss | **6–8** (4–10) | Never | Empty sac or large sac with minimal structures without fetal heart activity | Initial rise then fall |
| **Late** Pregnancy loss | **>12** (10–20) | Lost | Crown–rump length and fetal heart activity previously identified | Rise then static or fall |

and detail the event; for example, in case of fetal demise at 8 weeks, define it as fetal death at 8 weeks gestational age. In this way, possible pathophysiological mechanisms may be postulated and studied. Historically, clinicians have grouped all pregnancy losses that occur at a gestational age prior to theoretical viability under the umbrella of "abortion."

Between 1% and 2% of fertile women will experience recurring miscarriage (RM) [17]. Recently, among researchers in the field of RM, it has been recognized that the classification of pregnancy loss is more complex as the developing pregnancy undergoes various important stages, and different pathology at the time of pregnancy loss is exhibited at these different stages. As the majority of RM cases following investigation are classified as idiopathic [17], it is generally accepted that within the idiopathic group there is considerable heterogeneity and it is unlikely that one single pathological mechanism can be attributed to their RM history. Furthermore, there is considerable debate about cause and association as the exact pathophysiological mechanisms have not been elucidated. Current research is directed at theories related to implantation, trophoblast invasion and placentation, as well as factors which may be embryopathic.

No identifiable pregnancy on ultrasound examination in combination with a positive urine or serum beta hCG pregnancy test is named a pregnancy of unknown location (PUL). Biochemical pregnancy loss is a better description than trophoblast in regression or preclinical embryo loss. After ultrasound identification of pregnancy a miscarriage can be classified as early, before 12 weeks or late, after 12 weeks.

Heterotopic pregnancy is a combination of an intrauterine pregnancy and an ectopic pregnancy.

**Table 1.3** Pregnancy success prediction matrix [3]. Following idiopathic recurring miscarriage, the predicted probability (%) of successful pregnancy is determined by maternal age and previous miscarriage history (95% confidence interval <20% in bold).

| Age (years) | Number of previous miscarriages | | | |
|---|---|---|---|---|
| | **2** | **3** | **4** | **5** |
| 20 | 92 | 90 | 88 | 85 |
| 25 | 89 | 86 | 82 | 79 |
| 30 | 84 | 80 | 76 | 71 |
| 35 | 77 | 73 | 68 | 62 |
| 40 | 69 | 64 | 58 | 52 |
| 45 | 60 | 54 | 48 | 42 |

Hydatidiform mole pregnancies and partial mole would better replaced by the term gestational trophoblastic disease, complete or partial.

## Future direction

The revision of early pregnancy nomenclature is both desirable and essential in raising the standard of reporting (Table 1.2). To improve the accuracy of observational studies it is desirable to present a clear and consistent description of the pregnancy event that can be universally understood by the reader. For randomized controlled trials of treatments, it is essential to have a clear classification of pregnancy loss type for both fetal and very early loss events. In addition, there is a strong argument for mandatory karyotyping of all pregnancy losses to exclude a lethal trisomy karyotype or triploidy. This is because, irrespective of treatment intervention, pregnancy loss has

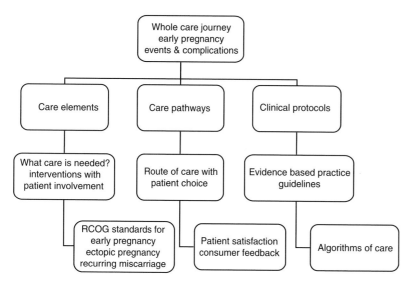

**Figure 1.1** Overview of clinical model for early pregnancy.

occurred and may have been ascribed as a "false" treatment failure. Recent papers testify to the high rate of abnormal chromosome type when pregnancy loss has occurred [16,18,19]. By actuarial analysis, the success rate for the next pregnancy can be reasonably predicted based on maternal age and number of losses (Table 1.3) [3].

The authors understand that a modernized classification system is not able to address every clinical scenario but the adoption of a revised terminology [19] is a better way forward than persisting with an antiquated description that precedes the universal use of transvaginal ultrasound findings or hCG levels. High-resolution transvaginal ultrasound provides surveillance and reassurance for the majority of women.

## Conclusions

- All women with early pregnancy complications should be evaluated in a dedicated early pregnancy unit (EPU).
- Management of patients should be conducted by trained and competent staff (Figure 1.1).
- Adequate facilities should exist to perform scans and for the measurement of hCG levels.
- Algorithms should be in place to guide management of spontaneous and recurrent miscarriage and ectopic pregnancy.
- Patients should be offered informed choice of management options.
- Patients should be furnished with written information in non-medical language.

- A quiet room conducive to breaking bad news should be located away from the work area.
- Bereavement counseling should be offered to all patients who suffer a pregnancy loss.
- Adherence to local and national standards should be audited regularly.

## References

1. Robinson HP. The diagnosis of early pregnancy failure by sonar. *Br J Obst Gynaecol* 1975; **82**: 849–57.

2. Everett C. Incidence and outcome of bleeding before the 20th week of pregnancy: prospective study from general practice. *Br Med J* 1997; **315**: 32–4.

3. Brigham S, Conlon C, Farquharson RG. A longitudinal study of pregnancy outcome following idiopathic recurring miscarriage. *Hum Reprod* 1999; **14**: 2868–71.

4. Ugwumadu A, Manyonda I, Reid F, Hay P. Effect of early oral clindamycin on late miscarriage and preterm delivery in asymptomatic women with abnormal vaginal flora and bacterial vaginosis: a randomized controlled trial. *Lancet* 2003; **361**: 983–8.

5. Farquharson RG, Jauniaux E, Exalto N, ESHRE Special Interest Group for Early Pregnancy (SIGEP). Updated and revised nomenclature for description of early pregnancy events :consensus statement. *Hum Reprod* 2005; **20**: 3008–11.

6. Royal College of Obstetricians and Gynaecologists. The Management of Early Pregnancy Loss. 2006, Greentop Guideline No 25.

7. Twigg J, Moshy R, Walker JJ, Evans J. Early pregnancy assessment units in the United Kingdom: an audit of current clinical practice. *J Clin Excell* 2002; **4**: 391–402.

8. Lewis G (ed.). *The Confidential Enquiry into Maternal and Child Health (CEMACH). Saving Mother's Lives: Reviewing Maternal Deaths to make Motherhood Safer – 2003–2005. The Seventh Report on Confidential Enquiries into Maternal Deaths in the UK*. London: CEMACH, 2007.

9. Kirk E, Condous G, Bourne T. Ectopic pregnancy deaths: what should we be doing? *Hosp Med* 2004; **65**: 657–60.

10. O'Rahilly R, Muller F. Developmental stages in human embryos: revised and new measurements. *Cells Tissues Organs* 2010; Feb 26 [Epub ahead of print].

11. Pedersen JF. Fetal crown rump length measurement by ultrasound in normal pregnancy. *BJOG* 1982; **89**: 926–30.

12. Bottomley C, Bourne T. Dating and growth in the first trimester, best practice & research. *Clin Obst Gynaecol* 2009; doi: 10.1016/j.bpobgyn.2009.01.011.

13. Jauniaux E, Kaminopetros P, El-Rafaey H. Early pregnancy loss. In CH Rodeck, MJ Whittle (eds.), *Fetal Medicine*. Churchill Livingstone, 1999; 835–47.

14. Royal College of Radiologists/ Royal College of Obstetricians and Gynaecologists. *Guidance and Ultrasound Procedures in Early Pregnancy*. London: RCOG Press, 1995.

15. Chittacharoen A, Herabutya Y. Slow fetal heart rate may predict pregnancy outcome in first-trimester threatened abortion. *Fertil Steril* 2004; **82**: 227–9.

16. Hutchon DJ, Cooper S. Missed abortion versus delayed miscarriage. *Br J Obstet Gynaecol* 1997; **104**: 73.

17. Stirrat GM. Recurrent miscarriage: definition and epidemiology. *Lancet* 1990; **336**: 673–5.

18. Philipp T, Philipp K, Reiner A, Beer F, Kalousek DK. Embryoscopic and cytogenetic analysis of 233 missed abortions: factors involved in the pathogenesis of developmental defects of early failed pregnancies. *Hum Reprod* 2003; **18**: 1724–32.

19. Bricker L, Farquharson RG. Types of pregnancy loss in recurrent miscarriage: implications for research and clinical practice. *Hum Reprod* 2002; **17**: 1345–50.

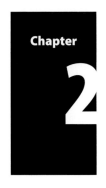

# Risk factors for miscarriage

Ruth Bender Atik, Barbara E. Hepworth-Jones and Pat Doyle

## What is a miscarriage and how common is it?

Miscarriage is the most common complication of early pregnancy. It is defined as the spontaneous end of a pregnancy at a time before fetal viability. In the UK the cut-off gestation defining a miscarriage is 24 weeks since the start of the last menstrual period (LMP). The death of a fetus at later gestations is referred to as a stillbirth.

Human reproduction is remarkably inefficient and only 30–50% of conceptions survive to a live birth (see Figure 2.1). Relatively little is known about embryo loss before the implantation stage (which happens around 20–23 days since LMP), but it is estimated from prospective studies of women attempting to conceive that around 1 in 3 pregnancies reaching the implantation stage will end in miscarriage[1–3]. The risk is strongly related to time since LMP, with around 25% of pregnancies ending in miscarriage between implantation and the 6th week since LMP [1–5]. Many of these early miscarriages go unnoticed because the woman may not know she is pregnant. After 6 weeks since LMP, the usual cut-off for defining a clinical pregnancy, recent epidemiological studies relying on self-report or linkage to clinical records find prevalences of 12–20% [6,7]. The vast majority of these occur between the 6th and 10th week since LMP, and in the second trimester of pregnancy (12–24 weeks since LMP) the likelihood of a pregnancy ending in miscarriage is only between 1 and 2%. Figure 2.1 illustrates how the risk of fetal loss varies by gestation.

The figures presented above describe the overall picture, and it is important to note that risk of miscarriage varies by individual maternal, paternal and fetal factors, which we summarize below. In this chapter we concentrate on risk factors for first-trimester miscarriage.

## Why does miscarriage happen?

The causes of miscarriage are still not wholly understood. This is surprising given how common, and distressing, the event is. The main explanation for this is that miscarriage is very difficult to study: there are few clinical registers of miscarriage, and miscarriages are often not even recorded in medical notes. Large prospective cohort studies of pregnancy are theoretically the ideal epidemiological design [8], but these take a lot of organization, take time and are expensive. A practical approach, used in many studies, is to use self-reported information, not only on the event itself but also on the suspected risk factors. Population-based surveys which ask the women themselves for their full reproductive history, including fetal losses at all gestations and relevant information on behaviors and exposures, are useful and informative if conducted with care and with attention to limiting potential biases.

In this chapter we summarize the current literature on risk factors for first-trimester miscarriage. We will concentrate on biological, social and lifestyle factors and will include findings from the National Women's Health Study (NWHS), a large UK population-based study of early miscarriage which was planned and initiated by the authors [7,9].

## Chromosomal abnormality in the fetus

There is good evidence that around a half of all miscarriages have some form of fetal chromosomal abnormality, with those ending at earlier gestations more likely to be affected than those ending later [10,11]. The largest single category of anomalies is autosomal trisomies, and molecular studies have shown that around 90% of these have their origin in maternal meiotic errors. Errors in paternal meiosis do occur and, for example, are responsible for 100% of monosomy X (Turner's syndrome) and around 50% of XXY

(Kleinfelter's syndrome) cases, but these conditions are rarer and possibly also less likely to end in miscarriage than other conditions [11].

## Maternal and paternal age

There is clear evidence that the risk of miscarriage increases with maternal age. Evidence from a large Danish study of over 1.2 million pregnancies, and from our UK study, shows a dramatic four-fold increase in risk between ages 20 and 40 [6,9] (see Figure 2.2). The risk of chromosomal anomaly is known to increase with maternal age, and this may explain much of the increase risk of miscarriage with advancing age. But it probably does not explain it all because there is some

evidence that miscarriages with normal karyotype also show a trend of increasing risk with maternal age [10]. Father's age has also been shown to be related to increased risk of miscarriage, albeit less dramatically than for mother's age [9,12,13].

## Previous reproductive history of the mother

A previous history of miscarriage has been shown to be associated with an increased risk of miscarriage in the next pregnancy [14]. We looked at this in some detail in our own study [9], and found that having a miscarriage almost doubled the risk of miscarriage in

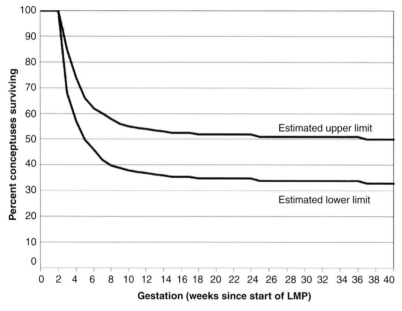

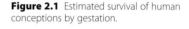
**Figure 2.1** Estimated survival of human conceptions by gestation.

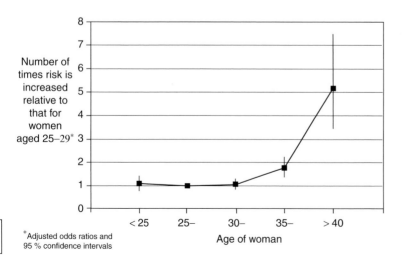

**Figure 2.2** Association between miscarriage and maternal age within National Womens Health Study [9].

*Adjusted odds ratios and 95 % confidence intervals

**Table 2.1** Summary of main findings from the National Women's Health Study [7].

| Factors associated with *increased* risk of first-trimester miscarriage | Factors associated with *decreased* risk of first-trimester miscarriage | *No evidence of association* with risk of first-trimester miscarriage |
|---|---|---|
| Socio-demographic factors | Obstetric factors | Socio-demographic factors |
| Maternal age over 35 years | Previous birth | Social class |
| Not living with the father of the baby | Nausea | Education |
| Pre-pregnancy BMI | Vitamins and diet | Obstetric factors |
| Being underweight | Taking vitamins (in particular folic acid, iron and multivitamins) | Pregnancy order (after accounting for previous pregnancy outcome) |
| Obstetric factors | Eating fresh fruit and vegetables daily | Short pregnancy interval |
| Previous miscarriage | Eating dairy products daily | Pre-eclampsia in previous pregnancies |
| Previous termination of pregnancy | Eating chocolate daily | Work |
| Longer time to conception | (Possibly eating white meat and fish twice weekly or more) | Full-time work |
| Infertility problems, particularly tubal infertility | Indicators of wellbeing | Sitting or standing for 6 hours or more per day at work |
| Assisted conception | Feeling happy and relaxed | Lifting heavy objects or people at work |
| Indicators of stress | Planned pregnancy | Diet |
| Being stressed or anxious | Air travel | Eating red meat, eggs, soya products and sugar substitutes |
| Experiencing one or more stressful/ traumatic events | Sexual intercourse (no bleeding) | Caffeine consumption (after accounting for nausea) |
| Having a stressful job | | Smoking and alcohol |
| Alcohol | | Smoking |
| Regularly drinking alcohol | | Moderate and occasional alcohol consumption (after accounting for nausea) |
| High alcohol consumption | | Exercise |
| Paternal factors | | Strenuous exercise |
| Changing partners | | Paternal smoking and alcohol |
| Paternal age over 45 years | | Paternal pre-conceptual alcohol |
| Other factors | | Paternal pre-conceptual smoking (and during the first 12 weeks) |
| Bleeding during sexual intercourse | | |

subsequent pregnancies, with the risk increasing with each additional miscarriage. By contrast, having a live birth reduced the risk of miscarriage in subsequent pregnancies by around 40% (see Table 2.1).

Although these findings may seem alarming, it is important to consider them in the context of the overall experience of women. Of the women aged 35 and over in this survey, one in six had experienced one miscarriage, one in 25 had experienced two miscarriages, and only one in 70 had experienced three or more miscarriages over their lives [9]. These data indicate that recurrent miscarriage, although a devastating outcome for women, is rare. The topic of recurrent miscarriage will be covered in more detail in a separate chapter.

There is some evidence that having a previous termination for non-medical reasons appears to increase the risk of subsequent miscarriage [9,15], although the evidence strongly suggests that this is only for surgical procedures, and not for medical procedures [16,17].

There is a strong relationship between infertility and miscarriage. The loss of an embryo before or just after implantation is probably very common, and the effect will be an apparent inability to become pregnant [18]. In our study, the risk of miscarriage was strongly associated with indicators of subfertility, such as taken to conceive or having a fertility problem diagnosed. For example, those who had taken over a year to conceive had more than double the risk of those who took less than 3 months to conceive. We also found an increased risk of miscarriage if the pregnancy had been conceived following treatment for infertility [9] (see Table 2.1).

## Socio-economic status

Studies have shown that risk of miscarriage varies by socio-economic position, but the trends are unclear [19] and most probably relate to exposure to environmental, occupational or behavioral risk factors [20] which we explore further in the sections below. In the NWHS we did not find any clear evidence of an effect of social class on risk, either when measured by the husband/partner's occupation or by the woman's own. There was, however, some suggestion of a shallow increasing trend in risk with increasing educational attainment, the opposite trend to that predicted. Interestingly, the risk of miscarriage was increased by around 73% if the couple were not married or living together, compared with those who were married or living together [9].

## Pre-pregnancy weight

Obesity before, as well as during and after, pregnancy has been highlighted as a major health issue in the developed world [21,22]. However, recent studies of miscarriage have emphasized the relationship with thinness, or low body mass index (BMI) [9,23,24]. This finding, although perhaps surprising at first sight, is biologically plausible and understandable when we consider the huge energy demands of pregnancy and breastfeeding. In the NWHS, women who were underweight at the start of their pregnancy (BMI less than 18.5) had a 75% increased risk compared with those who were within the normal BMI range. Those who were obese (BMI 30 or more) did not have an increased risk [9].

## Diet

There have been very few studies of diet in relation to miscarriage, but those that have been conducted have confirmed lower risks in women whose diets during early pregnancy were rich in green vegetables, fruit, milk, cheese, fish [9,25] and white meat [9]. Evidence for an effect of vitamin supplementation, particularly folic acid, on miscarriage risk is conflicting, but the few studies that adjust for confounding support a protective effect [9,26]. In the NWHS, taking vitamins reduced the risk of miscarriage by almost 50%. Compared with those taking no vitamins, women who took folic acid alone also had almost half the risk of miscarriage [9].

## Caffeine intake

Much has been written recently about the relationship between miscarriage risk and caffeine intake during pregnancy through coffee, tea, other caffeinated "energy" drinks, or chocolate [27–31]. But researchers have been concerned about the methods used in these surveys, including inaccurate recall or measurement of caffeine intake. Another important issue is the fact that nausea in pregnancy – which is an indicator of a successful ongoing pregnancy – may reduce coffee drinking and thus explain the effect seen [29,30]. In other words, it may be that the mothers with viable pregnancies have a *lower* level of caffeine intake, rather than mothers whose pregnancies are non-viable having a *higher* intake. In the NWHS we found a dose–response effect of estimated caffeine consumption during pregnancy on miscarriage risk, which disappeared when we controlled for the effect of nausea, indicating no independent effect of caffeine intake in our study [9].

## Alcohol intake

### Mother

Although high miscarriage rates have been reported for alcoholic women, the association between lower levels of maternal alcohol consumption and miscarriage is much less clear [27,32–41]. Two fairly recent studies from Denmark produced apparently contradictory findings: one reported that drinking in pregnancy, at 10 or more drinks per week, increased the risk by 2–3 times [39], but the other found no effect of binge drinking (five or more drinks on one occasion) on miscarriage [41]. The NWHS did not find an effect for moderate drinking (less than once a week), but there was evidence of an effect at drinking levels higher than this – most notably for those drinking every day [9].

### Father

Despite concern from animal studies about possible damaging effects of alcohol on semen characteristics, there is no convincing evidence to date that alcohol intake in the father increases the risk of miscarriage in offspring [9,32,33].

## Smoking

### Mother

Despite a widespread belief that smoking before or during pregnancy increases the risk of miscarriage, the evidence is in fact inconsistent [34,42–46]. This probably reflects differences in methodology, especially with regard to measuring smoking and the ability of the study to take confounding factors into consideration. In the NWHS we did not find strong evidence for a link between smoking in early pregnancy and risk of miscarriage [9].

### Father

The evidence here is more consistent. The few studies that have examined paternal smoking around the time of early pregnancy have not confirmed an effect on miscarriage risk [9,42,44,47].

## Physical and psychological stress

Evidence to link the classic occupational physical stressors of lifting, standing, noise and cold with miscarriage is not very strong [48,49]. The NWHS did not find evidence for a link between prolonged standing or lifting heavy objects in early pregnancy and miscarriage, and indeed found no impact of working in any capacity during pregnancy [9]. Two studies from Scandinavia have reported that exercise early in pregnancy [50], or physical strain of any type around the time of implantation [51], is associated with an increased risk of miscarriage, but the NWHS did not find an association between strenuous exercise in pregnancy and risk of miscarriage [9].

A very clear finding from the NWHS was the impact of stressful life events, a stressful job situation, and feelings of anxiety and depression on the risk of miscarriage [9]. Feelings of wellbeing were protective, which may explain the apparent reduced risk associated with having sexual intercourse during pregnancy [9]. Other literature has reported similar findings [24,52–54], and a recent study has confirmed a link between the level of maternal cortisol (the "stress" hormone) in the first 3 weeks following conception and probability of miscarrying that pregnancy [55].

## How can women and their partners be advised about miscarriage?

There remain many questions about risk factors for miscarriage and further good quality research is essential before it is possible to give unequivocal advice. In the meantime, how can advice be given to women and their partners in order to give their pregnancies the best possible chance of success, especially when studies continue to be reported in the lay media and often cause anxiety and concern? The next section of this chapter, based on the information in the earlier section, will look at this issue, including consideration of emotional reactions and strategies for coping.

## The concept of risk

The concept of risk is generally poorly understood, yet it is essential in order for relevant information to be imparted and acted upon. It is also crucial in order to reduce self-blame and guilt should the pregnancy miscarry.

It is important to stress that increased risk does not equate to cause. It may be helpful to give relevant examples of increased risk and cause, for example heavy smokers who never develop smoking-related diseases and light smokers who do. This is further complicated in the case of miscarriage as it is usually not possible to find a definite cause, so it is generally not possible to correlate miscarriage with a specific risk factor.

Those who experience miscarriage are generally eager to discover a cause, especially if it can reduce the risk in future pregnancies. Many find it hard to accept the usual protocol of investigations after three miscarriages and seek medical investigations after one or two miscarriages. In reality, however, identifying a specific problem is more likely to mean an increased, rather than a decreased risk.

## Which risks to discuss?

This needs to be tailored to the individual patient. Many of the potential and actual risk factors for miscarriage cannot be changed, so it may be important to provide a realistic picture of the likelihood of success of subsequent pregnancies. This should include sensitive but realistic discussion of immutable factors such as parental age and pregnancy history (Table 2.2).

**Table 2.2** Factors affecting the risk of miscarriage and over which there is little or no control.

| Factors associated with increased risk |
|---|
| Being over 35. The risk is greatest for women over 40, who are five times more likely to miscarry than those aged 25–29 |
| Having one or more previous miscarriages |
| Having a termination for non-medical reasons |
| Time to conceive. Women who take more than a year to conceive are twice as likely to miscarry as those who conceive within 3 months |
| Fertility problems, particularly those affecting the fallopian tubes |
| Assisted conception |
| Father over 45 |
| Factors associated with reduced risk |
| A previous live birth |
| A planned pregnancy |
| Nausea in early pregnancy |

**Table 2.3** Factors affecting the risk of miscarriage and over which there *may* be control.

| Factors associated with increased risk |
| --- |
| Being underweight, with a body mass index of less than 18.5 before pregnancy |
| Regular/heavy drinking. Risks are highest for women who drink every day and/or more than 14 units a week |
| Stress. Women under continuing stress (e.g. having a very stressful or demanding job) are more likely to miscarry. It may be possible to reduce some sources of stress e.g. moving jobs |
| Factors associated with reduced risk |
| Taking vitamins, particularly folic acid, iron or multivitamins containing them |
| Eating fruit and vegetables, dairy products and chocolate on most days and (possibly) eating fish or white meat twice weekly or more |
| Feeling happy, relaxed and in control |

**Table 2.4** Factors which do not appear to affect the risk of miscarriage.

| |
| --- |
| Pregnancy order i.e. whether it is a first or later pregnancy |
| Having a short interval since the last pregnancy |
| Having pre-eclampsia in a previous pregnancy |
| Eating red meat, eggs, soya products and sugar substitutes |
| Working full time |
| Work involving moderate physical activity |
| Partner's alcohol consumption in the 3 months before conception |
| Partner's smoking either before conception or during the pregnancy |
| Sex – as long as there is no bleeding |
| Air travel |

**Table 2.5** Factors where evidence of an associated increased risk appears contradictory and/or weak and where precaution may best be advised.

| |
| --- |
| Caffeine |
| Being overweight or obese |
| Smoking |
| Strenuous exercise |

It may be equally important to concentrate discussion on those factors over which there is some control, such as consumption of vitamins and fresh fruit and vegetables during the pregnancy, reducing drinking or reaching a BMI of at least 18.5 if underweight (Table 2.3). Consideration may also be given to discussing factors which may cause concern, but for which *either* there is no evidence of effect on risk, either negative or positive (Table 2.4) *or* where evidence is contradictory and/or weak (Table 2.5)

# Emotional reactions

Miscarriage can be a very unhappy and frightening experience. For many women, and their partners too, it represents the loss of a baby and the accompanying hopes, plans and dreams for that child. This can be true whether the miscarriage occurs early or late in the pregnancy and feelings of grief and loss may be considerable whatever the gestation. A range of personal, social and cultural factors, including previous pregnancy or fertility history, can also influence the emotional response to miscarriage.

For many women and their partners, miscarriage comes as a complete shock. Many will have spent years successfully controlling their fertility and thus assume that conception and pregnancy are also within their control. They may not know the true incidence of miscarriage or which of the reported risk factors – caffeine, age, air travel, diet – really do pose a risk. Even if they do, they rarely expect miscarriage to happen to them.

Women who have previously experienced miscarriage, especially repeated miscarriages, may have a heightened awareness of the risk of miscarriage. Many will be particularly anxious during pregnancy, especially in the weeks leading up to the gestation of their previous loss. But they too may be shocked by a recurrence, particularly if they passed their "vulnerable" date or already had a positive scan result – or, indeed, if they received treatment before or during the pregnancy for a diagnosed condition, such as antiphospholipid syndrome.

# Was it something I did?

In many cases, one of the first questions asked after miscarriage is *Why did it happen?* It is an understandable and common reaction to many medical problems. We seek to make sense of what has happened, to find an explanation, a clear cause and thus, potentially, a cure or at least a guide to preventing a recurrence. In a small minority of cases, you may be able to provide an answer but for most, the question remains unanswered. In the absence of an explanation, however, most women will seek to provide one, for example:

ACCEPTANCE: There must have been something the matter with the baby – these things happen.

BLAME: It might be because I didn't get a scan early enough, didn't get good care etc. . . .

GUILT/SELF-BLAME: It must be my fault – something I did or didn't do.

The third reaction, guilt, is the most common. Whether they are informed by friends and family, the media, Internet sites, medical and/or patient information, women cite a wide range of possible causes. High on the list are exercise, heavy lifting, eating spicy food, workplace stress, electromagnetic fields (pylons and mobile phone masts), drinking coffee and a previous termination. Some think that negative thoughts and feelings about the pregnancy, such as considering a termination, may have caused their miscarriage. If these or any other known risk factors apply, they will be seen as a likely cause.

# Information and support

When trying to make sense of cause and effect, women and their partners may need:

CLEAR EXPLANATIONS to enable them to understand the difference between risk and cause (it may be useful to use other examples, such as smoking and heart disease).

CLEAR INFORMATION so they recognize what might be in their power to change or moderate (drinking less alcohol, eating more fruit and vegetables) and what they cannot change (age, pregnancy history).

INFORMATION to help them understand that however much they reduce known risk factors, some factors (such as random chromosomal abnormalities) are beyond their – or your – control.

ACCURATE ASSESSMENT OF MEDIA REPORTS, as it is not uncommon for miscarriage to be featured in the lay press, with reports usually focusing on either a newly identified cause or a new/miracle treatment. These reports often refer back to specialist medical literature and it is important for health-care practitioners to obtain the original article or consult a trusted review source, in order to make an accurate judgment about the validity of such reports and hence advise accordingly.

INFORMATION ABOUT INVESTIGATIONS FOLLOWING RECURRENT MISCARRIAGE to help reduce unrealistic expectations. Unless counseled otherwise, most women or couples referred for investigations will expect tests to reveal the cause of their miscarriages and thus treatment to prevent recurrence. If no specific cause is identified, they may be greatly disappointed and some will continue to seek answers elsewhere. It is important, therefore, to explain the likelihood of identifying a cause or causes and to note that some conditions may not be subject to change. Most important of all is to provide reassurance – and evidence – that having no cause identified is actually the best news for future pregnancies, even though some patients will find this hard to accept.

SUPPORT AND UNDERSTANDING regarding a subsequent pregnancy/ies. This could include:

- Pre-conception care and advice (including information on maternal and paternal age).
- Access to early scanning if requested.
- Someone to talk to: health professional, counselor or support organization.

Levels of stress and anxiety in pregnancy after miscarriage are often high. There is good evidence that "tender loving care" for couples with idiopathic recurrent miscarriage can improve pregnancy outcomes [56,57]. It is noteworthy that in both studies cited here, the offer of open access for scanning and support in pregnancy after miscarriage was often enough in itself; it was not necessarily taken up.

REFERRAL for further support, care and/or information in the short and longer term, especially with help in coping with guilt and managing anxiety. This may include support in deciding whether or not to try again.

# Coping strategies when dealing with risk

Emotional reactions vary widely and so will coping strategies. For some people, actively changing factors over which there may be at least some measure of control may provide a coping strategy. Focusing on, for example, eating a healthy diet, taking vitamins, reaching a BMI of at least 18.5 if underweight, or delaying trying to become pregnant until stressful events are over may provide a sense of control. This measure of control may be fragile; it may be necessary to provide additional information and support (or signpost appropriate sources) in the event of threatened or actual pregnancy loss or recurrent miscarriage.

## Dealing with stress

There is increasing evidence that emotional wellbeing may be related to risk of miscarriage. Stress and traumatic events appear to increase risk and feeling relaxed and happy appears to decrease the risk. Risk appears to be greater with an increasing number of stressful or traumatic events, such as having a generally stressful or demanding job, loss of job/job insecurity (self or partner), separation or divorce, serious financial problems, accident, serious illness of self or someone close or death of someone close.

In some cases, it may be appropriate to suggest waiting for a while before conception in order to reduce the risk of miscarriage as much as possible, for example after a specific event such as a bereavement; or it may be possible to suggest changes to reduce stress, for example changing to a less stressful job. However, when advising in early pregnancy or where the stress is likely to persist for a long period, such as long-term illness of a close relative, and acknowledging the stress inherent in pregnancy after miscarriage, it is important to put the risk into context and to highlight other ways to minimize risk, for example taking vitamins and eating a healthy diet.

## Summary

First-trimester miscarriage is a common but distressing occurrence. Most people seek an explanation of the cause of their miscarriage and treatment or guidance to prevent a recurrence. Efforts to gather research evidence have been hampered in the past by methodological difficulties and the lack of understanding by health professionals that at least a proportion of miscarriages are preventable. While there is much that remains unclear, recent good quality research has highlighted several biological, behavioral and lifestyle risk factors for first-trimester miscarriage. The provision of accurate and up-to-date information on these risk factors, together with support and guidance in subsequent pregnancies, can make a positive difference to the physical and emotional health of miscarriage patients.

## Acknowledgments

We would like to thank Dr. Noreen Maconochie for her invaluable leadership as principal investigator of the National Women's Health Survey. We would also like to thank the contributions of the many women who took part in this survey. The project was funded by the Big Lottery Fund (through The Miscarriage Association) and by The Miscarriage Association.

## References

1. Wilcox AJ, Weinberg CR, O'Connor JF *et al*. Incidence of early loss of pregnancy. *New Engl J Med* 1988; **319**(4): 189–94.

2. Wilcox AJ, Baird DD, Weinberg CR. Time of implantation of the conceptus and loss of pregnancy. *New Engl J Med* 1999; **340**(23): 1796–9.

3. Wang X, Chen C, Wang L *et al.*. Conception, early pregnancy loss, and time to clinical pregnancy: a population-based prospective study. *Fertil Steril* 2003; **79**(3): 577–84.

4. Zinaman MJ, Clegg ED, Brown CC, O'Connor J, Selevan SG. Estimates of human fertility and pregnancy loss. *Fertil-Steril* 1996; **65**(3): 503–9.

5. Ellish NJ, Saboda K, O'Connor J *et al*. A prospective study of early pregnancy loss. *Hum Reprod* 1996; **11**(2): 406–12.

6. Nybo-Andersen A-M, Wohlfahrt J, Christens P, Olsen J, Melbye M. Maternal age and fetal loss: population based register linkage study. *Br Med J* 2000; **320**: 1708–12.

7. Maconochie N, Doyle P, Prior S. The National Women's Health Study: assembly and description of a population-based reproductive cohort. *BMC Public Health* 2004; **4**: 35.

8. Savitz DA, Hertz-Picciotto I, Poole C, Olshan AF. Epidemiologic measures of the course and outcome of pregnancy. *Epidemiol Rev* 2002; **24**(2): 91–101.

9. Maconochie N, Doyle P, Prior S, Simmons R. Risk factors for first trimester miscarriage – results from a UK-population-based case-control study. *BJOG* 2007; **114**(2): 170–86.

10. Hassold T, Abruzzo M, Adkins K *et al*. Human aneuploidy: incidence, origin, and etiology. *Environ Mol Mutagen* 1996; **28**(3): 167–75.

11. Warburton D, Byrne J, Canki N. *Chromosomal Anomalies and Prenatal Development: An Atlas. Oxford Monographs on Medical Genetics, No. 21*. New York: Oxford University Press, 1991.

12. Nybo Andersen AM, Hansen KD, Andersen PK, Davey Smith G. Advanced paternal age and risk of fetal death: a cohort study. *Am J Epidemiol* 2004; **160**(12): 1214–22.

13. Slama R, Bouyer J, Windham G et al. Influence of paternal age on the risk of spontaneous abortion. Am J Epidemiol 2005; **161**(9): 816–23.

14. Brown S. Miscarriage and its associations. Semin Reprod Med 2008; **26**(5): 391–400. Epub 2008 Sep 29.

15. Zhou W, Olsen J, Nielsen GL, Sabroe S. Risk of spontaneous abortion following induced abortion is only increased with short interpregnancy interval. J Obstet Gynaecol 2000; **20**(1): 49–54.

16. Sun Y, Che Y, Gao E, Olsen J, Zhou W. Induced abortion and risk of subsequent miscarriage. Int J Epidemiol 2003; **32**: 449–54.

17. Virk J, Zhang J, Olsen J. Medical abortion and the risk of subsequent adverse pregnancy outcomes. New Engl J Med 2007; **357**(7): 648–53.

18. Gan C, Zou Y, Wu S, Li Y, Liu Q. The influence of medical abortion compared with surgical abortion on subsequent pregnancy outcome. Int J Gynaecol Obstet 2008; **101**(3): 231–8.

19. Macklon NS, Geraedts JP, Fauser BC. Conception to ongoing pregnancy: the 'black box' of early pregnancy loss. Hum Reprod Update 2002; **8**(4): 333–43.

20. Hemminki K, Niemi ML, Saloniemi I, Vainio H, Hemminki E. Spontaneous abortions by occupation and social class in Finland. Int J Epidemiol 1980; **9**(2): 149–53.

21. Weck RL, Paulose T, Flaws JA. Impact of environmental factors and poverty on pregnancy outcomes. Clin Obstet Gynecol 2008; **51**(2): 349–59.

22. ESHRE Capri Workshop Group. Nutrition and reproduction in women. Hum Reprod Update 2006; **12**(3): 193–207.

23. Arendas K, Qiu Q, Gruslin A. Obesity in pregnancy: pre-conceptional to postpartum consequences. J Obstet Gynaecol Can 2008; **30**(6): 477–88.

24. Helgstrand S, Andersen AM. Maternal underweight and the risk of spontaneous abortion. Acta Obstet Gynecol Scand 2005; **84**(12): 1197–201.

25. Arck PC, Rücke M, Rose M et al. Early risk factors for miscarriage: a prospective cohort study in pregnant women. Reprod Biomed Online 2008; **17**(1): 101–13.

26. Di Cintio E, Parazzini F, Chatenoud L et al. Dietary factors and risk of spontaneous abortion. Eur J Obstet Gynecol Reprod Biol 2001; **95**(1): 132–6.

27. Bailey LB, Berry RJ. Folic acid supplementation and the occurrence of congenital heart defects,orofacial clefts, multiple births, and miscarriage. Am J Clin Nutr 2005; **81**(5): 1213S–17S.

28. Rasch V. Cigarette, alcohol and caffeine consumption: risk factors for spontaneous abortion. Acta Obstet Gynecol Scand 2003; **82**(2): 182–8.

29. Bech BH, Nohr EA, Vaeth M, Henriksen TB, Olsen J. Coffee and fetal death: a cohort study with prospective data. Am J Epidemiol 2005; **162**: 983–90.

30. Signorello LB, McLaughlin JK. Maternal caffeine consumption and spontaneous abortion: a review of the epidemiologic evidence. Epidemiology 2004; **15**: 229–39.

31. Savitz DA, Chan RL, Herring AH, Howards PP, Hartmann KE. Caffeine and miscarriage risk. Epidemiology 2008; **19**(1): 55–62.

32. Weng X, Odouli R, Li DK. Maternal caffeine consumption during pregnancy and the risk of miscarriage: a prospective cohort study. Am J Obstet Gynecol 2008; **198**(3): 279.e1–8.

33. Halmesmaki E, Valimaki M, Roine R, Ylikahri R, Ylikorkala O. Maternal and paternal alcohol consumption and miscarriage. Br J Obstet Gynaecol 1989; **96**(2): 188–91.

34. Parazzini F, Bocciolone L, La Vecchia C, Negri E, Fedele L. Maternal and paternal moderate daily alcohol consumption and unexplained miscarriages. Br J Obstet Gynaecol 1990; **97**(7): 618–22.

35. Armstrong BG, McDonald AD, Sloan M. Cigarette, alcohol, and coffee consumption and spontaneous abortion. Am J Public Health 1992; **82**(1): 85–7.

36. Parazzini F, Tozzi L, Chatenoud L et al. Alcohol and risk of spontaneous abortion. Hum Reprod 1994; **9**: 1950–3.

37. Long MG, Waterson EJ, MacRae KD et al. Alcohol consumption and the risk of first trimester miscarriage. J Obstet Gynecol 1994; **14**: 69–70.

38. Abel EL. Maternal alcohol consumption and spontaneous abortion. Alcohol 1997; **32**(3): 211–19.

39. Windham GC, Von Behren J, Fenster L, Schaefer C, Swan SH. Moderate maternal alcohol consumption and risk of spontaneous abortion. Epidemiology 1997; **8**(5): 509–14.

40. Henriksen TB, Hjollund NH, Jensen TK et al. Alcohol consumption at the time of conception and spontaneous abortion. Am J Epidemiol 2004; **160**(7): 661–7.

41. Strandberg-Larsen K, Nielsen NR, Grønbaek M et al. Binge drinking in pregnancy and risk of fetal death. Obstet Gynecol 2008; **111**(3): 602–9.

42. Windham GC, Swan SH, Fenster L. Parental cigarette smoking and the risk of spontaneous abortion. Epidemiology 1992; **135**(12): 1394–403.

43. Kline J, Levin B, Kinney A et al. Cigarette smoking and spontaneous abortion of known karyotype. Precise data but uncertain inferences. Am J Epidemiol 1995; **141**(5): 417–27.

44. Chatenoud L, Parazzini F, di Cintio E et al. Paternal and maternal smoking habits before conception and during the first trimester: relation to spontaneous abortion. Ann Epidemiol 1998; **8**(8): 520–6.

45. Wisborg K, Kesmodel U, Henriksen TB, Hedegaard M, Secher NJ. A prospective study of maternal smoking

and spontaneous abortion. *Acta Obstet Gynecol Scand* 2003; **82**(10): 936–41.

46. Nielsen A, Hannibal CG, Lindekilde BE *et al.* Maternal smoking predicts the risk of spontaneous abortion. *Acta Obstet Gynecol Scand* 2006; **85**(9): 1057–65.

47. Venners SA, Wang X, Chen C *et al.* Paternal smoking and pregnancy loss: a prospective study using a biomarker of pregnancy. *Am J Epidemiol* 2004; **159**(10): 993–1001.

48. McDonald AD, Armstrong B, Cherry NM *et al.* Spontaneous abortion and occupation. *J Occup Med* 1986; **28**(12): 1232–8.

49. Fenster L, Hubbard AE, Windham GC, Waller KO, Swan-SH. A prospective study of work-related physical exertion and spontaneous abortion. *Epidemiology* 1997; **8**(1): 66–74.

50. Madsen M, Jørgensen T, Jensen ML *et al.* Leisure time physical exercise during pregnancy and the risk of miscarriage: a study within the Danish National Birth Cohort. *BJOG* 2007; **114**(11): 1419–26.

51. Hjollund NH, Jensen TK, Bonde JP *et al.* Spontaneous abortion and physical strain around implantation: a follow-up study of first-pregnancy planners. *Epidemiology* 2000; **11**(1): 18–23.

52. O'Hare T, Creed F. Life events and miscarriage. *Br J Psychiatry* 1995; **167**(6): 799–805.

53. Neugebauer R, Kline J, Stein Z *et al.* Association of stressful life events with chromosomally normal spontaneous abortion. *Am J Epidemiol* 1996; **143**(6): 588–96.

54. Schenker MB, Eaton M, Green R, Samuels S. Self-reported stress and reproductive health of female lawyers. *J Occup Environ Med* 1997; **39**(6): 556–68.

55. Nepomnaschy PA, Welch KB, McConnell DS *et al.* Cortisol levels and very early pregnancy loss in humans. *Proc Natl Acad Sci USA* 2006; **103**(10): 3938–42.

56. Stray-Pedersen B, Stray-Pedersen S. Aetiologic factors and subsequent reproductive performance in 195 couples with a prior history of habitual abortion. *Am J Obstet Gynecol* 1984; **148**(2): 140–6.

57. Liddle HS, Pattinson NS, Zanderigo A. Recurrent miscarriage – outcome after supportive care in early pregnancy. *Aust N Z J Obstet Gynaecol* 1991; **31**(4): 320–2.

# Chapter 3

# Ectopic pregnancy

Emma Kirk and Tom H. Bourne

More than 10 000 ectopic pregnancies are diagnosed annually in the UK [1]. Although women may still present with the classic triad of symptoms: pain, vaginal bleeding and a period of amenorrhea, more women are now asymptomatic at the time of diagnosis. This has led to changes in the diagnosis and management of ectopic pregnancy in recent years. Historically, ectopic pregnancies were diagnosed and managed surgically in symptomatic women. The majority of ectopic pregnancies are now diagnosed non-surgically often in asymptomatic women, with the majority visualized on ultrasound prior to treatment. Management has also changed to reflect this with expectant and medical management now recognized alternatives to surgical management in appropriately selected women.

## Types of ectopic pregnancy

The majority of ectopic pregnancies occur within the Fallopian tube, with most implanted in the ampullary region [2]. Around 5% are non-tubal but they contribute to a disproportionate number of serious complications due to their anatomical location [3]. Interstitial ectopic pregnancies have been reported to account for between 1–6% of all ectopic pregnancies [4,5]. Ovarian pregnancies have an incidence of between 0.5–3.0% of all ectopic pregnancies [6]. Both cervical and abdominal pregnancies are rare and each account for less than 1% of all ectopic pregnancies [7,8]. Cesarean section scar pregnancy is considered to be the rarest form of ectopic pregnancy [9]. However, it has been reported to comprise 6% of all ectopic pregnancies in women with a previous cesarean section scar [10].

## Risk factors

A number of risk factors have been identified for ectopic pregnancy. These are detailed in Table 3.1. It is thought that a third of cases are caused by tubal infection or previous surgery [11]. The most common pathogen is *Chlamydia trachomatis*, although other organisms such as *Neisseria gonorrhoeae* may be responsible. Another third of cases are associated with smoking [11]. The exact mechanism whereby smoking has an effect is unknown but may include a combination of delayed ovulation, altered tubal and uterine motility and altered immunity. The risk of ectopic pregnancy also increases with advancing age [12]. This may be a reflection of a higher probability of exposure to most risk factors, an increase in chromosomal abnormalities in trophoblastic tissue and age-related changes in tubal function delaying ovum transport and resulting in tubal implantation.

## Diagnosis

### Surgical diagnosis

Historically, ectopic pregnancies were diagnosed at the time of surgery and today some are still not diagnosed until a laparoscopy or laparotomy has been performed. Macroscopically there may be hemoperitoneum, with a distended fallopian tube. Microscopically there will be chorionic villi within the tube. There may also be signs of rupture of the tube. However, although laparoscopy or laparotomy is thought to be the gold standard for diagnosis, not all ectopic pregnancies will be diagnosed at the time of surgery. Some may initially be missed due to their small size or anatomical location. Histological confirmation may also not be possible due to a failure to obtain any tissue.

### Ultrasound diagnosis

Transvaginal ultrasound (TVU) has now become the diagnostic technique of choice for ectopic pregnancy. Previously, ultrasound was used as a technique to

*Early Pregnancy*, ed. Roy G. Farquharson and Mary D. Stephenson. Published by Cambridge University Press.
© Cambridge University Press 2010.

**Table 3.1** Risk factors for ectopic pregnancy [12].

| Risk factor | Adjusted OR (95% CI) | OR (95% CI) |
|---|---|---|
| High risk | | |
| Previous tubal surgery | 4.0 (2.6–6.1) | 4.7–21.0 |
| Sterilization | | 9.3 (4.9–18.0) |
| Previous ectopic pregnancy | | 8.3 (6.0–11.5) |
| Diethylstilbestrol exposure | | 5.6 (2.4–13.0) |
| Current use of an IUCD | | 4.2–45.0 |
| Documented tubal pathology | 3.7 (1.2–4.8) | 3.8–21.0 |
| Moderate risk | | |
| Infertility | 2.1–2.7 | 2.5–21.0 |
| Previous genital infections | | 2.5–3.7 |
| Multiple sexual partners | | 2.1–2.5 |
| Previous termination | 2.8 (1.1–7.2) | |
| Previous miscarriage | 3.0 (>2) | |
| Age > 40 | 2.9 (1.4–6.1) | |
| Slight risk | | |
| Previous pelvic/ abdominal surgery | | 0.9–3.8 |
| Ruptured appendix | | 1.8 (1.2–2.7) |
| Cigarette smoking | 1.7–3.9 | 2.3–2.5 |
| Vaginal douching | | 1.1–3.1 |
| Age < 18 years at first intercourse | | 1.6 |

OR = odds ratio; CI = confidence interval; Adjusted OR = adjusted for previous pelvic infection, smoking, area, level of education and age; IUCD = intrauterine contraceptive device.

exclude an intrauterine pregnancy. Now TVU is used to diagnose an ectopic pregnancy by positively visualizing an extrauterine pregnancy. Using trans-abdominal ultrasonography (TAS) an intrauterine sac can be visualized when the hCG is >6500 U/L [13]. However with TVU an intrauterine sac should be visualized with hCG levels as low as 1000 U/L [14]. A number of studies have assessed the performance of TVU for the diagnosis of ectopic pregnancy. It has been shown to have an overall sensitivity of 87.0–99.0% for the detection of ectopic pregnancy [15–18]. However, results must be interpreted with caution as the diagnostic ultrasound examinations reported in these studies were often performed immediately prior to surgery and were not the only ultrasound examinations performed. A more recent study has shown that it should be possible to diagnose nearly 75% of ectopic pregnancies on the initial TVU examination performed at the time a patient first attends the clinic [19]. The other cases may initially be classified as a "pregnancy of unknown location" (PUL) and the majority of these with an ectopic pregnancy will have them visualized on subsequent ultrasound examinations. The reason why some ectopic pregnancies are missed on the initial TVU has been studied. It would appear that these ectopic pregnancies are just too small and too early in the disease process to be seen on the initial TVU [20]. In this study at the time of the initial TVU, women with ectopic pregnancies classified as a PUL had a significantly lower reported mean gestational age and mean hCG levels compared with those women who had their ectopic pregnancies visualized on the initial TVU [20].

Specific criteria for the ultrasound diagnosis of the different types of ectopic pregnancy have been described (Figure 3.1). However, although not diagnostic, other findings may also suggest the presence of an ectopic pregnancy. There may be anechoic or echogenic free fluid within the pelvis. Whilst anechoic fluid is unlikely to be significant, finding echogenic fluid within the Pouch of Douglas or Morison's Pouch may suggest hemoperitoneum secondary to a ruptured ectopic pregnancy or a tubal miscarriage, but it may also be seen with rupture of a hemorrhagic ovarian cyst. The finding of a collection of fluid within the endometrial cavity often referred to as a "pseudosac" is also widely discussed. However with TVU it is rarely difficult to distinguish this from an early intrauterine gestational sac, which is seen as an eccentrically placed hyperechoic ring within the endometrial cavity.

# Management

## Surgical management

Historically, laparotomy with salpingectomy was the standard treatment for ectopic pregnancy.

| Type | Criteria |
|---|---|
| **Tubal** 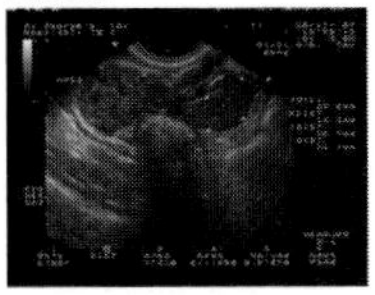 | An empty endometrial cavity with: (1) an inhomogeneous adnexal mass or (2) an empty extra-uterine sac or (3) a yolk sac or fetal pole cardiac activity in an extra-uterine sac. |
| **Interstitial** 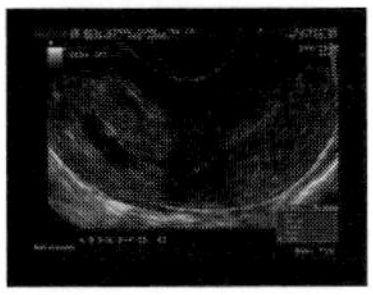 | An empty endometrial cavity with products of conception located outside of the endometrial echo, surrounded by a continuous rim of myometrium, within the interstitial area. |
| **Cervical** 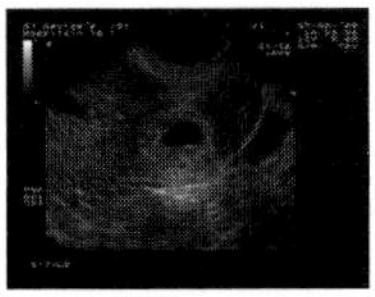 | An empty endometrial cavity, with a gestational sac present below the level of the internal os. An absent "sliding sign" and visible blood flow around the gestation sac using color Doppler. |
| **Cesarean section scar** 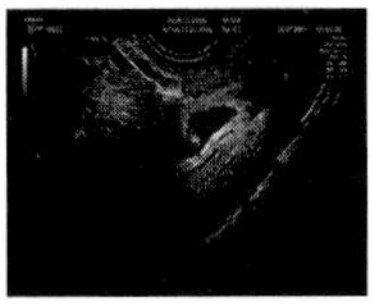 | An empty endometrial cavity and cervical canal with a gestational sac implanted within the lower anterior segment of uterine wall, with evidence of myometrial dehiscence. |
| **Ovarian** | No specific ultrasound criteria have been described, with ultrasound findings described in individual case reports. A study on six cases of ovarian pregnancies, reported that on ultrasound, these pregnancies appear as on or within the ovary as a cyst with a wide echogenic outside ring. |

**Figure 3.1** Sonographic criteria for the diagnosis of ectopic pregnancy.

Salpingostomy was then first performed in the 1950s [21] and in the 1970s laparoscopic procedures for the treatment of ectopic pregnancies were introduced [22,23].

Laparoscopic surgery has been shown to be superior to laparotomy, making it the surgical approach of choice. However, in the case of a hemodynamically unstable woman, surgery should be by the most expedient method, which in some cases will be laparotomy [24]. Reduced operating times, hospital stays, blood loss and analgesic requirements as well as shorter convalescence times and lower costs have been demonstrated in those undergoing laparoscopic procedures [25–29]. In these studies, subsequent intrauterine pregnancy rates were also found to be similar and there was a trend toward a lower repeat ectopic pregnancy rate if the laparoscopic approach was used.

There are some cohort studies that have compared laparoscopic salpingectomy with salpingostomy [30–33]. In one study of 266 women who were trying to conceive, the cumulative intrauterine pregnancy rate was found to be significantly higher after salpingostomy (88%) than after salpingectomy (66%) [33]. No difference was found in the recurrence rate of ectopic pregnancy between the treatments (16% vs 17%). In cases of contralateral tubal pathology, the chance of a future pregnancy was low. From this and other studies it seems reasonable to conclude that conservative surgery is superior to salpingectomy, although the condition of the other tube is important in determining the likelihood of a subsequent pregnancy.

However with salpingostomy, there is a risk that not all the functional trophoblast is removed. Persistent trophoblast has been reported in up to 8.1–8.3% of cases after laparoscopic salpingostomy and in 3.9–4.1% of cases after open salpingostomy [34–36]. It is therefore necessary to identify women with persistent disease by monitoring the postoperative hCG levels. There are no agreed protocols for the timing of hCG level measurements and when treatment should be instituted if levels fail to decrease. Treatment is, however, most commonly with a single dose of systemic methotrexate (see below). The ESEP study is currently under way with the aim to reveal the trade-off between both surgical options: whether the potential advantage of salpingostomy, i.e. a better fertility prognosis as compared with salpingectomy, outweighs the potential disadvantages, i.e. persistent trophoblast and an increased risk for a repeat ectopic pregnancy [37]. It is an international multicenter randomized controlled trial comparing salpingostomy versus salpingectomy in women with a tubal ectopic pregnancy without contralateral tubal pathology.

## Medical management

A number of drugs have been used for the treatment of ectopic pregnancy including potassium chloride, prostaglandins, hyperosmolar glucose, mifepristone and actinomycin D. However, the most commonly used drug in clinical practice for the treatment of ectopic pregnancy is methotrexate. It is a cytotoxic drug that binds to the enzyme dihydrofolate reductase,which is involved in the synthesis of purine nucleotides. As a consequence it interferes with DNA synthesis and disrupts cell multiplication. It can be used both systemically and locally for the treatment of both tubal and non-tubal ectopic pregnancies.

In the UK, methotrexate is most commonly given systemically as a single dose (Table 3.2) [38]. This involves giving a single dose of $50 \, mg/m^2$ on the day of presentation or diagnosis (day 1). Serum beta hCG levels are checked on days 4 and 7 post treatment. If the hCG level decreases by more than 15% between

**Table 3.2** Protocol for the use of single-dose methotrexate in unruptured ectopic pregnancy.

| Day | Management |
|-----|-----------|
| 0 | hCG, FBC, U&Es, LFTs, G&S |
| 1 | hCG<br>Intramuscular methotrexate $50 \, mg/m^2$ |
| 4 | hCG |
| 7 | hCG, FBC, LFT<br>Second dose of methotrexate if hCG decrease <15 % day 4–7<br>If hCG decrease >15 % repeat hCG weekly until <12 U/L |

FBC = full blood count; U&Es = urea and electrolytes; LFTs = liver function tests; G&S = group and serum storage

days 4 and 7, hCG levels are then checked on a weekly basis. If the hCG does not decrease by more than 15% a second dose can be given. The reported need for a second dose ranges from 3–27% of cases [38,39]. Absolute contraindications to its use include pain, signs of an acute hemoperitoneum, liver, kidney or bone marrow impairment. Relative contraindications include fetal cardiac activity, an ectopic mass greater than 3 cm in diameter and an hCG level greater than 5000 U/L. It is important that any woman receiving methotrexate is reliable, compliant and counseled appropriately before it is administered. Side effects from a single dose of methotrexate are rare but include nausea, gastric disturbance, tiredness and abdominal pain. Women should also be advised to avoid alcohol, folic acid and sexual intercourse during the period of treatment.

Reported success rates of single-dose methotrexate range from 65–95% [38,40,46]. The largest single study of single-dose methotrexate has been on 495 women with a success rate of 90% [44]. These success rates vary due to different inclusion criteria. Some studies include women with PULs and presumed, but not visualized ectopic pregnancies, and women already known to have failing pregnancies with decreasing hCG levels. Inclusion of these women can lead to an overestimation of the impact of methotrexate, as it is likely that these ectopic pregnancies may have resolved without any intervention. Other studies include women with fetal cardiac activity, hemoperitoneum and high initial hCG levels who may have been excluded from other studies. Success is lower when there is positive fetal cardiac activity [39]. This is probably a reflection of higher hCG levels and more active trophoblast. The presence of a hemoperitoneum could indicate either rupture of the ectopic pregnancy or tubal miscarriage. In the latter one would expect methotrexate to work well as the pregnancy has already failed. This might explain why one study showed a success rate of 62% in hemodynamically stable women with suspected ruptured ectopic pregnancy [47].

A recent systematic review has found that there is a substantial increase in the failure of medical management with single-dose methotrexate when the initial hCG level is >5000 IU/L [48]. The trend in hCG before and after methotrexate administration is also an indicator of treatment success and a predictor of possible tubal rupture. Serum beta hCG levels that increase more than 66% over 48 hours before diagnosis or persistently rising hCG concentrations after methotrexate administration may lower the threshold for surgical intervention [49]. The serum progesterone level has also been shown to be a predictor of the outcome of methotrexate treatment. If the serum progesterone level is more than 7–10 ng/ml there is a greater risk of failure with single-dose methotrexate [50,51]. A previous history of ectopic pregnancy also appears to be an independent risk factor for treatment failure [44]. Interestingly the likelihood of failure is not influenced by the previous method of treatment. In order to increase the efficacy of methotrexate, studies have looked at the addition of mifeprostone. A randomized study of over 200 ectopic pregnancies failed to demonstrate any benefit except when the serum progesterone was greater than 10 ng/L [52].

An alternative to single-dose methotrexate is the multiple-dose regimen. This involves giving 1 mg/kg on days 1, 3 and 5 with folinic acid rescue on days 2, 4 and 6. One randomized controlled trial has found that in selected cases methotrexate in a fixed multiple-dose intramuscular regimen has a non-significant tendency to a higher treatment success than laparoscopic salpingostomy [53]. A systematic review of over 1300 cases treated with either the single-dose or the multiple-dose regimens found that the multiple-dose regimen was more successful, but associated with significantly more side effects [54]. Side effects include stomatitis, conjunctivitis, gastritis, bone marrow depression, impaired liver function and photosensitivity. However, a Cochrane review on interventions for tubal ectopic pregnancy [55] quotes two randomized controlled studies on a total of 159 women, which showed no significant difference in primary treatment success between those receiving a single dose and those receiving fixed multiple doses [56,57]. Recently a novel-dosing regimen of methotrexate has been proposed. This involves giving intramuscular injections of $50\,mg/m^2$ on days 0 and day 4, with further injections on days 7 and/or day 11 if the hCG levels do not decrease by 15% during the follow-up period [58]. In a multicenter study on 101 women with ectopic pregnancies, the success of this regimen was 87%. The authors report that the treatment was well tolerated and that most of the side effects were reported as mild and transient. They concluded that this two-dose protocol minimizes the number of injections and surveillance visits compared with the multiple-dose regimen of methotrexate and has similar levels of treatment success [58].

Methotrexate can also be given locally, either at the time of laparoscopy or intra-amniotically under TVU guidance. Intra-amniotic methotrexate is more commonly used in the management of non-tubal ectopic pregnancies. In 2005, Monteagudo et al. reported on 18 cases of live ectopic pregnancy (ten cervical, four tubal, four cornual) managed with ultrasound-guided local injection of methotrexate or potassium chloride [59]. A commonly used regimen is intra-amniotic injection of 25–50 mg of methotrexate or intracardiac injection of 2 ml of potassium chloride [59,60].

Both single- and multiple-dose methotrexate regimens have been compared with surgical treatment. In a randomized trial involving 100 hemodynamically stable women with a laparoscopically confirmed tubal ectopic pregnancy, no significant differences were found in primary treatment success or tubal preservation following either multiple-dose systemic methotrexate or laparoscopic salpingostomy [53]. When comparing single-dose systemic methotrexate to laparoscopic surgery, two randomized studies have shown that single-dose methotrexate is as successful as salpingostomy in treating selected cases of ectopic pregnancy [41,61]. One study has shown that overall subsequent intrauterine pregnancy rates were higher and ectopic pregnancy rates lower after methotrexate [61]. However the issue with these studies is one of patient selection. Patients are generally only entered into the studies if they fulfill the criteria for medical treatment in any event. These studies do not say that medical management is as good as surgery for all women.

# Expectant management

Expectant management has been shown to be safe and effective for selected women with ectopic pregnancy. However close follow-up is required and emergency out-of-hours back-up essential. Some units report offering expectant management to over 60% of their cases of ectopic pregnancy [62].

The reported success rates for expectant management range between 48–100% [62–69]. In a study of 118 ectopic pregnancies managed expectantly, the overall success rate was 65% (77/118) [64]. In those with successful expectant management the initial hCG was much lower than in those who failed expectant management, 374 U/L (range, 20–10 762 U/L) compared with 741 U/L (range, 165–14 047 U/L). The success rate for a spontaneous resolution was 88% when the initial hCG level was <200 U/L but only 25% at levels >2000 U/L. Similar success rates have been shown in a more recent study, with 96% success when the hCG was <175 U/L [62]. In most units patients presenting with an ectopic pregnancy will have significantly higher hCG levels than the levels discussed in the literature and so it is hard to draw firm conclusions about the performance of expectant management outside a very carefully selected group of patients.

The data must therefore be interpreted with caution as success rates vary due to different inclusion criteria. Some include pregnancies of unknown location (PUL) rather than laparoscopically or sonographically visualized ectopic pregnancies. Other studies select women on the basis of hCG and progesterone levels, which are both likely to affect the overall success.

Lower initial hCG levels, a decreasing trend in hCG levels over time, the absence of an ectopic gestational sac visualized on ultrasound and a longer time from the last menstrual period have been shown to be predictors of successful expectant management [66,70].

There are only two randomized controlled trials comparing expectant management to other treatments, and because of this, a Cochrane review has concluded that expectant management of tubal ectopic pregnancy cannot yet be adequately evaluated [55]. One study involved 60 hemodynamically stable women who were treated for 5 days with either 2.5 mg/day oral methotrexate or placebo [71]. The overall success rate was 77% with no significant differences in primary treatment success between the two methods, however the median baseline hCG levels were low and the treatment used only low doses of methotrexate. Another study on 23 cases of tubal ectopic pregnancies with hCG levels of <2500 U/L has shown that expectant management is significantly less successful than prostaglandin therapy [72]. A multicenter trial is currently underway in the Netherlands to assess whether expectant management in women with ectopic pregnancy or a PUL with low but plateauing hCG concentrations is an alternative to methotrexate treatment in terms of treatment success, future pregnancy, health-related quality of life and costs [73].

Expectant management is not widely used in the management of non-tubal ectopic pregnancies. There are however various case reports about its use and successful outcomes in interstitial, cesarean section scar and cervical ectopic pregnancies [74–76].

# Subsequent fertility

This has been assessed directly by observing subsequent pregnancy rates and indirectly looking at tubal patency on post-treatment hysterosalpingograms in the case of non-surgical treatments and salpingotomy. Ipsilateral tubal patency rates of 77–82% have been reported after treatment with single-dose systemic methotrexate [38,77,78]. This is comparable to tubal patency rates after linear salpingostomy [78]. Subsequent pregnancy rates of over 80% have been reported following systemic methotrexate [38,79]. In one study 81% of the naturally conceived pregnancies were intrauterine and 18% were ectopic pregnancies [79].

Subsequent hysterosalpingography has shown patency for the affected tube in up to 93% of cases of ectopic pregnancy managed expectantly [80]. Subsequent intrauterine pregnancy rates vary from 63–88% [80–83]. Repeat ectopic pregnancy has been documented in 4–5% [80,81]. Helmy et al. (2007) have recently shown that the risk of recurrent ectopic pregnancy was not significantly different between those managed expectantly and those undergoing salpingectomy [83]. In one study of 180 ectopic pregnancies there were similar intrauterine pregnancy rates in those managed expectantly (63%) to those managed surgically (51%) [82]. Women undergoing delayed surgery due to failure of initial expectant management had similar subsequent intrauterine conception rates to those that underwent primary surgery [82]. A recent systematic review and meta-analysis on surgery, systemic methotrexate and expectant management for ectopic pregnancy concluded that subsequent fertility did not differ between the different treatments [84].

## Summary

Transvaginal ultrasound (TVU) is now the imaging modality of choice for the diagnosis of ectopic pregnancy. More than 90% of ectopic pregnancies should be visualized on TVU prior to treatment. The majority of these (~75%) will be visualized on the initial TVU examination at the time the woman first presents to the clinic. The remainder will initially be classified as a "pregnancy of unknown location." Ectopic pregnancies in these women are probably too small and too early in the disease process to be visualized on the initial TVU. Earlier diagnosis of ectopic pregnancy often in asymptomatic women means that surgical treatment is not always indicated. Medical treatment with methotrexate or expectant management is suitable for appropriately selected cases. Current evidence would suggest that there are no differences in subsequent fertility rates following the different treatments. Surgery remains an important management option for many women and the data suggest that salpingostomy is probably the best surgical approach, although a randomized study is being planned to answer this question.

## References

1. Lewis G (ed), The Confidential Enquiry into Maternal and Child Health (CEMACH). *Saving Mothers' Lives: reviewing maternal deaths to make motherhood safer–2003–2005. The Seventh Report into Maternal Deaths in the United Kingdom*. London: CEMACH, 2007.

2. Bouyer J, Coste J, Fernandez H, Pouly JL, Job-Spira N. Sites of ectopic pregnancy: a 10 year population-based study of 1800 cases. *Hum Reprod* 2002; **17**: 3224–30.

3. Condous G. The management of early pregnancy complications. *Best Pract Res Clin Obstet Gynaecol* 2004; **18**: 37–57.

4. Rock JA, Thompson JD (ed). *Telinde's Operative Gynecology*. 8th edition. Philadelphia: Lippincott-Raven, 1997, pp. 505–20.

5. Fernandez H, De Zeigler D, Bourget P, Feltain P, Frydman R. The place of methotrexate in the management of interstitial pregnancy. *Hum Reprod* 1991; **6**: 1271–9.

6. Itoh H, Ishihara A, Koita H et al. Ovarian pregnancy: report of four cases and review of the literature. *Pathol Int* 2003; **53**: 806–9.

7. Celik C, Bala A, Acar A, Gezgine K, Akyurek C. Methotrexate for cervical pregnancy. A case report. *J Reprod Med* 2003; **48**: 130–2.

8. Paternoster DM, Santarossa C. Primary abdominal pregnancy. A case report. *Minerva Ginecol* 1999; **51**: 251–3.

9. Fylstra DL. Ectopic pregnancy within a cesarean scar: a review. *Obstet Gynecol Surv* 2002; **57**: 537–43.

10. Seow KM, Huang LW, Lin YH et al. Cesarean scar pregnancy: issues in management. *Ultrasound Obstet Gynecol* 2004; **23**: 247–53.

11. Ankum WM, Mol BWJ, Van der Veen F, BNossuyt PMM. Risk factors for ectopic pregnancy: a meta analysis. *Fertil Steril* 1996; **65**: 1093–9.

12. Bouyer J, Coste J, Shojaei T et al. Risk factors for ectopic pregnancy: a comprehensive analysis based on a large case-control, population-based study in France. *Am J Epidemiol* 2003; **157**: 185–94.

13. Romero R, Kadar N, Jeanty P et al. Diagnosis of ectopic pregnancy: value of the discriminatory human chorionic gonadotropin zone. *Obstet Gynecol* 1985; **66**: 357–60.

14. Aleem FA, DeFazio M, Gintautas J. Endovaginal sonography for the early diagnosis of intrauterine and ectopic pregnancies. *Hum Reprod* 1990; **5**(6):755–8.

15. Braffman BH, Coleman BG, Ramchandani P et al. Emergency department screening for ectopic pregnancy: a prospective US study. *Radiology* 1994; **190**: 797–802.

16. Shalev E, Yarom I, Bustan M, Weiner E, Ben-Shlomo I. Transvaginal sonography as the ultimate diagnostic tool for the management of ectopic pregnancy: experience with 840 cases. *Fertil Steril* 1998; **69**: 62–5.

17. Atri M, Valenti DA, Bret PM, Gillett P. Effect of transvaginal sonography on the use of invasive procedures for evaluating patients with a clinical diagnosis of ectopic pregnancy. *J Clin Ultrasound* 2003; **31**: 1–8.

18. Condous G, Okaro E, Khalid A et al. The accuracy of transvaginal ultrasonography for the diagnosis of ectopic pregnancy prior to surgery. *Hum Reprod* 2005; **20**: 1404–9.

19. Kirk E, Papageorghiou AT, Condous G et al. The diagnostic effectiveness of an initial transvaginal scan in detecting ectopic pregnancy. *Hum Reprod* 2007; **22**: 2824–8.

20. Kirk E, Daemen A, Papageorghiou AT et al. Why are some ectopic pregnancies characterized as pregnancies of unknown location at the initial transvaginal ultrasound examination? *Acta Obstet Gynecol Scand* 2008; **87**: 1150–4.

21. Stromme WB. Salpingotomy for tubal pregnancy; report of a successful case. *Obstet Gynecol* 1953; **1**: 472–5.

22. Bruhat MA, Manhes H, Mage G, Pouly JL. Treatment of ectopic pregnancy by means of laparoscopy. *Fertil Steril* 1980; **33**: 411–14.

23. Garry R. The laparoscopic treatment of ectopic pregnancy: the long road to acceptance. *Gynaecol Endosc* 1996; **5**: 65–8.

24. Royal College of Obstetricians and Gynaecologists (RCOG). *Green-top Guideline No. 21. The Management of Tubal Pregnancy*. London: RCOG Press, 2004.

25. Murphy AA, Nager CW, Wujek JJ *et al.* Operative laparoscopy versus laparotomy for the management of ectopic pregnancy: a prospective trial. *Fertil Steril* 1991; **57**: 1180–5.

26. Vermesh M, Silva PD, Rosen GF *et al.* Management of unruptured ectopic gestation by linear salpingostomy: a prospective, randomized clinical trial of laparoscopy versus laparotomy. *Obstet Gynecol* 1989; **73**: 400–4.

27. Lundorff P, Thorburn J, Hahlin M, Kallfelt B, Lindblom B. Laparoscopic surgery in ectopic pregnancy. A randomized trial versus laparotomy. *Acta Obstet Gynecol Scand* 1991; **70**: 343–8.

28. Lundorff P, Thorburn J, Lindblom B. Fertility outcome after conservative surgical treatment of ectopic pregnancy evaluated in a randomized trial. *Fertil Steril* 1992; **57**: 998–1002.

29. Gray DT, Thorburn J, Lundorff P, Strandell A, Lindblom B. A cost-effectiveness study of a randomised trial of laparoscopy versus laparotomy for ectopic pregnancy. *Lancet* 1995; **345**: 1139–43.

30. Silva PD, Schaper AM, Rooney B. Reproductive outcome after 143 laparoscopic procedures for ectopic pregnancy. *Obstet Gynecol* 1993; **81**: 710–15.

31. Job-Spira N, Bouyer J, Pouly JL *et al.* Fertility after ectopic pregnancy: first results of a population-based cohort study in France. *Hum Reprod* 1996; **11**: 99–104.

32. Mol BW, Matthijsse HC, Tinga DJ *et al.* Fertility after conservative and radical surgery for tubal pregnancy. *Hum Reprod* 1998; **13**: 1804–9.

33. Bangsgaard N, Lund CO, Ottesen B, Nilas L. Improved fertility following conservative surgical treatment of ectopic pregnancy. *BJOG* 2003; **110**: 765–70.

34. Yao M, Tulandi T. Current status of surgical and non-surgical management of ectopic pregnancy. *Fertil Steril* 1997; **67**: 421–33.

35. Sowter M, Frappell J. The role of laparoscopy in the management of ectopic pregnancy. *Rev Gynaecol Practice* 2002; **2**: 73–82.

36. Hajenius PJ, Mol BW, Ankum WM *et al.* Clearance curves of serum human chorionic gonadotrophin for the diagnosis of persistent trophoblast. *Hum Reprod* 1995; **10**: 683–7.

37. Mol F, Strandell A, Jurkovic D *et al.* The ESEP study: salpingostomy versus salpingectomy for tubal ectopic pregnancy; the impact on future fertility: a randomised controlled trial. *BMC Womens Health* 2008; **26**(8): 11.

38. Stovall TG, Ling FW. Single dose methotrexate: an expanded clinical trial. *Am J Obstet Gynecol* 1993; **168**: 1759–65.

39. Erdem M, Erdem A, Arslan M *et al.* Single dose methotrexate for the treatment of unruptured ectopic pregnancy. *Arch Gynecol Obstet* 2004; **270**: 201–4.

40. Henry MA, Gentry WL. Single injection of methotrexate for treatment of ectopic pregnancies. *Am J Obstet Gynecol* 1994; **171**: 1584–7.

41. Sowter MC, Farquhar CM, Petrie KJ, Gudex G. A randomised trial comparing single dose systemic methotrexate and laparoscopic surgery for the treatment of unruptured tubal pregnancy. *BJOG* 2001; **108**: 192–203.

42. Stika CS, Anderson L, Frederiksen MC. Single-dose methotrexate for the treatment of ectopic pregnancy: Northwestern Memorial Hospital three-year experience. *Am J Obstet Gynecol* 1996; **174**: 1840–6.

43. Alshimmiri MM, Al-Saleh EA, Al-Harmi JA *et al.* Treatment of ectopic pregnancy with a single intramuscular dose of methotrexate. *Arch Gynecol Obstet* 2003; **268**: 181–3.

44. Lipscomb GH, Givens VA, Meyer NL, Bran D. Previous ectopic pregnancy as a predictor of failure of systemic methotrexate therapy. *Fertil Steril* 2004; **81**: 1221–4.

45. Lewis-Bliehall C, Rogers RG, Kammerer-Doak DN *et al.* Medical vs. surgical treatment of ectopic pregnancy. The University of New Mexico's six-year experience. *J Reprod Med* 2001; **46**: 983–8.

46. Srivichai K, Uttavichai C, Tongsong T. Medical treatment of ectopic pregnancy: a ten-year review of 106 cases at Maharaj Nakorn Chiang Mai Hospital. *J Med Assoc Thai* 2006; **89**: 1567–71.

47. Kumtepe Y, Kadanali S. Medical treatment of ruptured with haemodynamically stable and unruptured ectopic pregnancy patients. *Eur J Obstet Gynecol Reprod Biol* 2004; **116**: 221–5.

48. Menon S, Colins J, Barnhart KT. Establishing a human chorionic gonadotrophin cutoff to guide methotrexate treatment of ectopic pregnancy: a systematic review. *Fertil Steril* 2007; **87**: 481–4.

49. Dudley PS, Heard MJ, Sangi-Haghpeykar H, Carson SA, Buster JE. Characterizing ectopic pregnancies that rupture despite treatment with methotrexate. *Fertil Steril* 2004; **82**: 1374–8.

50. Ransom MX, Garcia AJ, Bohrer M, Corsan GH, Kemmann E. Serum progesterone as a predictor of success in the treatment of ectopic pregnancy. *Obstet Gynecol* 1994; **83**: 1033–7.

51. Corsan GH, Karacan M, Qasim S. Identification of hormonal parameters for successful systemic single-dose methotrexate therapy in ectopic pregnancy. *Hum Reprod* 1995; **10**: 2719–22.

52. Rozenberg P, Chevret S, Camus E. Medical treatment of ectopic pregnancies: a randomized clinical trial comparing methotrexate-mifeprostone and methotrexate-placebo. *Hum Reprod* 2003; **18**: 1802–8.

53. Hajenius PJ, Engelsbel S, Mol BW. Randomised trial of systemic methotrexate versus laparoscopic salpingostomy in tubal pregnancy. *Lancet* 1997; **13**(350): 774–9.

54. Barnhart KT, Gosman G, Ashby R, Sammel M. The medical management of ectopic pregnancy: a meta-analysis comparing 'single dose' and 'multidose' regimens. *Obstet Gynecol* 2003; **101**: 778–84.

55. Hajenius PJ, Mol F, Mol BW. Interventions for tubal ectopic pregnancy. *Cochrane Database Syst Rev* 2007; **24**: CD000324.

56. Klauser CK, May WL, Johnson VK, Cowan BD, Hines RS. Methotrexate for ectopic pregnancy: a randomized single dose compared with multiple dose. *Obstet and Gynaecol* 2005; **105**: 64S.

57. Alleyassin A, Khademi A, Aghahosseini M *et al.* Comparison of success rates in the medical management of ectopic pregnancy with single-dose and multiple-dose administration of methotrexate: a prospective, randomized clinical trial. *Fertil Steril* 2006; **85**: 1661–6.

58. Barnhart K, Hummel AC, Sammel MD *et al.* Use of "2-dose" regimen of methotrexate to treat ectopic pregnancy. *Fertil Steril* 2007; **87**: 250–6.

59. Monteagudo A, Minior VK, Stephenson C, Monda S, Timor-Tritsch IE. Non-surgical management of live ectopic pregnancy with ultrasound-guided local injection: a case series. *Ultrasound Obstet Gynecol* 2005; **25**: 282–8.

60. Jeng CJ, Ko ML, Shen J. Transvaginal ultrasound-guided treatment of cervical pregnancy. *Obstet Gynecol* 2007; **109**: 1076–82.

61. Fernandez H, Yves Vincent SC, Pauthier S, Audibert F, Frydman R. Randomized trial of conservative laparoscopic treatment and methotrexate administration in ectopic pregnancy and subsequent fertility. *Hum Reprod* 1998; **13**: 3239–43.

62. Elson J, Tailor A, Banerjee S *et al.* Expectant management of tubal ectopic pregnancy: prediction of successful outcome using decision tree analysis. *Ultrasound Obstet Gynecol* 2004; **23**: 552–6.

63. Ylostalo P, Cacciatore B, Sjoberg J *et al.* Expectant management of ectopic pregnancy. *Obstet Gynecol* 1992; **80**: 345–8.

64. Korhonen J, Stenman UH, Ylostalo P. Serum human chorionic gonadotrophin dynamics during spontaneous resolution of ectopic pregnancy. *Fertil Steril* 1994; **61**: 632–6.

65. Cacciatore B, Korhonen J, Stenman UH, Ylostalo P. Transvaginal sonography and serum hCG in monitoring of presumed ectopic pregnancies selected for expectant management. *Ultrasound Obstet Gynecol* 1995; **5**: 297–300.

66. Trio D, Strobelt N, Picciolo C, Lapinski RH, Ghidini A. Prognostic factors for successful expectant management of ectopic pregnancy. *Fertil Steril* 1995; **63**: 469–72.

67. Shalev E, Yarom I, Bustan M, Weiner E, Ben-Shlomo I. Transvaginal sonography as the ultimate diagnostic tool for the management of ectopic pregnancy: experience with 840 cases. *Fertil Steril* 1998; **69**: 62–5.

68. Lui A, D'Ottavio G, Rustico MA *et al.* [Conservative management of ectopic pregnancy] *Minerva Ginecol* 1997; **49**: 67–72.

69. Olofsson JI, Poromaa IS, Ottander U, Kjellberg L, Damber MG. Clinical and pregnancy outcome following ectopic pregnancy; a prospective study comparing expectancy, surgery and systemic methotrexate treatment. *Acta Obstet Gynecol Scand* 2001; **80**: 744–9.

70. Atri M, Valenti DA, Bret PM, Gillett P. Effect of transvaginal sonography on the use of invasive procedures for evaluating patients with a clinical diagnosis of ectopic pregnancy. *J Clin Ultrasound* 2003; **31**: 1–8.

71. Korhonen J, Stenman UH, Ylostalo P. Low-dose oral methotrexate with expectant management of ectopic pregnancy. *Obstet Gynecol* 1996; **88**: 775–8.

72. Egarter C, Kiss H, Husslein P. Prostaglandin versus expectant management in early pregnancy. *Prostaglandins Leukot Essent Fatty Acids* 1991; **42**: 177–9.

73. van Mello NM, Mol F, Adriaanse AH *et al.* The METEX study: methotrexate versus expectant management in women with ectopic pregnancy: a randomised controlled trial. *BMC Womens Health* 2008; **19**(8): 10.

74. Kirk E, Bourne T. The nonsurgical management of ectopic pregnancy. *Curr Opin Obstet Gynecol* 2006; **18**: 587–93.

75. Kirk E, Condous G, Haider Z *et al.* The conservative management of cervical ectopic pregnancies. *Ultrasound Obstet Gynecol* 2006; **27**: 430–7.

76. Jermy K, Thomas J, Doo A, Bourne T. The conservative management of interstitial pregnancy. *BJOG* 2004; **111**: 1283–8.

77. Glock JL, Johnson JV, Brumsted JR. Efficacy and safety of single-dose methotrexate in the treatment of ectopic pregnancy. *Fertil Steril* 1994; **62**: 716–21.

78. Tolaymat LL, Brown TL, Maher JE *et al.* Reproductive potential after methotrexate treatment of ectopic

gestation in a community hospital. *J Reprod Med* 1999; **44**: 335–8.

79. Gervaise A, Mason L, de Tayrac R, Frydman R, Fernandez H. Reproductive outcome after methotrexate treatment of tubal pregnancies. *Fertil Steril* 2004; **82**: 304–8.

80. Rantala M, Makinen J. Tubal patency and fertility outcome after expectant management of ectopic pregnancy. *Fertil Steril* 1997; **68**: 1043–6.

81. Zohav E, Gemer O, Segal S. Reproductive outcome after expectant management of ectopic pregnancy. *Eur J Obstet Gynecol Reprod Biol* 1996; **66**: 1–2.

82. Strobelt N, Mariani E, Ferrari L *et al.* Fertility after ectopic pregnancy. Effects of surgery and expectant management. *J Reprod Med* 2000; **45**(10): 803–7.

83. Helmy S, Sawyer E, Ofili-Yebovi D *et al.* Fertility outcomes following expectant management of tubal ectopic pregnancy. *Ultrasound Obstet Gynecol* 2007; **30**: 988–93.

84. Mol F, Mol BW, Ankum WM, van der Veen F, Hajenius PJ. Current evidence on surgery, systemic methotrexate and expectant management in the treatment of tubal ectopic pregnancy: a systematic review and meta-analysis. *Hum Reprod Update* 2008; **14**: 309–19.

# Ultrasound detection of congenital uterine anomalies

Dimitrios Mavrelos and Davor Jurkovic

## Introduction

Congenital uterine anomalies are relatively rare and there is no consensus about their clinical significance and optimal management. There is also no agreement about the classification of various types of uterine anomalies. Most authors follow the classification adopted by the American Fertility Society, which divides anomalies in seven different groups[1]. Although appealing, this classification is rather simplistic and does not allow for all the variations in uterine morphology. In addition, it does not include the criteria for differential diagnosis of the various anomalies as it is mainly based on the subjective examination of findings at open surgery. As such, the American Fertility Society Classification is not suited well for use in modern clinical practice, where the diagnosis of uterine anomalies is primarily made using non-invasive diagnostic methods. Nowadays, the assessment of women at high risk of having uterine anomalies, i.e. those who have a history of recurrent miscarriage or infertility, usually starts with an ultrasound scan. The scan is used to detect uterine morphological anomalies that could explain a woman's history of pregnancy losses. Ultrasound is also used in the investigation of many women with unrelated symptoms who, even though at low risk for a congenital uterine anomaly, are diagnosed with one incidentally. In this chapter we will describe the principles of ultrasound diagnosis of uterine anomalies and compare the results with other available diagnostic modalities.

## Background

The incidence of congenital uterine anomalies in the general population is between 0.4% and 3.2% [2–6]. They are caused by abnormalities in the embryological development of the uterus and vagina. Female reproductive organs develop between weeks 5 and 16 of fetal life and three main stages of development have been identified:

(1) Organogenesis: appearance after the 5th week of gestation of bilateral Müllerian (paramesonephric) ducts.
(2) Fusion: medial and caudal growth of the Müllerian ducts that fuse in the midline.
(3) Septal absorption: the most cranial parts of the Müllerian ducts form the fallopian tubes, the caudal segments fuse to form the uterus and part of the vagina.

The most cranial point of fusion of the Müllerian ducts forms the uterine fundus. Should failure of fusion occur an arcuate or bicornuate uterus is formed depending on the point of failure. Complete failure of fusion gives rise to a didelphic uterus. However, if failure of septal resorption occurs, a septate or subseptate uterus is formed, depending on the extent of failure [7–9]. Given this mechanism of formation, varying degrees of severity exist within a particular subtype of malformation.

## Diagnosis

### Two-dimensional ultrasound

#### Transabdominal ultrasound

The gold standard in the diagnosis of congenital uterine anomalies used to be a simultaneous laparotomy/laparoscopy and hysteroscopy to visualize the serosal surface of the uterus and the endometrial cavity. The surgery, however, is rather invasive, costly and it carries a risk of complications. For these reasons it is rarely used as a primary test to diagnose uterine anomalies. In routine clinical practice congenital uterine anomalies are usually detected by hysterosalpingography (HSG), which is performed as a part of the investigation protocols for infertility or recurrent miscarriage. This is also an invasive procedure, but much less so than surgery, which requires an injection of contrast media into the uterine cavity and the simultaneous exposure to radiation. Although HSG is widely used to diagnose uterine anomalies, there are few data describing its accuracy and reproducibility. Some studies reported poor accuracy of HSG in the diagnosis of uterine anomalies, ranging from 20–60% in comparison to surgical exploration [7,10,11]. This can be explained by the fact that HSG provides good views of the uterine cavity, but it does not allow for the imaging of the serosal surface of the uterus. The assessment of serosal surface of the uterus is critical for the differential diagnosis of between some common uterine anomalies, such as bicornuate and septate uterus. Hysterosalpingography is also unable to identify non-patent uterine structures such as a non-communicating rudimentary horn of a unicornuate uterus. Given the poor diagnostic performance of HSG investigators turned to ultrasound to improve diagnostic accuracy. In the late 1980s Reuter *et al.* [11] used transabdominal ultrasound as a second-stage test in women suspected to have a congenital uterine anomaly on HSG. This addition improved diagnostic accuracy to 90% (36/40) compared with 55% for HSG alone [11]. Despite these initially encouraging results transabdominal ultrasound did not perform so well when used alone as a first-line investigation. Nicolini *et al.* [12] used transabdominal ultrasound to scan 89 unselected patients being investigated for infertility. They diagnosed a unicornuate uterus when a small, laterally deviated uterus was seen and septate/bicornuate/didelphic uterus when they detected a duplication of the external contour of the uterine corpus or when the endometrial cavity demonstrated a septum seen as a separation of the endometrial cavity echoes on transverse section. The sensitivity of transabdominal ultrasound was poor (42.9%) with fairly good specificity (97.8%). They diagnosed nine of 15 major anomalies but missed all arcuate and subseptate uteri (6/6). They advocated examining patients in the luteal phase of the cycle when the visualization may be enhanced but nevertheless were unable to reliably examine 24 out of 69 patients, which is a high failure rate[12]. A year later Fedele *et al.* [13] used transabdominal ultrasound to attempt to diagnose specific malformations in 39 women with a known history of "double uterus" diagnosed by HSG. They used the following variables to attempt to classify these anomalies:

(1) The presence or absence of a sagittal notch in the serosal surface of the uterus and its depth in millimeters.
(2) The presence or absence of a sagittal notch in the endometrial cavity.
(3) The width in degrees in the angle between the two endometrial hemicavities.
(4) The length of the myometrial spur separating the two hemicavities and the level of this apex.

A diagnosis of bicornuate uterus was made when the sagittal notch in the serosal surface of the uterus was >10 mm, a sagittal notch was visible in the endometrial cavity and the angle between the two hemicavities was >60°. The level of the apex was used to separate didelphic from bicornuate uteri and septate from subseptate uteri. Using these criteria they were able to achieve sensitivity of 92.3% with specificity 100% for the accurate characterization of congenital uterine anomalies [13]. These results demonstrate that even though transabdominal ultrasound can be useful in cases where a suspicion of congenital uterine anomaly exists it is not a sensitive method to screen for congenital uterine anomalies. As we will see later, it was the advent of high-frequency transvaginal probes that paved the way for the development of a sensitive screening test for uterine malformations. Nevertheless clinicians should maintain their skill in transabdominal ultrasound as in some cases a transvaginal scan is not practical or possible.

## Transvaginal ultrasound

Pellerito *et al.* [10] first used transvaginal ultrasound in a series of 26 patients with a surgical diagnosis of Müllerian anomaly. They managed to perform transvaginal ultrasound in only 14 patients but they showed that the accuracies of transvaginal ultrasound and MR imaging for the diagnosis of congenital uterine anomalies are very similar (92% vs 100%). Both modalities performed significantly better than HSG which correctly classified anomalies in only 29% of cases [10]. Clifford *et al.* [14] in a series of 500 women with recurrent miscarriage used transvaginal ultrasound as a screening test for congenital uterine anomalies. They detected nine women with malformations, all of which were confirmed on hysteroscopy or HSG. This represents a low prevalence of congenital uterine anomalies for a high-risk population which cast some doubts on the sensitivity of this test. In a study of 61 women with a previous HSG, the results of which were unknown to the operator at the time of the scan, Jurkovic et al. [15] found that two-dimensional transvaginal ultrasound was able to detect all congenital uterine anomalies. However, it was not reliable in the distinction between the various types of anomalies because of its inability to obtain transverse sections through the long axis of the uterus. They concluded that two-dimensional ultrasound is useful as a screening test but not as a diagnostic test. In a later study by the same group [4] of 1046 low-risk women, the usefulness of two-dimensional transvaginal ultrasound as a screening test was demonstrated. In this study a congenital uterine anomaly was suspected when there was duplication or splitting of the endometrial echo on two-dimensional transvaginal ultrasound (Figure 4.1). Fifty-five women were screen positive and a uterine malformation was confirmed in all of them by three-dimensional transvaginal ultrasound. Some authors have used saline infusion sonohysterography to improve the diagnostic accuracy of two-dimensional transvaginal ultrasound [16–20]. These reports are contradictory as some claim that it is not possible to distinguish between septate and bicornuate uteri without visualization of the serosal contour of the uterus by laparoscopy [17] whilst others [16,18–20] claim that sonohysterography can be 100% accurate in the diagnosis of specific uterine

anomalies. Certainly it is difficult to see how the infusion of saline in the endometrial cavity would improve visualization of the serosal surface of the uterus. It is unlikely therefore the sonohysterography would significantly improve the diagnostic accuracy of unenhanced, two-dimensional transvaginal ultrasound.

We believe that unenhanced two-dimensional transvaginal ultrasound is a sensitive screening method for congenital uterine anomalies provided the examination is performed in a systematic way. In our practice we advocate a careful examination of the uterine cavity in the transverse plane in order to detect uterine cavity malformations. A series of parallel transverse planes are examined starting from the level of the internal os until the uterine fundus is reached. This will identify all duplication anomalies as well as arcuate uteri and uterine septa. As part of the examination we advocate a routine visualization of both interstitial portions of the fallopian tubes as the diagnosis of a unicornuate uterus is based on the detection of a single interstitial portion of the fallopian tube (Figure 4.2). The diagnosis is facilitated by the presence of pronounced uterine lateroflexion, which is common in cases of unicornuate uterus. If a unicornuate uterus is suspected careful examination of contralateral adnexa is indicated as 75% will have a rudimentary cornu [21]. With good scanning technique it is almost always possible to ascertain whether the rudimentary cornu is communicating with the rest of the uterus and whether it contains functional endometrium. The diagnosis of T-shaped uterus is very difficult and is usually not possible to achieve on two-dimensional ultrasound scan alone. Even though two-dimensional transvaginal scanning is a good screening method for congenital

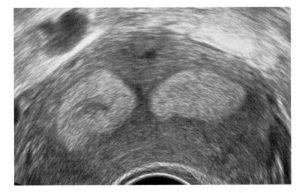

**Figure 4.1** A transvaginal two-dimensional ultrasound image demonstrating a duplication of the endometrial cavity in the transverse section of the uterus. This is a typical finding, which is obtained during routine ultrasound scan in cases of congenital uterine anomalies. This finding should prompt a – three-dimensional ultrasound examination of the uterus to clarify the type of congenital uterine anomaly.

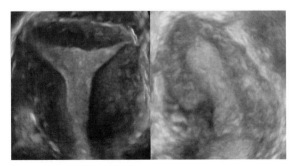

**Figure 4.2** Three-dimensional ultrasound images of a normal uterus (left) and a unicornuate uterus (right). Two interstitial portions of fallopian tube are visible in the normal uterus in contrast to a single interstitial portion of fallopian tube in the unicornuate uterus.

**Table 4.1** Morphological criteria for differential diagnosis of uterine anomalies using three-dimensional ultrasound. From Woelfer *et al.* [22] with permission.

| Uterine morphology | Fundal contour | External contour |
|---|---|---|
| Normal | Straight/ convex | Uniformly convex or indentation <10 mm |
| Arcuate | Concave fundal indentation with central point of indentation at obtuse angle (>90) | Uniformly convex or indentation <10 mm |
| Subseptate | Presence of septum which does not extend to cervix with central point of septum at acute angle (<90) | Uniformly convex or indentation <10 mm |
| Septate | Presence of uterine septum that completely divides cavity from fundus to cervix | Uniformly convex or indentation <10 mm |
| Bicornuate | Two well-formed uterine cornua | Fundal indentation >10 mm dividing the two cornua |
| Unicornuate with or without rudimentary horn | Single well-formed uterine cavity with a single interstitial portion of fallopian tube and concave fundal contour | |

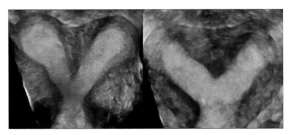

**Figure 4.3** Three-dimensional transvaginal ultrasound images of a bicornuate uterus (left) and a subseptate uterus (right).

uterine anomalies it is not possible to routinely visualize the serosal surface of the uterus which, as we have seen, is an essential plane for the differentiation of different anomaly types. It was the development of three-dimensional scanning that overcame the anatomical constraints that limit the diagnostic power of two-dimensional transvaginal ultrasound.

## Three-dimensional ultrasound

The real breakthrough in ultrasound assessment of congenital uterine anomalies was the development of three-dimensional transvaginal probes. This technique involves the acquisition and storage of a volume of ultrasound information which can then be analyzed at a later date. The major advantage of this technique is that it allows the examination of the acquired volume in any arbitrary plane that the operator may select (Figure 4.3). This overcomes the limitation of conventional two-dimensional ultrasound that allows examination of the uterus in either the longitudinal or the transverse plane and which relies on proxy indicators, such as the presence of loops of

bowel between the uterine horns [13], to assess the serosal uterine contour. Jurkovic *et al.* in 1995 [15] demonstrated that it is possible to obtain an adequate-quality three-dimensional ultrasound volume for the assessment of congenital uterine anomalies in up to 95% of cases. They also showed that three-dimensional ultrasound performs very well with no false positives or false negative results even for minor anomalies such as an arcuate uterus compared with HSG. However, it soon became clear that the current AFS classification is not suitable for use with three-dimensional scanning. The ability to examine the uterus in great detail and to measure the extent of the distortion of uterine anomaly required a modification of AFS classification to include quantitative criteria for the differential diagnoses. Woelfer *et al.* in 2001 [22] published expanded criteria for the diagnosis for congenital uterine anomalies using three-dimensional ultrasound. Although this modified classification was largely based on the AFS, the use of numerical cut-off was essential to ensure reproducibility (Table 4.1). The reproducibility of the classification was tested by Salim *et al.* in 2003 [23] in a study of 89 pre-selected malformations that were classified independently by two expert operators. They demonstrated complete agreement between the two operators in classifying the uteri as normal or abnormal and did not find any significant difference between the measurements of the two observers. To date transvaginal three-dimensional ultrasound is the only diagnostic modality which has been tested for its reproducibility in the diagnosis of uterine anomalies.

Raga *et al.* [24] in 1996 used transvaginal three-dimensional ultrasound to examine 42 women, 12 of which had a Müllerian anomaly confirmed by laparoscopy and HSG. They confirmed the excellent sensitivity of three-dimensional ultrasound for the detection of congenital uterine anomalies. They also correctly classified 11/12 anomalies but did not publish their diagnostic criteria and used the unmodified AFS classification which does not include objective diagnostic criteria. Similar results were published by Wu *et al.* [25] a year later who studied 40 high-risk women. More recently Ghi *et al.* [26] used the modified criteria published by Woelfer *et al.* (Table 4.1) in a series of 284 high-risk patients. They achieved 92.4% concordance between three-dimensional transvaginal ultrasound and endoscopy (52/54). It should be noted that they performed laparoscopy/hysteroscopy in cases of suspected anomaly whilst they performed only office hysteroscopy in cases where the ultrasound was reported as normal. Given the inability of hysteroscopy to assess the serosal surface of the uterus it is possible that mild anomalies were missed on office hysteroscopy thereby overestimating the accuracy of ultrasound.

Despite the high positive and negative predictive value of three-dimensional ultrasound for the detection of congenital uterine anomalies all authors point out pitfalls that may give rise to errors. Jurkovic *et al.* [15] and Raga *et al.* [24] point out that care has to be taken when fibroids are present in the uterus as they may distort the uterine cavity or the serosal surface of the uterus. Ghi *et al.* [26] misdiagnosed a septate uterus as bicornuate uterus early in their patient series. They suggest that the error was made because the serosal surface of the uterine fundus was examined whilst the uterine body was not perpendicular to the examination plane, giving rise to the false impression of a cleft. This error is commensurate with our experience and can be avoided if the operator ensures that the initial plane of examination includes both interstitial portions of the fallopian tubes and the internal cervical os and that the scrolling plane is perpendicular to this.

## Magnetic resonance imaging

Magnetic resonance imaging (MRI) has been shown to be effective [10,27,28] for the diagnosis of congenital uterine anomalies with sensitivity and specificity up to 100%. This is because of the ability of MRI imaging to depict the serosal surface of the uterus and therefore allow the differentiation between bicornuate and septate uterus. This differentiation is not as straightforward as might be assumed as in some cases a fundal indentation co-exists with a uterine septum. Fedele *et al.* [28] established some arbitrary criteria for this differentiation, namely a fundal indentation >10 mm with an angle >60° between the medial margins of the hemicavities. An MRI scan may obviate the need for diagnostic laparoscopy or laparotomy in women suspected to have a congenital uterine anomaly. However, MRI is not an investigation readily available and in most hospitals it is rationed as it is associated with a high financial cost. It cannot therefore serve as a screening test or first-line investigation.

## Clinical consequences

### Reproductive performance

The commonest uterine anomaly found in a large screening study of an asymptomatic population was an arcuate uterus (71%), followed by septate/subseptate uteri (29%), bicornuate (7%), unicornuate (4%) and uterine agenesis (2%) [4]. The main clinical consequence of a congenital uterine anomaly is the effect it can have on a woman's reproductive performance. Amongst women with recurrent pregnancy loss the incidence of congenital uterine anomalies is up to three times higher (1.8–7.2%) compared with a population of women with no history of recurrent pregnancy loss [14,29–31]). However the distribution of anomaly subtypes in women with recurrent miscarriage is similar to that found in women with no history of pregnancy loss [29]. This would suggest that symptomatic women have more severe malformations rather than a particular subtype being responsible for pregnancy loss. Because the AFS classification system is based on the subjective assessment of the diagnosing clinician [22] and does not specify objective criteria, it cannot distinguish between mild and severe malformations within a particular subtype. So anomalies classified by the AFS under the same category can have different clinical consequences in terms of a woman's reproductive performance which causes obvious problems when counseling women and planning interventions [29]. In order to identify objective factors that predict the reproductive performance of women with congenital uterine anomalies, Woelfer *et al.* [22] performed a screening study on a large group of low-risk women using

**Table 4.2** Criteria for differential diagnosis between intrauterine pregnancy in an anomalous uterus and various forms of ectopic pregnancy. From Mavrelos et al. [32].

| | Uterine shape | Uterine cavity | Number of interstitial tubes | Communication between gestational sac and uterine cavity | Myometrial mantle continuous with the uterus | Mobility | Vascular pedicle |
|---|---|---|---|---|---|---|---|
| Intrauterine pregnancy in anomalous uterus | Abnormal | Abnormal | 2 | Wide | Yes | – | No |
| Tubal ectopic | Normal | Normal | 2 | Absent | No | + | No |
| Interstitial | Normal | Normal | 2 | Narrow | Yes | – | No |
| Abdominal | Normal | Normal | 2 | Absent | No | – | No |
| Cornual | Abnormal | Abnormal | 1 | Absent | No | ++ | Yes |

two-dimensional transvaginal ultrasound with three-dimensional ultrasound used as a diagnostic test. They found that women with subseptate uteri had a significantly higher proportion of first-trimester miscarriages compared with women with a normal uterus. In the same study women with arcuate uteri had a higher rate of second trimester loss and preterm labor. In a follow-up study, Salim et al. [29] using three-dimensional transvaginal ultrasound sought to further investigate objective measures of the severity of congenital uterine anomalies. They compared the uterine morphological characteristics of 121 women with recurrent miscarriage to those of 105 low-risk women who were diagnosed with congenital uterine anomalies. They found that the ratio of the length of the septum to the total length of the uterine cavity (distortion index) is significantly higher in women with recurrent miscarriage (0.60 vs 0.40 in subseptate uteri). They also found a prevalence of arcuate uterus of 17% among women with recurrent pregnancy loss compared with 3.2% in low-risk women. This study showed that not only type, but also severity of uterine anomaly is important when assessing the effect of uterine morphology on reproductive outcomes. This was the first demonstration of the value of quantitative measurement in classification of congenital uterine anomalies.

## Uterine anomalies in early pregnancy

Secondary effects of uterine malformations include complications surrounding the diagnosis of pregnancy as well as complications at the time of uterine instrumentation, for example for termination. With the advent of early pregnancy scanning often the diagnosis of a congenital uterine anomaly is made on two-dimensional transvaginal ultrasound in the first trimester. The diagnostic methodology is similar to that for non-pregnant women but the presence of a congenital uterine anomaly can give rise to confusion as to whether the pregnancy is intrauterine or not. Misdiagnosis of an intrauterine pregnancy as an ectopic could potentially result in termination of a wanted pregnancy, which is a serious adverse clinical outcome. The main difficulty is differential diagnosis between an intrauterine pregnancy in a bicornuate/subseptate uterus and an interstitial pregnancy. Problems may also arise in cases of a pregnancy in the non-communicating rudimentary horn of a unicornuate uterus (cornual pregnancy). Ultrasound diagnostic criteria to achieve these differential diagnoses were recently published [32] (Table 4.2) but some of these remain to be prospectively tested. According to these criteria a pregnancy in the horn of a bicornuate uterus is differentiated from an interstitial pregnancy by the caliber of communication between the pregnancy and the endometrial cavity. In an interstitial pregnancy this communication is narrow, representing the interstitial portion of the fallopian tube medial to the pregnancy [33,34]; in contrast in an intrauterine pregnancy in a bicornuate uterus the communication is wide [35] (Figure 4.4). A cornual pregnancy (pregnancy in the non

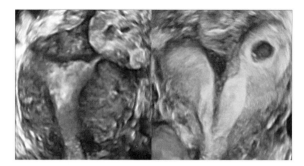

**Figure 4.4** Three-dimensional transvaginal ultrasound images of a left interstitial tubal pregnancy (left) and an intrauterine pregnancy in the left horn of a bicornuate uterus (right). The images contrast the narrow connection between pregnancy and endometrial cavity in the interstitial pregnancy and the wide connection in the intrauterine pregnancy in the bicornuate uterus.

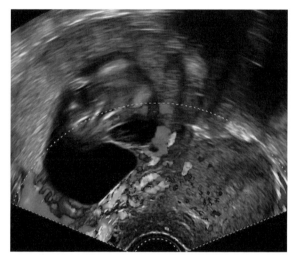

**Figure 4.5** Two-dimensional transvaginal ultrasound image of a 13 week cornual pregnancy. The image demonstrates the ultrasound diagnostic criteria including a left unicornuate uterus, a gestation sac surrounded by myometrium and a vascular pedicle connecting the gestation sac and the unicornuate uterus.

communicating horn of a unicornuate uterus) can be differentiated from a tubal or abdominal ectopic if the following ultrasound diagnostic criteria are applied (Figure 4.5):

(1) A single interstitial portion of fallopian tube in the uterine corpus (unicornuate uterus).
(2) A gestation sac surrounded by myometrium.
(3) A vascular pedicle connecting the gestation sac to the uterine corpus [32].

In a reported series of eight cornual pregnancies there were no false positive results using these criteria. Achieving this rare diagnosis is important not only because of the high morbidity associated with cornual

pregnancies but also because of the different treatment required for these different types of ectopic pregnancy [36–38].

Congenital uterine anomalies increase the risk of failed termination 90-fold [39] usually because the congenital uterine anomaly is missed on ultrasound and an evacuation of one side of the uterus only is performed. The relatively low sensitivity of transabdominal ultrasound for the detection of congenital uterine anomalies is likely to be contributing to congenital uterine anomalies being missed at the initial screening ultrasound. The use of transvaginal ultrasound, with its higher sensitivity, at this initial screening would reduce the potential for such errors. If a congenital uterine anomaly is detected the evacuation should be performed under ultrasound guidance which would ensure that the gestation sac is reached [40].

## Conclusion

The advent of three-dimensional ultrasound has greatly enhanced our ability to diagnose congenital uterine anomalies in an outpatient setting. It has also enabled more detailed studies of the uterine morphology and reproducible measurement of various morphological features such as length of the septum or depth of fundal indentation. These advancements in diagnosis are likely to improve our understanding of clinical significance of various uterine anomalies and improve selection of women who are likely to benefit from surgical correction of uterine anomaly.

## References

1. The American Fertility Society classifications of adnexal adhesions, distal tubal occlusion, tubal occlusion secondary to tubal ligation, tubal pregnancies, mullerian anomalies and intrauterine adhesions. *Fertil Steril* 1988; **49**: 944–55.

2. Simon C, Martinez L, Pardo F *et al.* Mullerian defects in women with normal reproductive outcome. *Fertil Steril* 1991; **56**: 1192–3.

3. Cooper JM, Houck RM, Rigberg HS. The incidence of intrauterine abnormalities found at hysteroscopy in patients undergoing elective hysteroscopic sterilization. *J Reprod Med* 1983; **28**: 659–61.

4. Jurkovic D, Gruboeck K, Tailor A *et al.* Ultrasound screening for congenital uterine anomalies. *Br J Obstet Gynaecol* 1997; **104**: 1320–1.

5. Byrne J, Nussbaum-Blask A, Taylor WS *et al.* Prevalence of Mullerian duct anomalies detected at ultrasound. *Am J Med Genet* 2000; **94**: 9–12.

6.  Ashton D, Amin HK, Richart RM *et al.* The incidence of asymptomatic uterine anomalies in women undergoing transcervical tubal sterilization. *Obstet Gynecol* 1988; **72**: 28–30.

7.  Braun P, Grau FV, Pons RM *et al.* Is hysterosalpingography able to diagnose all uterine malformations correctly? A retrospective study. *Eur J Radiol* 2005; **53**: 274–9.

8.  Acien P. Embryological observations on the female genital tract. *Hum Reprod* 1992; **7**: 437–45.

9.  Rock JA, Breech L. Surgery for anomalies of the Mullerian ducts. In JA Rock, HWI Jones (eds), *Te Linde's Operative Gynecology*. 10th edition. Philadelphia: Wolters Kluwer, Lippincott, Williams & Wilkins, 2008, pp. 541–7.

10. Pellerito JS, McCarthy SM, Doyle MB *et al.* Diagnosis of uterine anomalies: relative accuracy of MR imaging, endovaginal sonography, and hysterosalpingography. *Radiology* 1992; **183**: 795–800.

11. Reuter KL, Daly DC, Cohen SM. Septate versus bicornuate uteri: errors in imaging diagnosis. *Radiology* 1989; **172**: 749–52.

12. Nicolini U, Bellotti M, Bonazzi B *et al.* Can ultrasound be used to screen uterine malformations? *Fertil Steril* 1987; **47**: 89–93.

13. Fedele L, Ferrazzi E, Dorta M *et al.* Ultrasonography in the differential diagnosis of "double" uteri. *Fertil Steril* 1988; **50**: 361–4.

14. Clifford K, Rai R, Watson H *et al.* An informative protocol for the investigation of recurrent miscarriage: preliminary experience of 500 consecutive cases. *Hum Reprod* 1994; **9**: 1328–32.

15. Jurkovic D, Geipel A, Gruboeck K *et al.* Three-dimensional ultrasound for the assessment of uterine anatomy and detection of congenital anomalies: a comparison with hysterosalpingography and two-dimensional sonography. *Ultrasound Obstet Gynecol* 1995; **5**: 233–7.

16. Keltz MD, Olive DL, Kim AH *et al.* Sonohysterography for screening in recurrent pregnancy loss. *Fertil Steril* 1997; **67**: 670–4.

17. Goldberg JM, Falcone T, Attaran M. Sonohysterographic evaluation of uterine abnormalities noted on hysterosalpingography. *Hum Reprod* 1997; **12**: 2151–3.

18. Alborzi S, Dehbashi S, Parsanezhad ME. Differential diagnosis of septate and bicornuate uterus by sonohysterography eliminates the need for laparoscopy. *Fertil Steril* 2002; **78**: 176–8.

19. Valenzano MM, Mistrangelo E, Lijoi D *et al.* Transvaginal sonohysterographic evaluation of uterine malformations. *Eur J Obstet Gynecol Reprod Biol* 2006; **124**: 246–9.

20. Alatas C, Aksoy E, Akarsu C *et al.* Evaluation of intrauterine abnormalities in infertile patients by sonohysterography. *Hum Reprod* 1997; **12**: 487–90.

21. Jayasinghe Y, Rane A, Stalewski H *et al.* The presentation and early diagnosis of the rudimentary uterine horn. *Obstet Gynecol* 2005; **105**: 1456–67.

22. Woelfer B, Salim R, Banerjee S *et al.* Reproductive outcomes in women with congenital uterine anomalies detected by three-dimensional ultrasound screening. *Obstet Gynecol* 2001; **98**: 1099–103.

23. Salim R, Woelfer B, Backos M *et al.* Reproducibility of three-dimensional ultrasound diagnosis of congenital uterine anomalies. *Ultrasound Obstet Gynecol* 2003; **21**: 578–82.

24. Raga F, Bonilla-Musoles F, Blanes J *et al.* Congenital Mullerian anomalies: diagnostic accuracy of three-dimensional ultrasound. *Fertil Steril* 1996; **65**: 523–8.

25. Wu MH, Hsu CC, Huang KE. Detection of congenital mullerian duct anomalies using three-dimensional ultrasound. *J Clin Ultrasound* 1997; **25**: 487–92.

26. Ghi T, Casadio P, Kuleva M *et al.* Accuracy of three-dimensional ultrasound in diagnosis and classification of congenital uterine anomalies. *Fertil Steril* 2008; **8**: 1–6.

27. Carrington BM, Hricak H, Nuruddin RN *et al.* Mullerian duct anomalies: MR imaging evaluation. *Radiology* 1990; **176**: 715–20.

28. Fedele L, Dorta M, Brioschi D *et al.* Magnetic resonance evaluation of double uteri. *Obstet Gynecol* 1989; **74**: 844–7.

29. Salim R, Regan L, Woelfer B *et al.* A comparative study of the morphology of congenital uterine anomalies in women with and without a history of recurrent first trimester miscarriage. *Hum Reprod* 2003; **18**: 162–6.

30. Tulppala M, Palosuo T, Ramsay T *et al.* A prospective study of 63 couples with a history of recurrent spontaneous abortion: contributing factors and outcome of subsequent pregnancies. *Hum Reprod* 1993; **8**: 764–70.

31. Makino T, Umeuchi M, Nakada K *et al.* Incidence of congenital uterine anomalies in repeated reproductive wastage and prognosis for pregnancy after metroplasty. *Int J Fertil* 1992; **37**: 167–70.

32. Mavrelos D, Sawyer E, Helmy S *et al.* Ultrasound diagnosis of ectopic pregnancy in the non-communicating horn of a unicornuate uterus (cornual pregnancy). *Ultrasound Obstet Gynecol* 2007; **30**: 765–70.

33. Ackerman TE, Levi CS, Dashefsky SM *et al.* Interstitial line: sonographic finding in interstitial (cornual) ectopic pregnancy. *Radiology* 1993; **189**: 83–7.

34. Hafner T, Aslam N, Ross JA *et al.* The effectiveness of non-surgical management of early interstitial

pregnancy: a report of ten cases and review of the literature. *Ultrasound Obstet Gynecol* 1999; **13**: 131–6.

35. Jurkovic D, Mavrelos D. Catch me if you scan: ultrasound diagnosis of ectopic pregnancy. *Ultrasound Obstet Gynecol* 2007; **30**: 1–7.

36. Martin JN, Jr., McCaul JFt. Emergent management of abdominal pregnancy. *Clin Obstet Gynecol* 1990; **33**: 438–47.

37. Jermy K, Thomas J, Doo A *et al.* The conservative management of interstitial pregnancy. *BJOG* 2004; **111**: 1283–8.

38. Cutner A, Saridogan E, Hart R *et al.* Laparoscopic management of pregnancies occurring in non-communicating accessory uterine horns. *Eur J Obstet Gynecol Reprod Biol* 2004; **113**: 106–9.

39. Bradshaw H, Stewart P. Failed medical termination of pregnancy associated with implantation in a non-communicating uterine horn. *J Fam Plann Reprod Health Care* 2004; **30**: 178.

40. Pennes DR, Bowerman RA, Silver TM *et al.* Failed first trimester pregnancy termination: uterine anomaly as etiologic factor. *J Clin Ultrasound* 1987; **15**: 165–70.

# Ultrasound and early pregnancy

Nicole S. Winkler and Anne Kennedy

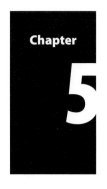

## Introduction

This book is a resource for individuals setting up, or working in, early pregnancy assessment units (EPUs). The goal of these units is to provide timely management to patients in the first trimester of pregnancy. Ultrasound is an integral part of early pregnancy assessment; this chapter will cover normal findings in early pregnancy, the ultrasound diagnosis of early pregnancy failure, the spectrum of appearances of perigestational hemorrhage and the first-trimester evaluation of chorionicity and amnionicity in multiple gestations.

Other chapters will discuss ectopic pregnancy, gestational trophoblastic disease and sonographic detection of uterine anomalies, therefore these topics will not be discussed in detail. As EPUs are for triage of acute problems in the first trimester, a detailed discussion of first-trimester screening is beyond the scope of this text. Some examples of anomalies detectable within the first trimester are included in order to aid with recognition and appropriate referral to specialist centers.

Ultrasound in the first trimester can be performed via the transabdominal (TA) or transvaginal (TV) route. Transabdominal sonography is adequate to confirm cardiac activity for maternal reassurance and may adequately demonstrate perigestational hemorrhage but in general TV sonography is preferred for detailed evaluation. The higher frequency of the TV transducer results in much higher image resolution and maternal habitus is less of a factor than for TA imaging. One important caveat to the use of TV scans is the patient in whom torsion is a consideration. A large ovarian mass which has undergone torsion may be high in the pelvis beyond the range of the vaginal transducer. If the ovaries are not seen with the vaginal transducer, reassessment with the abdominal transducer will prevent delayed or missed diagnosis of a large ovarian mass +/− torsion.

The goals of ultrasound in early pregnancy are outlined in Table 5.1.

## Normal findings in early pregnancy

A clear understanding of normal pregnancy development is essential in order to diagnose first-trimester complications. The first trimester is the best time to obtain accurate dates and confirm expected date of delivery (EDD) based on the last menstrual period (LMP). Biological variation takes effect after the 13th week of gestation therefore in the first trimester all normal pregnancies can be expected to develop in a defined way. An EDD is generally revised if there is more than a one-week discrepancy between menstrual and sonographic dates. There are two exceptions to this rule. If a patient is certain of menstrual dates or has used ovulation prediction an early size/date discrepancy may indicate early pregnancy failure and short-interval follow-up is more appropriate than revision of the EDD. Another is in patients with recurrent pregnancy loss. In our practice we wait until an embryo is identified in order to revise menstrual dating in this group of patients.

Sonographic signs described in very early pregnancy include the intradecidual sac sign (IDSS) and the double decidual sac sign (DDSS). The DDSS was the first sonographic sign of intrauterine pregnancy (IUP) to be described. Following the DDSS, development of a yolk sac within the gestation sac confirms IUP. Thereafter, the embryo appears and demonstration of cardiac activity confirms the existence of a live IUP. The term "viable," though often used, is inappropriate as a first-trimester embryo clearly cannot survive independent of the mother.

**Table 5.1** Goals of ultrasound in early pregnancy.

Is there an intrauterine pregnancy?

Is it normally located?

Is size appropriate for dates?

How many embryos are there?

Is there cardiac activity?

Is the heart rate normal?

Look for any uterine abnormality

Exclude adnexal mass

Because first-trimester pregnancies develop in a predictable manner there are "milestones" for normal development. These are important for serial evaluation. Failure to meet milestones can allow a definitive diagnosis of early pregnancy failure on a single scan. In dubious cases follow-up can be arranged at an interval such that confident diagnosis of failure vs normal development can be made.

## Normal early pregnancy milestones

Knowledge of these normal developmental milestones is essential for the accurate assessment of patients in the first trimester. Failure to meet any of the following milestones is associated with failed pregnancy. A yolk sac should be visible within a gestational sac once the mean sac diameter (MSD) reaches 10 mm on transvaginal scans. An embryo should be visible when the MSD reaches 18 mm. An embryo measuring ≥5 mm should demonstrate cardiac activity. A recent study by Aziz et al. [1] found that identification of an embryo 5 mm or smaller (as small as 2 mm in length) without demonstrated cardiac activity in women with vaginal bleeding was associated with pregnancy failure in every case. This is a single study but worthy of repetition as, until now, additional follow-up is recommended if the embryo is <5 mm in size. In the authors' experience cardiac activity has certainly been seen to develop on follow-up of 3 and 4 mm embryos in a population with asymptomatic recurrent pregnancy loss.

The MSD reflects the mean diameter of the gestational sac. It is accurately assessed by taking measurement of the anechoic sac only (without including the echogenic rim) in three planes and taking the average of these three measurements. The MSD increases by about 1 mm per day. The crown–rump length (CRL) is a measurement of the embryonic length. It is the most accurate measurement to date a pregnancy and should be used from the initial visualization of the embryo until about 12 weeks. Figures 5.1 and 5.2 illustrate various normal findings on first-trimester ultrasound and Table 5.2 summarizes normal early pregnancy measurements and milestones.

## Intradecidual sac sign

First described in 1986 by Yeh et al. [2], the IDSS refers to the sonographic appearance seen after the fertilized ovum implants into the decidualized endometrium. Transvaginal sonography demonstrates an echogenic ring completely embedded within thickened decidua on one side of the intrauterine cavity such that the central cavity is not yet deformed [3]. The IDSS is observed by 4–4.5 weeks post LMP. The sensitivity and specificity of this sign in the diagnosis of intrauterine pregnancy has been debated. The most recent study by Chiang et al. demonstrated a sensitivity of 60–68%, specificity of 97–100% with increased sensitivity of >80% associated with MSD >3 mm or hCG levels greater than or equal to 2000 IU/L [4].

The IDSS is not a stand-alone sign of IUP as endometrial cysts can cause a similar appearance. Follow-up should be obtained in all cases to ensure progressive enlargement of the sac and development of normal structures.

## Double decidual sac sign

Two concentric echogenic rings surrounding an anechoic sac within the endometrial cavity comprise the DDSS. This finding is the earliest transabdominal sign of an IUP and may be seen by 5 weeks post LMP. The inner echogenic ring represents the decidua capsularis and basalis, which covers the anechoic gestational sac. The decidua parietalis corresponds to the outer echogenic ring, which is made up of decidualized endometrium. A thin crescent of endometrial fluid can be seen between the inner and outer ring up to 9 weeks gestational age when coaptation of the decidua capsularis and parietalis occurs, obliterating this fluid space [5]. This sign is helpful if the yolk sac is not yet visible, however a yolk sac should be seen by 5–5.5 weeks, limiting the utility of this sign in the diagnosis of intrauterine pregnancy [6].

## Gestation sac with yolk sac

Visualization of the yolk sac confirms IUP. The yolk sac should be visible once the MSD reaches 10 mm. This structure is seen by 5–5.5 weeks as a small round

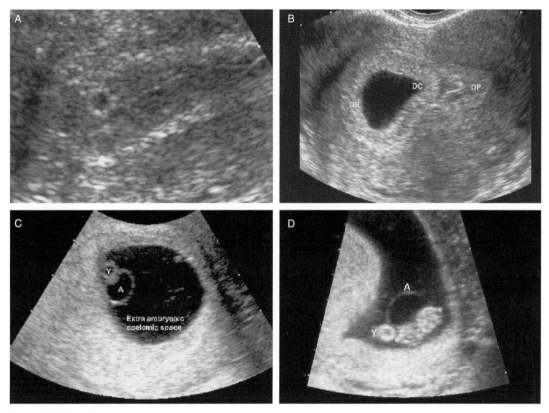

**Figure 5.1** Normal very early pregnancy.
A. The small echogenic ring burrowed into the decidualized endometrium is the earliest sign of IUP on TV sonography. This is the intradecidual sac sign (IDSS).
B. The next stage of development, the double decidual sac sign (DDSS), occurs as the gestation sac enlarges. The decidual capsularis (DC) creates one echogenic ring and the decidua parietalis (DP) creates the second. The decidual basalis (DB) is also noted.
C. The double bleb appearance is created by the yolk sac (Y) beside the amniotic sac (A). The embryo lies between the two "blebs" and the echogenic material surrounding the amniotic sac is the proteinaceous fluid in the extra-embryonic coelomic space.
D. As the pregnancy progresses, the embryo enlarges and lies within the amniotic cavity. A = amniotic membrane. The yolk sac (Y) lies outside the amniotic cavity. The asterisks show how to measure the crown–rump length. The yolk sac should not be included in the measurement which should be obtained through the longest axis of the embryo.

echogenic ring within the anechoic gestational sac. Each yolk sac has a corresponding amnion and though the amnion has already developed at this point, it is more difficult to see. The normal yolk measures 6 mm. It is visible between the amnion and chorion until about 14 weeks when it is obliterated by the coaptation of the membranes.

A focal thickening on one part of the circumference of the yolk sac represents the earliest sonographic evidence of embryonic development, sometimes described as the "diamond ring" sign in which the ring is the yolk sac and the embryo is the diamond.

## Visualization of the amnion

The amnion is seen as a thin, delicate membrane inside the echogenic chorionic ring. The amnionicity is equal to the number of yolk sacs in multiple gestations. By 14–16 weeks the membranes are no longer visible as separate layers. Amniotic fluid is produced by the membranes in the first trimester and renal function does not account for the majority of fluid volume until 16–17 weeks. Amniotic fluid is anechoic but the fluid around the amnion, between it and the chorion, is proteinaceous and may appear quite echogenic. This extra embryonic coelomic space is normal and should not be confused with perigestational/subchorionic hemorrhage in which there is bleeding deep to the chorion.

## Normal embryonic development

An embryo should be seen when the MSD reaches 18 mm. The "diamond ring sign" describes the

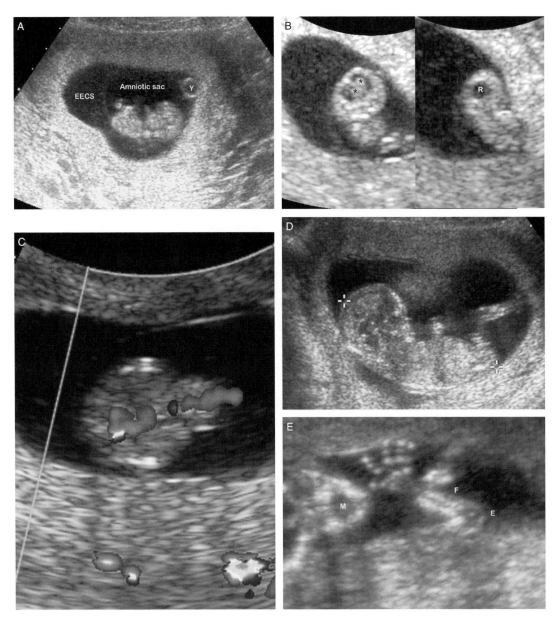

**Figure 5.2** Normal early pregnancy at 9–13 weeks.

A. By 9 weeks the embryo has a recognizable "head end" seen adjacent to the yolk sac (Y) and the limb buds are also enlarging. The embryo is clearly within the amniotic sac and the extra embryonic coelomic space (EECS) is decreasing in volume with respect to the amniotic cavity.

B. The rhombencephalon (R) is a normal precursor to the posterior fossa brain structures. This should not be confused with holoprosencephaly or neural tube defect. In this case normal choroid plexus (asterisk) is seen on either side of an intact midline confirming the presence of two cerebral hemispheres at 9 weeks.

C. In this transverse view through the torso echogenic bowel loops are seen protruding into the base of the umbilical cord; the so-called physiological omphalocele. This appearance is abnormal after 12 weeks or when the crown–rump length is >44 mm.

D. By 12 weeks the fetus is recognizably human with head, chest, abdomen and extremities all easily visible even on transabdominal scans.

E. This is a 13 week fetus; note that it is possible to count fingers even at this early stage. E = elbow, F = forearm, M = mouth. The fingers are in plane and the thumb is partly adducted, therefore not seen in its entirety in this image.

**Table 5.2** Normal early pregnancy milestones and measurements.

| |
|---|
| MSD 10 mm, must see yolk sac |
| MSD 18 mm, should see embryo |
| Crown–rump length 5 mm, must see cardiac activity |
| MSD increase by about 1 mm per day |
| CRL increase by about 1 mm per day |
| Sac diameter should be about 1 cm > CRL |
| Cord length approximates embryo length |

MSD = mean sac diameter; CRL = crown–rump length.

sonographic finding of an early embryo (diamond) as an echogenic focus atop the yolk sac (ring). An embryo with a CRL ≥ 5 mm should demonstrate cardiac activity by TV ultrasound. The trilaminar embryo is a linear structure which lies between the amnion and the adjacent yolk sac, creating the "double bleb" sign. As the embryo enlarges it first becomes C-shaped then undergoes rapid growth and a complex folding process which results in development of the neural tube and closure of the anterior abdominal wall. The limb buds develop by 9 weeks and the hands and feet are fully formed by 13 weeks. Physiological bowel herniation occurs because the growth of the gastrointestinal tract exceeds the capacity of the peritoneal cavity and bowel herniates into the base of the umbilical cord. The bowel rotates 270 degrees and returns to the abdomen by 11 weeks. This normal process should not be confused with omphalocele or gastroschisis.

## Placental development

The placenta arises from the chorion frondosum which develops as focal thickening in the wall of the chorionic sac. This process starts at 8 weeks. Normal placenta thickness is about 1 mm per week gestational age. The umbilical cord normally inserts into the center of the chorion frondosum.

## First trimester findings in multiple gestations

Chorionicity is the most important prognostic indicator in multiple gestations therefore it is vital to make an accurate determination of this any time a multiple pregnancy is seen. The best time to assess chorionicity and amnionicity is the first trimester (Figure 5.3).

After fertilization there is rapid growth of the zygote. If two separate ova are fertilized the twins are dizygotic. By definition, dizygotic twins are dichorionic. If a single zygote splits the type of twinning depends on when the split occurs. A split within 3 days of conception results in dichorionic diamniotic twins; each twin has a separate chorion and amnion surrounding the embryo. When the inner cell mass of the blastocyst splits between days 4 and 8 after conception monochorionic diamniotic (MCDA) twinning occurs. Chorionic tissue has already been formed; the split results in two amnions and two embryos. A split at days 9–13 results in monochorionic monoamniotic (MCMA) twinning. Chorion and amnion have already been formed therefore the twin embryos are inside a single amniotic sac. A split after 13 days results in conjoined twinning of which there are several anatomical subtypes.

The chorion is visualized as a thick echogenic ring. The double layer of chorion and amnion creates the "thick membrane" seen in later pregnancy. The echogenic chorionic tissue at the base of the membrane creates the "twin peak" or "lambda" sign. In the first trimester, dichorionic twins are easily diagnosed based on the presence of two brightly echogenic rings [7]. As pregnancy progresses each bright ring should contain a yolk sac, a thin amniotic membrane and an embryo.

Monochorionic diamniotic twins can be confused with monoamniotic twins by the unwary. In both types there is a single echogenic chorionic ring. Although embryologically, the amnion forms before the yolk sac, it is such a thin delicate membrane that it is not easily seen. The yolk sac is a small, distinct, round structure with an echolucent center and should be seen within the chorion once the MSD is >10 mm. The number of yolk sacs parallels the number of amnions. Therefore if two embryos are seen within a single chorionic sac but two yolk sacs are also seen the pregnancy is almost certainly monochorionic diamniotic.

The "thin membrane" is composed of two layers of opposed amnion. The membrane abuts the placental surface as a "T" shape without a wedge of echogenic chorionic tissue at the base. If only one yolk sac is seen this increases suspicion for MCMA twins. Serial evaluation will show that the embryos are within one sac without an intervening membrane.

Monochorionic diamniotic twins are at risk for specific complications such as twin–twin transfusion

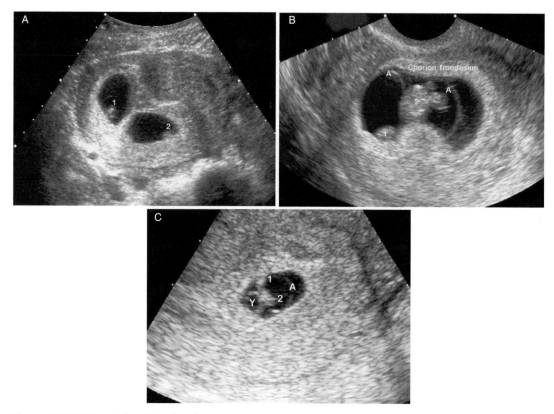

**Figure 5.3** Multiple gestations in the first trimester.

A. Dichorionic twins are each surrounded by a separate, thick chorionic membrane. Two yolk sacs were seen on other imaging planes.

B. Contrast the appearance of dichorionic twins with this example of monochorionic, diamniotic twins. There is a single echogenic chorionic ring; the focal thickening of the chorion frondosum indicates the site of placental development. Within the chorionic sac, there are two embryos each surrounded by a thin amniotic membrane (A). Two yolk sacs were seen on other imaging planes.

C. Monochorionic twins may be monoamniotic as well (i.e. the fertilized ovum splits later in embryogenesis) and there is no dividing membrane. Both embryos are within a single amniotic cavity. In this very early example of monoamniotic twinning at the "double bleb" stage two embryos are seen between a single yolk sac (Y) and a single amnion (A). Cardiac activity was demonstrable in both.

syndrome; this makes the prognosis worse than for dichorionic twins. Monochorionic monoamniotic twins are at risk for all of the complications of MCDA twins as well as cord entanglement which can result in demise of one or both fetuses. Thus all MCDA and MCMA twins should be referred to specialist centers as soon as the diagnosis is made.

## Ultrasound findings in early pregnancy failure

As with all patient interaction, history and physical findings are as important as the imaging findings. In the first trimester of pregnancy evaluation of serum hormonal levels such as hCG and progesterone are often useful for triage.

Progesterone is produced by the corpus luteum; it maintains the early pregnancy until the placenta takes over production. Low serum progesterone has been associated with pregnancy failure and ectopic pregnancy. Though a firm cut-off value has not been established, multiple studies have used values <40 nmol/L [8].

The quantitative hCG is defined as the serum level at which an IUP should be identified sonographically. The exact level is somewhat controversial [9]. At the authors' institution a level of ± 2000 IU/L (3rd international reference preparation) is used. The serum level doubles every 48 hours in normal early pregnancy.

Figure 5.4 illustrates some abnormal findings on first-trimester ultrasound.

## Failure to meet milestones

As normal early pregnancies follow a predictable growth pattern, deviation from normal interval growth

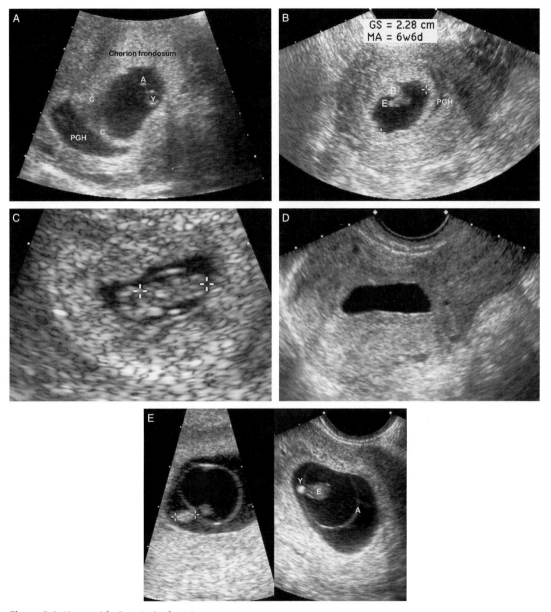

**Figure 5.4**  Abnormal findings in the first trimester.

A. Perigestational hemorrhage (PGH) occurs deep to the chorion (C). A live embryo was seen on other scan planes. The yolk sac (Y) and the edge of the amnion (A) are visible in this plane. This was a large PGH but the pregnancy went to term. The fact that the chorion frondosum remained well attached to the myometrium may have contributed to the good outcome.

B. The cursors mark the correct location for measurement of sac size to calculate the mean sac diameter. No cardiac activity was seen in a 9 mm embryo (E) indicating embryonic demise. This was a follow-up on a case with a chorionic bump (B); a focal protrusion of chorionic tissue thought to represent focal hematoma. Note also that the sac shape is irregular and that there is a sliver of PGH. Most failed pregnancies will exhibit multiple abnormal findings.

C. In this case a live embryo (calipers) was seen within a very small amniotic sac; note that the amniotic membrane appears shrink-wrapped around the embryo. The embryo was dead on follow-up one week later.

D. In this case of embryonic demise note the flattened, oval appearance of the gestation sac and the lack of brightly echogenic decidual reaction/chorionic tissue surrounding the sac.

E. Composite image showing two abnormal yolk sacs. The first (calipers) is flattened and was mistaken for the embryo, however it cannot be an embryo as it is outside the amnion. The second (Y) is calcified hence brightly echogenic. A dead embryo (E) was seen inside the amniotic cavity (A).

indicates a problem. If a single scan shows a size/date discrepancy, but is not definitive for pregnancy failure, short-interval follow-up can be timed such that milestones should have been achieved. For example a gestation sac with MSD of 11 mm, containing a yolk sac is sonographically "normal" even if size is less than expected for LMP. On follow-up 7–10 days later embryonic development should be apparent if the pregnancy is normal. Lack of an embryo would indicate failed early pregnancy due to failure to meet normal milestones. Similarly, even if cardiac activity is present, lack of normal embryonic growth is associated with pregnancy failure.

Once the MSD reaches or exceeds 18 mm the lack of an embryo indicates anembryonic pregnancy. It is possible to demonstrate the amniotic cavity as an anechoic fluid-filled space within the gestational sac. The yolk sac is outside the amnion, between it and the chorion. The term "empty amnion" is used to describe this appearance in anembryonic gestations.

## Abnormal sac

The normal gestational sac is seen as a brightly echogenic ring within the echogenic decidualized endometrium. If the tissue surrounding the sac is thin, irregular or poorly echogenic this correlates with abnormal pregnancy and poor prognosis. The normal gestation sac is a rapidly growing structure with convex contours; flattened shape or irregular margins are abnormal and sac position low in the uterus also correlates with poor outcome [10]. In the absence of a live embryo, abortion in progress is part of the differential for low sac position. In cases where there is a live embryo in a sac implanted low in the uterus the examiner should always exclude cervical and cesarean scar ectopic pregnancy.

Although ectopic pregnancy is not part of this discussion all operators examining women in the first trimester of pregnancy should be aware of the pseudosac seen in the uterus of patients with ectopic pregnancy. Pregnancy hormones result in decidualization of the endometrium regardless of the site of implantation. Accumulation of small amounts of blood product within the endometrial cavity produces a hypoechoic structure with an echogenic rim. The pseudosac differs from a normal early IUP in a number of different ways. It is central within the uterine cavity rather than burrowed or implanted into one layer of decidualized endometrium. There is a single echogenic ring surrounding it, composed of the separated layers of decidualized endometrium.

A normal IUP is eccentrically located and has a double echogenic ring composed of the decidua parietalis and capsularis surrounding the sac. The pseudosac is flattened or oval in shape whereas a normal IUP is spherical or oblate spheroid in shape.

## Embryo to sac size discrepancy

The sac diameter is generally about 1 cm > CRL. A smaller sac leads to a "shrink wrapped" appearance of the embryo; this is described as first trimester oligohydramnios [11].

If the sac is much larger than it should be in relation to CRL this suggests arrest of embryonic development. Biometric tables are available to correlate CRL and menstrual age.

## Embryonic demise

If cardiac activity is absent after prior demonstration that is unequivocal evidence of demise and embryonic failure. Lack of cardiac activity in an embryo >5 mm in length also indicates demise. A recent study by Aziz et al. [1] showed that even with embryos smaller than 5 mm lack of cardiac activity indicated embryonic demise in the subset of patients with vaginal bleeding.

## Empty uterus

In the patient with a positive pregnancy test but an empty uterus there are three possible options: ectopic pregnancy, complete spontaneous abortion or very early IUP. The history and physical findings may enable a clinical diagnosis but more often than not the diagnosis is unclear. Correlation with quantitative beta hCG is very helpful in this situation (Table 5.3).

## Retained products of conception

The term retained products of conception (RPOC) refers to the finding of residual placental tissue within the endometrial cavity after delivery or abortion (spontaneous or therapeutic) resulting in immediate or delayed bleeding. The classic sonographic finding is an echogenic mass with high-velocity, low-resistance blood flow within the endometrial cavity. Unfortunately this finding is associated with an overall false positive rate of 34% due to significant overlap with the normal postpartum uterus after a term delivery [12]. In the first trimester RPOC can

**Table 5.3** What to do when the uterus is empty but the pregnancy test is positive.

| |
|---|
| Careful history |
| Is menstrual history firm? |
| What is cycle length? |
| Risk factors for ectopic pregnancy? |
| Passage of tissue? |
| Clinical examination |
| Pulse, blood pressure |
| Os open/closed |
| Cervical motion tenderness |
| Palpable adnexal mass |
| Additional evaluation |
| Consider serum progesterone measurement |
| Serum beta hCG |
| If above threshold level and uterus is empty suspicion for ectopic increases |
| If below threshold level repeat at 48 hours and rescan if increasing |

Remember, that if the patient is unstable, inability to demonstrate an ectopic does not exclude the diagnosis, especially in the presence of intraperitoneal bleeding. Operative intervention should not be delayed.

occur after an incomplete abortion and the differential diagnosis includes gestational trophoblastic disease and residual blood clot.

The presence of blood clot can be confusing; however clot is avascular and is usually hypoechoic. Lack of perfusion decreases suspicion for RPOC but does not categorically rule out the diagnosis. A follow-up scan can be performed in 24–48 hours in equivocal cases, while cases of obvious RPOC should undergo dilation and curettage to prevent prolonged hemorrhage and infection.

# Abnormal findings in first-trimester pregnancy

## Abnormal yolk sac

A normal yolk sac is thin-walled, spherical and <6 mm in diameter. The yolk sac is outside the amnion but inside the chorion. A collapsed yolk sac should not be mistaken for an embryo as the embryo lies inside the amniotic cavity. Large or calcified yolk sacs are associated with poor prognosis [13].

## Chorionic bump

The chorionic "bump" is an irregular, convex protrusion from the choriodecidual surface into the adjacent gestational sac. This was associated with a >50% loss rate in infertility patients [14]. The authors' experience in a population with recurrent pregnancy loss corroborates this finding (unpublished). The etiology of this focal irregularity is unclear, but it may represent focal hemorrhage. Chorionic bump has also been associated with partial mole.

## Embryonic bradycardia

Embryonic bradycardia is defined as a heart rate <90 beats per minute (bpm) at any gestational age [15–17]. Bradycardia is associated with a high rate of demise. The normal embryonic heart rate is >100 bpm by 6 weeks, increasing to an average of 143 at 8 weeks. A plateau occurs at 9 weeks with heart rates ranging from 137–144 [18]. Most pregnancies abort within a week of diagnosis of embryonic bradycardia, therefore follow-up ultrasound in about 1 week is recommended to avoid delayed diagnosis. The prognosis of

**Table 5.4** Embryonic heart rates in the first trimester [20].

| Normal |
| --- |
| ≥100 at <6.3 weeks |
| ≥120 at 6.3–7 weeks |
| Borderline |
| 90–99 at <6.3 weeks |
| 110–119 at 6.3–7 weeks |
| Abnormal |
| <90 at <6.3 weeks |
| <110 at 6.3–7 weeks |

embryos surviving beyond a week after diagnosis remains guarded even if the heart rate increases to >100 bpm until at least 11 weeks (Table 5.4) [19,20]. There is a two-fold increased risk of structural and chromosomal anomalies in newborns with bradycardia diagnosed in the first trimester [21].

## Echogenic fluid in the cul de sac

Physiological fluid is a common finding in pelvic ultrasound. A small volume of anechoic fluid is a normal finding, however, echogenic fluid correlates strongly with intraperitoneal hemorrhage. In the pregnant patient this is especially concerning if an IUP cannot be identified and increases suspicion for a ruptured ectopic [22].

## Gestational trophoblastic disease

Gestational trophoblastic disease is covered in detail elsewhere. Sonographically a complete mole has a typical appearance, completely filling the uterine cavity with an echogenic, multicystic, hypervascular mass. However, only about 56% of first-trimester cases show this typical appearance [23]. In the first trimester, a complete mole may present with thickened cystic endometrium, or as an apparent anembryonic pregnancy [24].

Ovarian theca lutein cysts are also rare in the first trimester as the hCG levels are not yet sufficiently high enough to cause them.

## Perigestational hemorrhage

The term perigestational hemorrhage (PGH) is synonymous with subchorionic hemorrhage. The estimated sonographic prevalence in women presenting with vaginal bleeding in the first trimester is 18% [25]. A fluid collection separate from, but adjacent to the gestational sac is the sonographic finding. This fluid collection may have a curvilinear appearance, which follows the uterine contour or a mass-like appearance that may distort the gestational sac. The fluid collection is always deep to (i.e. on the myometrial side of) the chorion. The normal echogenic fluid in the extra embryonic coelomic space should not be mistaken for a PGH. Additional features vary depending on the age and extent of hemorrhage.

The vast majority of pregnant women presenting with vaginal bleeding in the first trimester will have a good outcome. The presence of a live embryo is the most reassuring sign associated with an excellent prognosis of >90% survival when the PGH is small.

A less favorable prognosis is associated with large PGH, advanced maternal age, fetal bradycardia and gestational sac size <16 mm [26,27]. Follow-up imaging in 5–7 days can be helpful in early cases bearing in mind that blood evolves quickly, decreasing in echogenicity and size over time and the gestational sac should grow 1 mm/day.

Color Doppler can help differentiate an isoechoic PGH from chorionic frondosum. No blood flow will be seen in a PGH.

Although the gestational sac may appear to be "floating" within a large PGH, the term placental abruption should not be used in the first trimester. The diagnosis of placenta previa should also be avoided in the first trimester because the placenta often covers the internal os at this stage of pregnancy. As the pregnancy progresses and the lower uterine segment elongates the placenta appears to migrate superiorly. This process is known as placental trophotropism.

Despite the overall good prognosis in the majority of first-trimester PGH cases, there is an associated increased risk of morbidity within the second and third trimesters. Fetal growth restriction, pre-eclampsia, pre-term delivery, pregnancy-induced hypertension and a five-fold risk of placental abruption have all been described in association with PGH in the first trimester. Therefore, careful attention on follow-up second- and third-trimester imaging is recommended.

Be aware that twin gestation can mimic PGH particularly in cases where one twin fails early in pregnancy.

## Fetal anomalies

Detection and characterization of fetal anomalies is beyond the scope of this text but the examiner should be aware of the appearances of certain malformations in order to expedite referral and avoid undue delay in diagnosis (Figure 5.5). Similarly the normal appearance of the rhombencephalon and physiological bowel herniation should not be confused with pathological processes [28].

Normal choroid plexus fills the ventricles in the first trimester; this is called the "butterfly" sign and when seen excludes anencephaly and alobar or semi-lobar forms of holoprosencephaly. This is particularly reassuring to patients with a history of a prior affected fetus. Exencephaly can also be diagnosed in the first trimester as the uncovered brain causes an unusual head shape.

Cystic hygroma is a multiseptated fluid collection extending from the fetal neck, often associated with diffuse skin edema. This is associated with Turner's and Down's syndrome and carries a poor prognosis even in euploid fetuses.

The limbs are fully formed by 13 weeks including fingers and toes; inability to visualize four extremities is abnormal and should raise concern for limb reduction defects [29].

Conjoined twins can be diagnosed with confidence if two heartbeats are seen within a conglomerate tissue mass. Twin reverse arterial perfusion sequence is

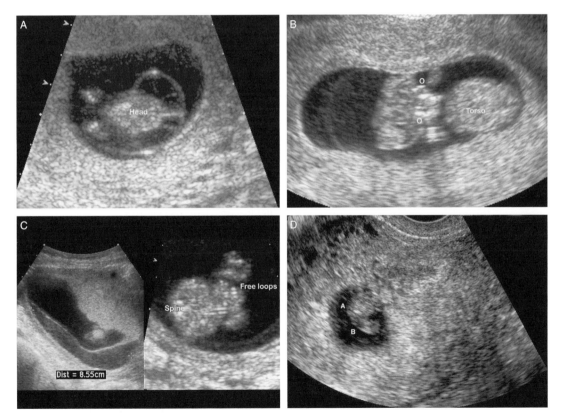

**Figure 5.5** Anomalies visible in the first trimester.

A. Transverse image through the fetal head at 12 weeks shows a septated fluid collection consistent with a cystic hygroma. Chorionic villus sampling showed Turner syndrome.

B. Coronal image through the fetal head and torso at 12 weeks shows exencencephaly. Bony detail is seen in the orbital area (O) but there is no evidence of an ossified skull vault and the brain tissues form an amorphous mass above the orbits. This is a lethal malformation.

C. Composite image shows large PGH (calipers) at 12 weeks 6 days. Additional images showed gastroschisis with free loops of bowel in the amniotic fluid (Spine = fetal spine). Ductus venosus flow was also abnormal and the patient elected termination of pregnancy.

D. Two embryos (A, B) are seen within a single amniotic cavity. Additional images showed only one yolk sac but confirmed two foci of cardiac activity within the conglomerate tissue mass indicating conjoined twins.

present when the direction of flow in the umbilical artery is toward an anomalous twin rather than toward the placenta.

## Adnexal mass

Routine use of TV sonography in evaluation of the first-trimester pregnancy will result in the detection of incidental adnexal masses. It goes without saying that any patient with pain in the first trimester should be carefully evaluated for ectopic pregnancy. The finding of an IUP greatly decreases suspicion for ectopic gestation unless there are risk factors for heterotopic pregnancy. However, hemorrhagic cyst, cyst rupture, ovarian torsion appendicitis and ureteric calculi can all occur and present with pelvic pain [30].

Amongst the incidental masses seen in the first trimester ovarian lesions are commonest. Use of transducer pressure and manual abdominal pressure helps to determine if the mass moves with the ovary, i.e. is ovarian in origin, or slides over the ovary indicating a non-ovarian, adnexal origin. Pedunculated fibroids tend to be hypoechoic; careful evaluation with color Doppler will often demonstrate vessels extending from the myometrium into the fibroid.

The normal corpus luteum has a thick, echogenic wall with a "ring of fire" appearance on color Doppler interrogation. Hemorrhage is not uncommon; lacy reticular internal echoes are present although on occasion homogeneous internal echoes may simulate a solid mass. Lack of internal vascularity and increased through-transmission of sound should suggest the diagnosis. Endometriomata may be seen particularly in patients with a history of assisted reproduction; they typically contain multiple, fine, low-level internal echoes and exhibit increased through-transmission. Punctate echogenic foci with comet tail artifacts in the walls are a characteristic finding. Theca lutein cysts are seen with ovarian stimulation, hyperreactio luteinalis and gestational trophoblastic disease. Associated ascites and pleural effusion indicate ovarian hyperstimulation syndrome which necessitates careful monitoring of fluid balance and renal function.

The most common ovarian neoplasm in the reproductive age group is the benign ovarian teratoma (dermoid cyst). The typical findings include a shadowing, echogenic "plug," hair, teeth, fat-fluid levels and echogenic fat. The fat content may cause significant distal acoustic shadowing. This "tip of the iceberg" phenomenon may result in significant underestimation of the size of teratomas. Malignant ovarian neoplasms are uncommon but can occur. A solid mass lesion with papillary projections and vascular internal septations, or a persistent large cystic mass should be further evaluated by gynecological oncology.

## Conclusion

Ultrasound is a key component of early pregnancy assessment. Knowledge of the normal imaging findings and expected developmental milestones is vital for accurate interpretation. Recognition of monochorionic pregnancies and significant anomalies will allow for appropriate early referral for specialist evaluation. Ultrasound is the most accurate way to triage patients with pain and/or bleeding in the first trimester.

## References

1. Aziz S, Cho RC, Baker DB *et al*. Five-millimeter and smaller embryos without embryonic cardiac activity: outcomes in women with vaginal bleeding. *J Ultrasound Med* 2008; **27**(11): 1559–61.

2. Yeh HS, Goodman JD, Carr L *et al*. Intradecidual sign: a US criterion of early intrauterine pregnancy. *Radiology* 1986; **161**: 463–7.

3. Laing FC, Brown DL, Price JF, Teeger S, Wong ML. Intradecidual sign: is it effective in diagnosis of an early intrauterine pregnancy? *Radiology* 1997; **204**: 655–60.

4. Chiang G, Levine D, Swire M, McNamara A, Mehta T. The intradecidual sign: is it reliable for diagnosis of early intrauterine pregnancy? *AJR* 2004; **183**: 725–31.

5. Bradley WG, Fiske CE, Filly RA. The double sac sign of early intrauterine pregnancy: use in exclusion of ectopic pregnancy. *Radiology* 1982; **143**: 223–6.

6. Yeh HS. Efficacy of the intradecidual sign and fallacy of the double decidual sac sign in the diagnosis of early intrauterine pregnancy. *Radiology* 1999; **210**: 579–81.

7. Shetty A, Smith AP. The sonographic diagnosis of chorionicity. *Prenat Diagn* 2005; **25**(9): 735–9.

8. Chetty M, Elson J. Biochemistry in the diagnosis and management of abnormal early pregnancy. *Clin Obstet Gynecol* 2007; **50**: 55–66.

9. Peisner DB, Timor-Tritsch IE. The discriminatory zone of beta-hCG for vaginal probes. *J Clin Ultrasound* 1990; **18**(4): 280–5.

10. Nyberg DA, Laing FC, Filly RA. Threatened abortion: sonographic distinction of normal and abnormal gestation sacs. *Radiology* 1986; **158**(2): 397–400.

11. Stabile I, Campbell S, Grudzinskas JG. Ultrasonic assessment of complications during first trimester of pregnancy. *Lancet* 1987; **2**(8570): 1237–40.

12. Sadan, O, Golan, A, Girtler, O *et al.* Role of sonography in the diagnosis of retained products of conception. *J Ultrasound Med* 2004; **23**: 371–4.

13. Cho FN, Chen SN, Tai MH, Yang TL. The quality and size of yolk sac in early pregnancy loss. *Aust N Z J Obstet Gynaecol* 2006; **46**(5): 413–18.

14. Harris RD, Couto C, Karpovsky C, Porter MM, Ouhilal S. The chorionic bump: a first-trimester pregnancy sonographic finding associated with a guarded prognosis. *J Ultrasound Med* 2006; **25**(6): 757–63.

15. Doubilet PM, Benson CB. Embryonic heart rate in early first trimester: what rate is normal? *J Ultrasound Med* 1995; **14**(6): 431–4.

16. Achiron R, Tadmor O, Mashiach S. Heart rate as a predictor of first trimester spontaneous abortion after ultrasound-proven viability. *Obstet Gynecol* 1991; **78**: 330–4.

17. Leboda LA, Estroff, JA, Benacerraf BR. First trimester bradycardia: a sign of impending fetal loss. *J Ultrasound Med* 1989; **8**: 561–3.

18. Hertzberg BS, Mahony BS, Bowie JD. First trimester fetal cardiac activity. Sonographic documentation of a progressive early rise in heart rate. *J Ultrasound Med* 1988; **7**: 573–5.

19. Benson, C, Doubilet P. Slow embryonic heart rate in early first trimester: indicator of poor pregnancy outcome. *Radiology* 1994; **192**: 343–4.

20. Doubilet P, Benson, C. Outcome of first-trimester pregnancies with slow embryonic heart rate at 6–7 weeks gestation and normal heart rate by 8 weeks at US. *Radiology* 2005; **236**: 643–6.

21. Doubilet PM, Benson, CB, Chow JS. Long-term prognosis of pregnancies complicated by slow embryonic heart rates in the early first trimester. *J Ultrasound Med* 1999; **18**(8): 537–41.

22. Nyberg DA, Hughes MP, Mack LA, Wang KY. Extrauterine findings of ectopic pregnancy of transvaginal US: importance of echogenic fluid. *Radiology* 1991; **178**(3): 823–6.

23. Benson CB, Genest DR, Bernstein MR *et al.* Sonographic appearance of first trimester complete hydatidiform moles. *Ultrasound Obstet Gynecol* 2000; **16**(2): 188–91.

24. Lazarus E, Hulka C, Siewert B, Levine D. Sonographic appearance of early complete molar pregnancies. *J Ultrasound Med* 1999; **18**(9): 589–94.

25. Maso G, D'Ottavio G, de Seta F *et al.* First trimester intrauterine hematoma and outcome of pregnancy. *Obstet Gynecol* 2005; **105**: 339–44.

26. Pedersen JF, Mantoni M. Prevalence and significance of subchorionic hemorrhage in threatened abortion: a sonographic study. *AJR* 1990; **154**: 353–7.

27. Bennett GL, Bromley B, Lieberman E, Benacerraf BR. Subchorionic hemorrhage in the first trimester pregnancies: prediction of pregnancy outcome with sonography. *Radiology* 1996; **200**: 803–6.

28. Sonek J. First trimester ultrasonography in screening and detection of fetal anomalies. *Am J Med Genet C Semin Med Genet* 2007; **145**C(1): 45–61.

29. Castro-Aragon I, Levine D. Ultrasound detection of first trimester malformations: a pictorial essay. *Radiol Clin North Am* 2003; **41**(4): 681–93.

30. Eyvazzadeh AD, Levine D. Imaging of pelvic pain in the first trimester of pregnancy. *Radiol Clin North Am* 2006; **44**(6): 863–77.

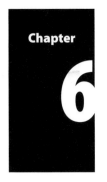

# Management of pregnancy loss

Willem M. Ankum

## Introduction

On a global scale, overpopulation is one of mankind's major challenges. On the individual level, however, human reproduction is a relatively inefficient process [1,2]. Only about 30% of successfully fertilized oocytes result in the delivery of a living child. Approximately 60% of successful conceptions, however, do not even reach the stage of a clinically recognized pregnancy. This phenomenon has earlier been referred to as the "black box" of early pregnancy loss [3]. These occult miscarriages result from immediate demise or failed implantation, which is followed by a normal period at the expected time. The rate of pre-clinical losses can only be detected by close biochemical surveillance, and ultimately defines the upper success rates of human reproduction, not only in spontaneous cycles but also during treatment with artificial reproductive technologies. Pre-clinical losses, therefore, are mainly of scientific importance for those trying to understand reproductive biology rather than being a clinical problem encountered at the early pregnancy unit (EPU).

After the missed period, another 10–15% of successful conceptions are bound to fail during the first trimester as clinically recognized miscarriages. These women constitute a large proportion of those visiting an EPU. This chapter focuses on these patients, and summarizes current knowledge on the epidemiology, diagnosis and treatment of first-trimester pregnancy loss.

## Epidemiology

First-trimester pregnancy loss is a common event, experienced by about 25% of all women during their reproductive career. The vast majority of first-trimester miscarriages are sporadic events, half being accounted for by cytogenetic abnormalities,

i.e. numerical or structural chromosomal anomalies and mosaicism as demonstrated by classical techniques. It seems likely that, with improving cytogenetic techniques, the unexplained part might also turn out to represent hitherto unrecognized – more subtle – chromosomal anomalies (see Chapter 10).

In daily practice it is generally acknowledged that parental cytogenetic screening is unnecessary in sporadic miscarriages, which should be restricted to couples with recurrent miscarriages, a topic beyond the scope of this chapter (see Chapter 7).

Because the occurrence of miscarriages is a highly age-dependent phenomenon, incidence rates vary widely from 10% for women aged 20–24 years, to a staggering 90–100% for those between 45 and 50 years of age [4]. Increased age is not only associated with an elevated risk of Down's syndrome, as is generally known and acknowledged, but also predisposes for other chromosomal anomalies which explain the increased risk of (repeated) miscarriages in these women [5–7].

Risk factors for the occurrence of miscarriages are addressed in more detail elsewhere (see Chapter 2).

## Natural course and clinical findings

In the majority of cases, vaginal bleeding is the first clinical symptom of impending miscarriage. This symptom is by no means specific, since about 50% of these pregnancies will prove to be viable on sonographic examination, most of which are likely to progress without serious consequences. In these women, the exact origin of bleeding usually remains unknown. When other causes, especially cervical Chlamydia infection, cervical carcinoma or a bleeding ectropion have been ruled out, this type of bleeding is ascribed to the process of placental invasion of the endometrium. Straightforward evidence to

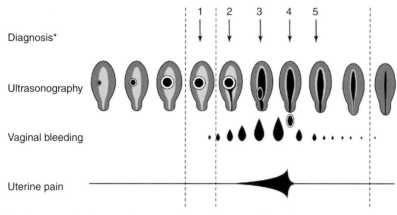

Diagnosis*

Ultrasonography

Vaginal bleeding

Uterine pain

**Figure 6.1** Natural course of miscarriage with clinical and sonographic findings. Courtesy of Br Med J Publishers; from Ankum *et al.* 2001 [8].

*1, ultrasonography shows early anembryonic pregnancy or fetal death (missed miscarriage);
 2, vaginal bleeding occurs (threatened miscarriage);
 3, open cervical os (inevitable miscarriage);
 4, miscarrriage (products of conception are expelled, and cramps and bleeding soon subside);
 5, ultrasonography may show uterine contents - decidua, blood, and some villi.

substantiate this origin, though plausible from a biological viewpoint, is lacking from the literature.

Sooner or later, women with first-trimester miscarriages are bound to experience painful uterine contractions as an accompanying symptom (Figure 6.1). During the process of expulsion of uterine contents which follows, i.e. the actual miscarriage, vaginal bleeding increases and blood clots may be lost. The cervix gradually dilates to allow passage of the nonvital pregnancy, which usually is passed as a complete gestational sac which can easily be distinguished from accompanying blood clots. If the miscarriage is complete, pain and bleeding decrease promptly to the level of a regular menstrual period [8].

Some bleeding may persist for several weeks, and is followed by a normal period some 4–7 weeks after the actual miscarriage took place [9].

In case of an incomplete miscarriage, where a portion of the gestational sac is retained in the uterus, persistent cramping pain and excessive bleeding should indicate the need for surgical evacuation, rather than mere sonographic findings.

Knowledge about the natural course of miscarriages is important whenever expectant management is aimed for. If patients have not been informed about things to come, they may easily be alarmed by the natural course of events and end up undergoing unnecessary surgical evacuation in the final stages of the process. Unawareness of these matters might easily result in disillusionment with the entire experience, not only for the patient but also for the healthcare providers.

Another problem arises when a spontaneous miscarriage simply does not happen within a reasonable period of time, a situation which occurs in about half of those cases undergoing expectant management. After 2 weeks of waiting in vain, even well-motivated women lose their faith, change their minds, and tend to ask for surgical evacuation. Obviously, this scenario should also be addressed when counseling women about treatment options.

## Diagnostic management

Clinical characteristics of women presenting with first-trimester bleeding are of little value in correctly predicting a miscarriage, and cannot be relied upon in daily practice [10]. The only exception is the presence of an expelled gestational sac, found at vaginal examination. This is a highly specific finding, but because of its rarity (4%), sensitivity is low [11,12]. There is no doubt that transvaginal sonography is the most reliable tool in the diagnosis of first-trimester miscarriages at present. Sonographic equipment and expertise, therefore, are indispensable prerequisites for any unit providing care for women with first-trimester pregnancies and their complications (see Chapter 5).

The most constant sonographic findings indicative of a miscarriage are those of an empty gestational sac, where no yolk sac and no embryonic pole are present, or the finding of an embryo or fetus without cardiac activity. There are caveats in the interpretation of these findings, and both need further specification especially if one relies on information obtained from a single scan.

- Firstly, a gestational sac can only be called empty with acceptable certainty if its mean diameter exceeds 15 mm.
- Secondly, the absence of fetal cardiac activity can only be diagnosed with certainty if the fetal crown–rump length exceeds 5 mm.
- If these criteria are not met, the pregnancy may turn out to be vital when sonography is repeated after a week [13].

Some authors have advocated the additional use of serum progesterone measurements in differentiating between viable and non-viable pregnancies in these cases with encouraging results [14]. The usefulness of a single progesterone measurement without further sonographic evaluation, however, is limited, since it does not discriminate between miscarriages and ectopic pregnancies.

Apart from sonographic observations indicative of a miscarriage or a vital pregnancy, another sonographic finding deserves attention, i.e. when sonography fails to show any signs of an intrauterine gestation. In the absence of a clear history of a recent spontaneous miscarriage, this finding is suggestive of an ectopic pregnancy. Obviously, the absence of a gestational sac also complies with the non-pregnant state; therefore, a pregnancy test should be done immediately to exclude this possibility. Many ectopic pregnancies are easily detected by transvaginal sonography and should be looked for carefully. A gestational sac outside the uterus is a very specific finding, but some free fluid in the cul-de-sac and an ectopic mass are less reliable in diagnosing ectopic pregnancy. The addition of hCG measurements is useful when sonography fails to identify an intra-uterine gestation, or whenever no ectopic pregnancy is detected or findings are dubious, i.e. in case of a "pregnancy of unknown location" (PUL). In these circumstances, hCG levels >1500–2000, or plateauing hCG concentrations at a lower level on follow-up (persisting PUL), are indicative of ectopic pregnancy [15–21]. Both serum beta hCG and serum progesterone measurements may be used in monitoring the expectant management of self-limiting ectopic pregnancies, which resolve spontaneously in the majority of cases without need for further invasive procedures (see Chapter 3).

# Prevention of early pregnancy loss

In the past, several drugs have been clinically applied in attempts to prevent miscarriages.

Diethylstilbestrol (DES) is the oldest example, and was used between 1948 and 1974 for this purpose. The drug, an orally active synthetic estrogen, was completely ineffective in preventing miscarriages, as was shown in a randomized study in 1953 [22]. Despite these findings, its use remained widely embraced by the medical community, and DES was prescribed to millions of pregnant women. Unfortunately, DES increased the risk of cervical and vaginal clear cell carcinoma in DES-exposed female offspring of treated women, and also turned out to be strongly associated with the occurrence of ectopic pregnancy in these women [23,24]. Its use during pregnancy was banned in 1971 by the US Food and Drug Administration.

More recently, progesterone has also been applied in the prevention of miscarriages. This topic has recently been systematically reviewed in The Cochrane Library [25]. No evidence of effectiveness with the use of vaginal progesterone compared with placebo was found in reducing the risk of miscarriage (relative risk 0.47; 95% CI 0.17–1.30). The authors concluded that: "Based on scarce data from two methodologically poor trials, there is no evidence to support the routine use of progestogens for the treatment of threatened miscarriage. Information about potential harms to the mother or child, or both, with the use of progestogens is lacking. Further, larger, randomized controlled trials on the effect of progestogens on the treatment of threatened miscarriage, which investigate potential harms as well as benefits, are needed."

These findings are no surprise in view of the assumption that many early losses are the result of chromosomal aneuploidies. But even pre-implantation genetic screening (PGS) for chromosomal aneuploidies in women undergoing artificial reproductive technology was unable to solve this problem. In contrast to its theoretical advantages, instead of increasing a woman's chances of having a baby, PGS increased the risk of early pregnancy loss [26].

If anything, these earlier attempts to prevent early pregnancy loss illustrate the lack of knowledge and understanding in this field. The debacles with the application of DES during the 1950s, 1960s and 1970s and, more recently, with PGS, underline the importance of rigorous evaluation and should remind us of the dangers of any medical intervention carried out in early pregnancy.

## Therapeutic management

At present, three different treatment options are being used in managing first-trimester miscarriages: expectant, surgical and medical management.

Expectant management, i.e. awaiting the natural course as described earlier, represents the oldest form of management in first-trimester miscarriages. Obviously, expectant management originates from a time when no other options were available, circumstances which still apply for less privileged parts of the world. During the first half of the twentieth century, surgical evacuation became the preferred treatment option for managing miscarriages in many countries. This strategy was prompted by the high incidence of sepsis and mortality associated with miscarriages in cases of retained products of conception. Many complicated cases resulted from criminal attempts to terminate undesired pregnancies, rather than being complications of spontaneous miscarriages [27,28]. Expectant management remained in use, albeit modestly, in some Western societies where general practitioners were involved in providing routine obstetrical care [29–31]. More recently, expectant management of spontaneous miscarriages experienced a revival in many Western countries where its use had been abolished earlier. Ironically, again terminations of pregnancies played a pivotal role in this process of change. The revived interest in non-surgical management of miscarriages followed the encouraging results of medical terminations of pregnancy induced by the combined use of the anti-progestagen mifepristone and the prostaglandin misoprostol [32].

The available knowledge from randomized controlled trials comparing various treatment options for miscarriages has been systematically reviewed [33–35]. In these reviews, formal meta-analysis is hampered by heterogeneity of the available studies on various subjects, which often differ in the type of patients, setting, dosages and route of administration, and time frames allowed in expectantly and medically managed patients. According to these reviews, aspiration curettage results in the highest complete evacuation rate in comparison to non-surgical management options. Medical management (i.e. misoprostol administered orally or vaginally) reduces the need for curettage by 81–99%, whereas expectant management reduces the need for surgery by 28–94%, depending on the type of pregnancy loss, i.e. incomplete miscarriages or those with a gestational sac still being present, and on the time frame of expectancy. The vast majority of incomplete miscarriages were managed safely without the need for additional surgical intervention. The incidence of pelvic inflammatory disease as a complication of treatment did not differ between women undergoing surgical curettage and those managed non-invasively.

In studies comparing medical versus expectant management, misoprostol was more effective in reaching complete evacuation of the uterus, at the expense, however, of minor gastrointestinal side effects and an increased need of analgesics. These findings were confirmed in a later paper, not included in the systematic reviews, which compared expectant and medical treatment in a randomized placebo-controlled trial [36]. In that study, a regimen of daily 600 μg misoprostol, administered vaginally in up to two doses, had similar side effects compared with placebo.

Recently the MIST trial, a large multicenter randomized study, compared all three available options: expectant, medical (800 μg misoprostol vaginally) and surgical management [37]. No difference was found in infection rates between the three strategies (2–3%), nor in the need for blood transfusions (0–1%). More women undergoing expectant management (50%) than those treated medically (38%) needed a curettage. The risk of unplanned hospital admissions was highest in expectantly managed women. Despite this, the net societal costs were lowest in the expectantly managed group at £1086, versus £1410 in the medical group and £1585 in the surgery group [38].

The MIST trial used a combination of mifepristone followed by misoprostol in medically managed patients. A later study found no difference between mifepristone followed by misoprostol versus misoprostol alone [39]. Indeed, many clinics now use misoprostol as a single agent, thereby further reducing costs. Probably the vaginal administration of misoprostol 600 μg, which can be repeated after 24 hours, now offers the optimal balance between effectiveness and side effects.

As an alternative to immediate treatment, a delayed management option has also been studied. This randomized trial compared the vaginal administration of misoprostol and curettage, after a week of failed expectant management. Here again the non-invasive strategy was found to be more cost-effective [40,41].

In view of the available evidence, non-invasive treatment modalities can now be offered with confidence to women with first-trimester pregnancy loss who wish to avoid surgery. This is important, since freedom of treatment choice improves quality of life in these unfortunate women [42–44].

## Future research

Several subjects in the field of early pregnancy loss have not been addressed as yet, and need further attention in clinical studies. For instance, the option of self-administered vaginal misoprostol deserves to be explored. Self-administration seems feasible for most women, and would render the miscarriage process easier to plan at a convenient time and place for the patient. This probably would increase patients' satisfaction in comparison to the administration of medication by healthcare professionals, and would probably reduce costs.

Another topic to be explored in future research concerns the role of vacuum curettage under combined local anesthesia /conscious sedation. This approach should be explored in comparison to general anesthesia, both in terms of patient satisfaction and costs.

## Acknowledgment

Parts of this chapter have been published earlier and are used with kind permission of the *British Journal of Hospital Medicine* [45].

## References

1. Wilcox AJ, Weinberg CR, O'Connor JF *et al.* Incidence of early loss of pregnancy. *New Engl J Med* 1988; **319**: 189–94.

2. Chard T. Frequency of implantation and early pregnancy loss in natural cycles. *Baillière's Clin Obstet Gynaecol* 1991; **5**: 179–89.

3. Macklon NS, Geraedts JPM, Fauser BCJM.Conception to ongoing pregnancy: the 'black box' of early pregnancy loss. *Hum Reprod Update* 2002; **8**: 333–43.

4. Nybo-Andersen AM, Wohlfahrt J, Christens P, Olsen J, Melbye M. Maternal age and fetal loss: population based register linkage study. *Br Med J* 2000; **320**: 1708–12.

5. Heffner LJ. Advanced maternal age – how old is too old? *New Engl J Med* 2004; **351**: 1927–9.

6. Goddijn M, Lesschot NJ. Genetic aspects of miscarriage. *Baillière's Clin Obstet Gynaecol* 2000; **14**: 855–65.

7. Franssen MTM, Korevaar JC, van der Veen F *et al.* Reproductive outcome after chromosome analysis in couples with two or more miscarriages: case-control study. *Br Med J* 2006; **332**: 759–63.

8. Ankum WM, Wieringa-de Waard M, Bindels PJE. Management of spontaneous miscarriage in the first trimester. *Br Med J* 2001; **322**: 1343–6.

9. Wieringa-de Waard M, Ankum WM, Bonsel GJ *et al.* The natural course of spontaneous miscarriage: analysis of signs and symptoms in 188 expectantly managed women. *Br J Gen Pract* 2003; **53**: 704–8.

10. Wieringa-de Waard M, Bonsel GJ, Ankum WM, Vos J, Bindels, PJE. Threatened miscarriage in general practice: diagnostic value of history taking and physical examination. *Br J Gen Pract* 2002; **52**: 825–9.

11. Chung TKH, Sahota DS, Lau TK *et al.* Threatened abortion: prediction of viability based on signs and symptoms. *Aust N Z J Obstet Gynaecol* 1999; **4**: 443–7.

12. Buckley RG, King KJ, Disney JD, Gorman JD, Klausen JH. History and physical examination to estimate the risk of ectopic pregnancy: validation of a clinical prediction model. *Ann Emerg Med* 1999; **34**: 589–94.

13. Schouwink MH, Fong BF, Mol BWJ, Veen F van der. Ultrasonographic criteria for non-viability of first trimester intra-uterine pregnancy. *Early Pregnancy Biol Med* 2000; **IV**: 203–13.

14. Mol BWJ, Lijmer JG, Ankum WM, Van der Veen F, Bossuyt PMM. The accuracy of single progesterone measurement in the diagnosis of ectopic pregnancy: a meta-analysis. *Hum Reprod* 1998; **13**: 3220–7.

15. Ankum WM. Editorial: Diagnosing suspected ectopic pregnancy; HCG monitoring and transvaginal ultrasound lead the way. *Br Med J* 2000; **321**: 1235–6.

16. Ankum WM, Van der Veen F, Hamerlynck JVThH, Lammes FB. Laparoscopy: a dispensable tool in the diagnosis of ectopic pregnancy? *Hum Reprod* 1993; **8**: 1301–6.

17. Ankum WM, Van der Veen F, Hamerlynck JVThH, Lammes FB. Transvaginal sonography and human chorionic gonadotrophin measurements in suspected ectopic pregnancy; a detailed analysis of a diagnostic approach. *Hum Reprod* 1993; **8**: 1307–11.

18. Ankum WM, Van der Veen F, Hamerlynck JVThH, Lammes FB. Ectopic pregnancy: what to do when HCG levels are below the discriminatory zone? *J Reprod Med* 1995; **40**: 525–8.

19. Condous G, Okaro E, Khalid A *et al.* The use of a new logistic regression model for predicting the outcome of pregnancies of unknown location. *Hum Reprod* 2004; **19**: 1900–10.

20. Condous G, Kirk E, Lu C et al. There is no role for uterine curettage in the contemporary diagnostic workup of women with a pregnancy of unknown location. *Hum Reprod* 2006; **21**: 2706–10.

21. Elson J, Tailor A, Banerjee S et al. Expectant management of tubal ectopic pregnancy: prediction of successful outcome using decision tree analysis. *Ultrasound Obstet Gynaecol* 2004; **23**: 552–6.

22. Dieckmann WJ, Davies ME, Rynkiewicz LM, Pottinger RE. Does the administration of diethylstilbestrol during pregnancy have therapeutic value? *Am J Obstet Gynecol* 1953; **66**: 1062–81.

23. Rubin MM. Antenatal exposure to DES: lessons learned … future concerns. *Obstet Gynecol Surv* 2007; **62**: 548–55.

24. Ankum WM, Mol BWJ, Bossuyt PMM van der Veen F. Risk factors for ectopic pregnancy: a meta-analysis. *Fertil Steril* 1996; **65**: 1093–9.

25. Wahabi HA, Abed Althagafi NF, Elawad M. Progestogen for treating threatened miscarriage. *Cochrane Database of Syst Rev* 2008; **4**.

26. Mastenbroek S, Scriven P, Twisk M et al. What next for preimplantation genetic screening? More randomized controlled trials needed? *Hum Reprod* 2008; **23**: 2626–8.

27. Balagh SA, Harris HA, Demasio K. Is curettage needed in uncomplicated incomplete spontaneous abortion? *Am J Obstet Gynecol* 1998; **179**: 1279–82.

28. Irving J. *The Cider House Rules.*. London: Black Swan, 1985.

29. Ambulatory Sentinel Practice Network. Spontaneous abortion in primary care. *J Am Board Fam Pract* 1988; **1**: 15–23.

30. Ankum WM, van der Veen F. Management of first trimester abortion. *Lancet* 1995; **345**: 1179.

31. Chipchase J, James D. Randomised trial of expectant versus surgical management of spontaneous miscarriage. *Br J Obstet Gynaecol* 1997; **104**: 840–1.

32. Henshaw RC, Naji SA, Russell IT, Templeton AA. Comparison of medical abortion with surgical vacuum aspiration: women's preferences and acceptability of treatment. *Br Med J* 1993; **307**: 714–17.

33. Graziosi GCM, Mol BW, Ankum WM, Bruinse HW. Management of early pregnancy failure. *Int J Gynaecol Obstet* 2004; **86**: 337–46.

34. Nanda K, Peloggia A, Grimes D, Lopez L, Nanda G. Expectant care versus surgical treatment for miscarriage. *Cochrane Database of Syst Rev* 2006; **2**.

35. Neilson JP, Hickey M, Vazquez J. Medical treatment for early fetal death (less than 24 weeks). *Cochrane Database of Syst Rev* 2008; **4**.

36. Bagratee JS, Khullar V, Regan L, Moodley J, Kagoro H. A randomised controlled trial comparing medical and expectant management of first trimester miscarriage. *Hum Reprod* 2004; **19**: 266–71.

37. Trinder J, Brocklehurst P, Porter R, Read M, Vyas S, Smith L. Management of miscarriage: expectant, medical, or surgical? Results of randomised controlled trial (miscarriage treatment (MIST) trial). *Br Med J* 2006; **332**: 1235–40.

38. Petrou S, Trinder J, Brocklehurst P, Smith L. Economic evaluation of alternative management methods of first-trimester miscarriage based on results from the MIST-trial. *Br J Obestet Gynaecol* 2006; **113**: 879–89.

39. Stockheim D, Machtinger R, Wiser A et al. A randomized prospective study of misoprostol or mifedipine followed by misoprostol when needed for the treatment of women with early pregnancy failure. *Fertil Steril* 2006; **86**: 956–60.

40. Graziosi GC, Mol BW, Reuwer PJ, Drogtrop A, Bruinse HW. Misoprostol versus curettage in women with early pregnancy failure after initial expectant management: a randomised trial. *Hum Reprod* 2004; **19**: 1894–9.

41. Graziosi GC, van der Steeg JW, Reuwer PJ et al. Economic evaluation of misoprostol in the treatment of early pregnancy failure compared to curettage after an expectant management. *Hum Reprod* 2005; **20**: 1067–71.

42. Wieringa-de Waard M, Vos J, Bonsel GJ, Bindels, PJE, Ankum WM. Management of miscarriage: a randomized controlled trial of expectant management versus surgical evacuation. *Human Reprod* 2002; **17**: 2445–50.

43. Wieringa-de Waard M, Hartman EE, Ankum WM et al. Expectant management versus surgical evacuation in first trimester miscarriage: health related quality of life in randomized and non-randomized patients. *Human Reprod* 2002; **17**: 1638–42.

44. Petrou S, McIntosh E. Women's preferences for attributes of first-trimester miscarriage management: A stated preference discrete-choice experiment. *Value in Health* 2009; **12**(4): 551–9.

45. Ankum W M. Management of first trimester miscarriage. *Br J Hosp Med* 2008; **69**: 380–3.

# Investigation of recurrent miscarriage

Feroza Dawood, Roy G. Farquharson and Mary D. Stephenson

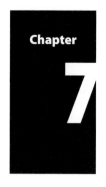

Recurrent miscarriage (RM) affects between 1–2% of fertile couples and is a clinical condition of heterogeneous etiology. The traditional definition of a miscarriage has been pregnancy loss prior to 20 weeks and RM is defined as three or more consecutive miscarriages [1]. However, the gestational period spanning the first 20 weeks of pregnancy encompasses several developmental stages and milestones and hence there is a need for pregnancy loss to be more specifically defined. Classification of RM is of fundamental importance in the investigation and exploration of the pathophysiological mechanisms underlying RM. There is a need to embrace current theories of abnormalities in implantation, trophoblast invasion and placentation when defining pregnancy loss.

A crucial tool in investigating RM is the stratification of the type of pregnancy loss. A clear delineation of pregnancy losses will also yield a framework for comparison of RM studies. Indeed, the inconsistent use of the definition of RM, as well as the divergent nomenclature in describing pregnancy loss in various studies, looking at causation in recurrent miscarriage has led to much debate and controversy.

It is increasingly evident that uniformity in nomenclature would enhance the dissemination of knowledge and ultimately improve our understanding of RM. In Europe, the ESHRE Special Interest Group for Early Pregnancy (SIGEP) [2] has suggested a clarification of terminology for pregnancy loss prior to 20 weeks' gestation, while in North America, a slightly different terminology is proposed (Table 7.1) [3].

## Investigative algorithm

### History

The investigation of recurrent miscarriage commences with a meticulous history which should elicit details of the sequential events surrounding the prior miscarriages. Ideally, this should include serial ultrasound assessment of gestational age, documented presence of fetal heart activity and crown–rump length (CRL) at the time of demise [4]. The two most important determinants of future pregnancy success are maternal age and number of miscarriages [5]. The risk of a subsequent miscarriage following a history of RM increases with maternal age and number of previous successive losses [6].

It is also prudent to take a smoking, alcohol and caffeine history, because all of these substances are associated with an increased risk of miscarriage. There is increasing evidence that excessive caffeine consumption [7,8] is associated with clinical miscarriage. Furthermore, exposure to occupational hazards such as ionizing radiation, organic solvents and compounds such as mercury and lead have been found to be linked with miscarriage [9]. There is also evidence that the chemical compound bisphenol A, which binds to estrogen receptors, may increase the risk of RM by an autoimmune mechanism [10].

## Infective screen

Routine screening for toxoplasmosis, rubella, cytomegalovirus and herpes simplex virus (TORCH) and listeria infections are currently deemed unnecessary [11]. However, they should be performed in women with RM history if an acute infectious episode is suspected [12]. If acute or chronic endometritis is suspected it is prudent to perform an endometrial biopsy [13].

## Endocrinological investigations

Obesity has emerged as an important endocrinological factor for RM and has been linked with a statistically

**Table 7.1** Classification of miscarriage, based on hCG levels and/or ultrasound findings.

| Type of miscarriage | European definitions ESHRE SIG Early Pregnancy [2] | North American definitions [3] |
|---|---|---|
| Biochemical miscarriage | Falling low positive serum/urinary hCG, pregnancy not located on ultrasound (typically <6 weeks) | Falling low positive serum/urinary hCG, no ultrasound performed |
| Anembryonic or empty sac miscarriage | Gestational sac with absent structures or minimal embryonic debris without heart rate activity (typically 6–8 weeks) | An empty gestational sac, with a mean sac diameter of >8 mm |
| Yolk sac miscarriage | Term not used | A gestational sac with a yolk sac only, with a mean sac diameter of >16 mm |
| Embryonic miscarriage | Gestation sac with embryo >6 mm without cardiac activity (typically 6–8 weeks) | Embryo ≥5 mm without cardiac activity |
| Fetal miscarriage | Previous identification of crown–rump length and fetal heart activity followed by loss of heart activity (typically >12 weeks) | Fetus measuring ≥33 mm without cardiac activity |

significant increased risk of recurrent miscarriage (odds ratio 3.5, 95% CI 1.03–12.01) [14].

Although the presence of polycystic ovaries has been reported as having a higher prevalence in RM women compared with the general population [15], the association may be due to obesity and/or insulin resistance, rather than the ovarian features [16].

Another contentious issue is that hypersecretion of luteinizing hormone (LH) is associated with an increased risk for RM; however, wide variations in the levels of LH have been found in women with RM [17]. Presently, there is little evidence to justify routine testing in RM patients.

There is limited evidence supporting a causal relationship between hyperprolactinemia and RM [18].

The value of routine screening for underlying diabetes and thyroid disease in asymptomatic patients has recently been questioned, as the prevalence of these endocrinopathies have been found to be similar in women with RM and the general population [11]. Uncontrolled diabetes has been associated with an increased risk of pregnancy loss and complications, therefore, tight control preconceptually is recommended. Thyroid function and diabetes screening are relatively inexpensive and evidence suggests they should be normalized in early pregnancy [4,19], therefore, such screening is advocated as part of the investigative protocol for RM [19].

Luteal phase deficiency, defined by mid luteal phase progesterone <10 ng/mL, has been associated with RM in the past [4]. More recently, there has been a suggestion that polymorphisms on the progesterone receptor gene may contribute to impaired reproductive function and consequently to recurrent pregnancy losses, so there may be some benefit in testing mid luteal phase progesterone levels [20].

# Genetic investigations

## Parental cytogenetic analysis

Parental structural chromosome rearrangements are reported in 3–8% of couples suffering recurrent miscarriage and testing of both partners is therefore recommended [11] (see Chapter 11). The commonest rearrangements appear to be balanced reciprocal and Robertsonian translocations [4,21]. There is an increased probability of a structural chromosome rearrangement in young women with recurrent miscarriage who have a parent or sibling with a history of recurrent miscarriage; this risk is increased further if the parents of the partner also report a history of recurrent miscarriage [22]. The identification of a parental structural chromosome rearrangement should prompt referral to a clinical geneticist. Subsequent pregnancy outcome depends on the specific rearrangement, but overall, is associated with a 70% live-birth rate, without treatment [23].

## Cytogenetic analysis of miscarriage tissue

Conventional cytogenetic analysis of miscarriage tissue from women with a history of RM has detected a 26–57% abnormality rate [22,24]. However, when age is taken into account there appears to be little difference in the distribution of cytogenetically abnormal miscarriages in couples with RM compared with controls [25].

Although cytogenetic analysis of miscarriage tissue is not routinely performed in most miscarriage clinics, for financial reasons, there is a cogent justification for performing such testing, because it differentiates miscarriage associated with a numeric chromosome abnormality, thought to be a random event [26] from those which may be due to an underlying parental factor (see Chapter 10). Indeed, without chromosome assessment of miscarriage tissue, it is impossible to determine whether the miscarriage resulted from a failure of the treatment or as a result of a lethal trisomy, monosomy or polyploidy.

## Detection of anatomical abnormalities

Uterine anomalies have been traditionally associated with mid-trimester losses; however they may also be implicated in recurrent early (<10 weeks) miscarriage. In the RM population, the prevalence of reported uterine malformations range widely from between 1.8% to 37.6% [11], largely due to inherent differences in methodology. The septate uterus is the commonest congenital structural abnormality. A recent review of approximately 24 studies suggests that the prevalence of congenital uterine anomalies in the RM population is probably as high as 16.7% compared with 6.7% in the general population [27]; hence screening for uterine anomalies is definitely warranted. Diagnostic tools for detecting uterine anomalies include two- and three-dimensional ultrasound, hysteroscopy, laparoscopy and magnetic resonance imaging (MRI). Office hysteroscopy allows direct visualization and avoids general anesthesia. Ultrasound and magnetic resonance imaging are non-invasive and avoid radiation exposure.

## Thrombophilia testing

The antiphospholipid syndrome (APS) remains entrenched as one of the most studied factors associated with RM. Pregnancy losses that have been associated with APS include recurrent early miscarriage, fetal miscarriage of ≥10 weeks' gestation, and second and third trimester complications associated with placental insufficiency resulting in intrauterine growth restriction, placental abruption or sudden intrauterine fetal demise [28]. Antiphospholipid syndrome is characterized by thrombotic and/or obstetric events together with the presence of laboratory criteria. Strict clinical and laboratory criteria need to be adhered to before a diagnosis of antiphospholipid syndrome can be made. The criteria for diagnosis were revised at a consensus conference in Sydney in 2006.

Antiphospholipid syndrome is present if at least one of the following clinical criteria and one of the laboratory criteria are met:

Clinical criteria:

One or more clinical episodes of arterial, venous or small vessel thrombosis, in any tissue or organ. The thrombotic event must be confirmed by objective validated criteria (i.e. unequivocal findings of appropriate imaging studies or histopathology). Histopathologic findings should show thrombosis without significant evidence of inflammation in vessel wall.

Pregnancy morbidity:

(a) One or more unexplained deaths of a morphologically normal fetus (ultrasound evidence or direct examination) at or beyond the 10th week of gestation.

(b) One or more premature births of a morphologically normal neonate before the 34th week of gestation secondary to: (i) eclampsia or severe pre-eclampsia defined according to standard definitions, or (ii) recognized features of placental insufficiency.

(c) Three or more unexplained consecutive spontaneous miscarriages before the 10th week of gestation, with maternal anatomic or hormonal abnormalities and paternal and maternal chromosomal causes excluded.

Laboratory criteria:

(1) Lupus anticoagulant (LA) present in plasma on two or more occasions at least 12 weeks apart.

(2) Anticardiolipin antibody (aCL) antibody of IgG and/or IgM isotype in serum or plasma, present in medium or high titre (i.e. >40 GPL or MPL, or >99th percentile), on two occasions, at least 12 weeks apart, measured by a standardized ELISA.

(3) Anti-beta 2-glycoprotein I antibody of IgG and/or IgM isotype in serum or plasma, present in medium or high titre (i.e. >40 GPL or MPL, or >99th percentile), on two occasions, at least 12 weeks apart, measured by a standardized ELISA.

## Other thrombophilias

More recently attention has focused on the significance of other genetic and acquired thrombophilias as potential putative factors in RM. Amongst these are the factor V Leiden mutation, activated protein C resistance (APCR), protein S deficiency, protein C deficiency, prothrombin gene mutation and antithrombin III deficiency, which have been proven to be independent risk factors for venous thromboembolism [29,30]. It has been hypothesized that these thrombophilias may be associated with recurrent miscarriage as a result of decreased uteroplacental perfusion [31,32]. However, studies exploring the association between RM and thrombophilias have revealed discordant results. Some studies have espoused a link between thrombophilia and RM [33,34] whereas other studies have refuted any significant association between the two [35]. However, the incongruity of results from different studies may lie in inherent differences in study design, lack of uniformity regarding pregnancy classification and wide variation in patient numbers. Multicentered randomized controlled trials are certainly warranted to elucidate whether or not thrombophilia testing should be routinely incorporated in the investigative work-up for RM.

Recently, two meta-analyses [34,35,36] and a review of 69 studies [37] have strengthened the case for testing for factor V Leiden, activated protein C resistance and the prothrombin gene.

## Immunologic investigations

### Natural killer cells

Natural killer (NK) cells are found in peripheral blood and within the endometrium and have been associated with recurrent miscarriage. Different subpopulations of NK cells with various functional roles may directly interact with trophoblasts in the developing placenta [38].

It has also been postulated that NK cell cytotoxicity is altered in peripheral blood of women with RM and that increased cytotoxicity and increased levels of interleukin-2 may be considered risk factors for women with RM [39]. There is some evidence that immunosuppressive therapy may reduce high numbers of uterine NK cells thereby improving reproductive outcome in women with RM [40].

However, the evidence for a definite putative mechanism of NK cells and RM is not yet robust enough. There are phenotypic and functional differences between peripheral and uterine NK cells [41] and some case–control studies have revealed no statistically significant differences between NK cell counts

and pregnancy failure [42]. Furthermore, peripheral NK cell measurement carried out using flow cytometry revealed no significant difference in the number of peripheral natural killer cells and their subsets in women with recurrent miscarriage compared with controls [43].

Further prospective trials are needed to explore whether the cytokine expression of NK cells affects pregnancy outcome. There appears to be limited value in the routine measurement of peripheral NK cells in women with RM and endometrial sampling for uterine NK cells should currently be confined to research programs.

## Mannan-binding lectin

Mannan-binding lectin (MBL; also known as mannose-binding lectin) is an opsonic C-type lectin plasma protein that is synthesized in the liver. It elicits activation of the complement system and plays an important role in innate immune defence [44]. Low levels of MBL predispose to various infectious and inflammatory disorders. There is emerging evidence that MBL deficiency has a significant association with recurrent miscarriage [45,46].

More recently, the genetics of MBL has been further explored. Mannan-binding lectin levels are genetically determined by a combination of complex haplotypes and the presence of several possible point mutations in the structural gene has the greatest influence on phenotype [46].

Mannan-binding lectin concentration is determined by three major single-nucleotide polymorphisms (SNPs) in exon 1 of the *MBL2* gene on chromosome 10q11 and by three SNPs in the promoter region of the gene [47]. A very recent study has investigated polymorphisms in the *MBL2* gene associated with plasma MBL levels in women with RM. They found significantly more low-producing *MBL2* genotypes in women with RM compared with controls [47].

Isolated MBL deficiency may induce a predisposition to RM in conjunction with other immunological disturbances which remain to be investigated. At the present time, there is not enough evidence to recommend testing for MBL on a clinical basis.

## Other investigations

### Hyperhomocysteinemia

Homocysteine is metabolized by either the transsulphuration pathway (excess homocysteine is

**Table 7.2** Predicted probability of a future successful pregnancy in women with a history of idiopathic miscarriages (95% CI). From Brigham *et al.*, 1999 with permission [5].

| Age (years) | Number of previous miscarriages | | | |
|---|---|---|---|---|
| | 2 | 3 | 4 | 5 |
| 20 | 92 | 90 | 88 | 85 |
| 25 | 89 | 86 | 82 | 79 |
| 30 | 84 | 80 | 76 | 71 |
| 35 | 77 | 73 | 68 | 62 |
| 40 | 69 | 64 | 58 | 52 |
| 45 | 60 | 54 | 48 | 42 |

converted to methionine) or the remethylation pathway (recycling of homocysteine to form methionine). Hyperhomocysteinemia has a reported prevalence of around 5–16% in the general population and is an independent risk factor for venous thromboembolism [48].

Hyperhomocysteinemia is most commonly due to a dietary deficiency of folate, although it is sometimes associated with the 667 C T MTHFR mutation, that results in a thermolabile enzyme with reduced activity for the remethylation of homocysteine. The homozygous form of the mutation may infrequently induce a state of hyperhomocysteinemia.

Of the few documented studies that assessed the association of MTHFR mutation in recurrent miscarriage, none was statistically significant [49,50,51]. However, another study has reported an association between maternal hyperhomocysteinemia and recurrent early pregnancy loss [52]. Therefore, there is little evidence at this time to incorporate homocysteine testing into the investigative work-up of RM.

## Human leukocyte antigen testing

The potential role of human leukocyte antigen (HLA) genes and the etiology of RM remain debatable. It was previously thought that maternal immune recognition of HLA antigens expressed by the fetus determined maternal–fetal tolerance in pregnancy. Some studies have identified an association between RM and the human leukocyte antigen G, which is the dominant HLA at the materno–fetal interface [53]. HLA–G single nucleotide polymorphisms have been found to be linked with pregnancy losses [54]. However the contribution of the human HLA complex in the pathophysiology of RM needs to be better defined.

There is presently no benefit derived from routine testing for HLA or anti-paternal cytotoxic antibodies in an RM population.

## Idiopathic recurrent miscarriage

It is important to be cognisant that the heterogeneous nature of RM implies that while there may well be a convergence of etiologies, in about 50% of cases the etiology remains elusive, the so-called "idiopathic" RM.

Idiopathic recurrent miscarriage is a diagnosis of exclusion, meaning that known factors associated with RM have been ruled out [13]. Maternal age and number of previous miscarriages are the most important parameters in predicting subsequent live birth. Supportive therapy with regular ultrasound surveillance and reassurance, in a dedicated early pregnancy clinic, has been shown to be effective in improving subsequent pregnancy outcome (74% vs 51%, *P* = 0.002 [55]. Using statistical actuarial analysis [5], the likelihood of a live birth, stratified for maternal age, for women with a history of idiopathic RM is shown in Table 7.2.

## Summary

Recurrent miscarriage is a challenging reproductive issue for the clinician. Determining the gestational age and chromosome results of prior miscarriages is useful in determining whether further evaluation is required. Presently, many of the RM investigations are controversial because of limited studies, inconsistent terminology and small and poorly designed treatment studies. Over the next decade, we will probably see major advances in the evaluation and management of recurrent miscarriage, based on well-defined cohorts of patients and trials.

## References

1. Stirrat GM. Recurrent miscarriage: definition and epidemiology. *Lancet* 1990; **336**: 673–5.
2. Farquharson RG, Jauniaux E on behalf of the ESHRE Special Interest Group for Early Pregnancy (SIGEP). Updated and revised nomenclature for description of early pregnancy events. *Hum Reprod* 2005; **20**(11): 3008–11.
3. Stephenson MD. Management of recurrent early pregnancy loss. *J Reprod Med* 2006; **51**: 303–10.
4. Stephenson MD, Kutteh W. Evaluation and management of recurrent early pregnancy loss. *Clin Obstet Gynaecol* 2007; **50**(1): 132–45.

5.  Brigham SA, Conlon C, Farquharson RG. A longitudinal study of pregnancy outcome following idiopathic recurrent miscarriage. *Hum Reprod* 1999; **14**: 2868–71.

6.  Andersen AMN, Wohlfahrt J, Christens P, Olsen J, Melbye M. Maternal age and fetal loss: population based register linkage study. *Br Med J* 2000; **320**: 1708–12.

7.  Rasch V. Cigarette, alcohol and caffeine consumption: risk factors for spontaneous abortion. *Acta Obstet Gynecol Scand* 2003; **82**: 182–8.

8.  Infante-Rivard C, Fernandez A, Gauthier R *et al.* Fetal loss associated with caffeine intake before and during pregnancy. *J Am Med Assoc* 1993; **270**: 2940–3.

9.  Gardella JR, Hill JA. Environmental toxins associated with recurrent pregnancy loss. *Semin Reprod Med* 2000; **18**: 407–24.

10. Mayumi SO, Yasuhiko O, Shin-ichi S *et al.* Exposure to bisphenol A is associated with recurrent miscarriage. *Hum Reprod* 2005; **20**(8): 2325–9.

11. Royal College of Obstetricians and Gynaecologists (RCOG). *Guideline 17: the Management of Recurrent Miscarriage.* London: RCOG Press, 1998.

12. Li TC, Makris M, Tomsu M, Tuckerman E, Laird S. Recurrent miscarriage: aetiology, management and prognosis. *Hum Reprod Update* 2002; **8**: 463–81.

13. Stephenson MD. Frequency of factors associated with habitual abortion in 197 couples. *Fertil Steril* 1996; **66**: 24–9.

14. Lashen H, Fear K, Sturdee DW. Obesity is associated with increased risk of first trimester and recurrent miscarriage: matched case-control study. *Hum Reprod* 2004; **19**: 1644–6.

15. Rai R, Backos M, Rushworth F, Regan L. Polycystic ovaries and recurrent miscarriage: a reappraisal. *Hum Reprod* 2000; **15**: 612–15.

16. Fedorcsak P, Dale PO, Storeng R, Tanbo T, Abyholm T. The impact of obesity and insulin resistance on the outcome of IVF or ICSI in women with polycystic ovarian syndrome. *Hum Reprod* 2001; **16**: 1086–91.

17. Li TC, Spuijbroek E, Tuckerman B *et al.* Endocrinological and endometrial factors in recurrent miscarriage. *BJOG* 2000; **107**: 1975–80.

18. Hirahara F, Andoh N, Sawai K *et al.* Hyperprolactinemic recurrent miscarriage and results of randomized bromocriptine treatment trials. *Fertil Steril* 1998; **70**(2): 253–5.

19. Christiansen OB, Andersen AMN, Bosch E *et al.* Evidence-based investigations and treatments of recurrent pregnancy loss. *Fertil Steril* 2005; **83**: 821–39.

20. Sweikert A, Rau T, Berkholz A *et al.* Association of progesterone receptor polymorphism with recurrent abortions. *Eur J Obstet Gynecol Reprod Bio* 2004; **113**: 67–72.

21. Braekeleer de M, Dao TN. Cytogenetic studies in couples experiencing repeated pregnancy losses. *Hum Reprod* 1990; **5**: 519–28.

22. Franssen MTM, Korevaar JC, Leschot NJ *et al.* Selective chromosome analysis in couples with two or more miscarriages: case-control study. *Br Med J* 2005; **331**: 137–9.

23. Stephenson MD, Sierra S. Reproductive outcomes in recurrent pregnancy loss associated with a parental carrier of a structural chromosome rearrangement. *Hum Reprod* 2006; **21**: 1076–82.

[24] Ogasawara M, Aoki K, Okada S, Suzumori K. Embryonic karyotype of abortuses in relation to the number of previous miscarriages. *Fertil Steril* 2000; **73**: 300–4

25. Stephenson MD, Awartani KA, Robinson WP. Cytogenetic analysis of miscarriages from couples with recurrent miscarriage: a case-control study. *Hum Reprod* 2002; **17**: 446–51.

26. Hassold T, Chiu D. Maternal age specific rates of numerical chromosome abnormalities with special reference to trisomy. *Hum Genet* 1985; **70**: 11–17.

27. Saravelos SH, Cocksedge KA, Li TC. Prevalence and diagnosis of congenital uterine anomalies in women with reproductive failure: a critical appraisal. *Hum Reprod Update* 2008; **14**(5): 415–29.

28. Miyakis S, Lockshin MD, Atsumi T *et al.* International consensus statement on an update of the classification criteria for definite antiphospholipid syndrome (APS). *J Thromb Haemost* 2006; **4**(2): 295–306.

29. Zoller B, Dahlback B. Linkage between inherited resistance to activated protein C and factor V gene mutation in venous thrombosis. *Lancet* 1994; **343**: 1536–8.

30. Van Boven HH, Reitsma PPH, Rosendaal FR *et al.* Factor V Leiden (FVR506Q) in families with inherited antithrombin deficiency. *Thromb Haemost* 1996; **75**: 417–21.

31. Kupferminc MJ, Eldor A, Steiman N *et al.* Increased frequency of genetic thrombophilia in women with complications of pregnancy. *New Engl J Med* 1999; **340**: 9–13.

32. Dizon-Townson DS, Meline L, Nelson LM *et al.* Fetal carriers of the factor V Leiden mutation are prone to miscarriage and placental infarction. *Am J Obstet Gynecol* 1997; **177**: 402–5.

33. Dawood F, Farquharson R, Quenby S, Toh CH. Acquired activated protein C resistance may be a risk factor for recurrent fetal loss. *Fertil Steril* 2003; **80**: 649–50.

34. Rey E, Kahn SR, David M, Shrier I. Thrombophilic disorders and fetal loss: a meta-analysis. *Lancet* 2003; **361**: 901–8.

35. Roque H, Paidas MJ, Funai EF, Kuczynski E, Lockwood CJ. Maternal thrombophilias are not associated with early pregnancy loss. *Thromb Haemost* 2004; **91**: 290–5.

36. Kovalevsky G, Gracia CR, Berlin JA *et al.* Evaluation of the association between hereditary thrombophilias and recurrent pregnancy loss: a meta-analysis. *Arch Intern Med* 2004; **164**; 558–63.

37. Krabbendam I, Franx A, Bots ML *et al.* Thrombophilias and recurrent pregnancy loss: a critical appraisal of the literature. *Eur J Obstet Gynecol Reprod Biol* 2005; **118**: 143–53.

38. Kwak-Kim J, Gilman-Sachs A. Clinical implication of natural killer cells and reproduction. *Am J Reprod Immunol* 2008; **59**: 388–400.

39. Hadinedoushan H, Mirahmadian M, Aflatounian A. Increased natural killer cell cytotoxicity and IL-2 production in recurrent spontaneous abortion. *Am J Reprod Immunol* 2007; **58**(5): 409–14.

40. Quenby S, Kalumbi C, Bates M, Farquharson R, Vince G. Prednisolone reduces preconceptual natural killer cells in women with recurrent miscarriage. *Fertil Steril* 2005; **84**: 980–4.

41. Moffett A, Regan L, Braude P. Natural killer cells, miscarriage, and infertility. *Br Med J* 2004; **329**: 1283–5.

42. Ozcimen EE, Kiyici H, Uckuyu A, Yanik FF. Are CD57+ natural killer cells really important in early pregnancy failure? *Arch Gynecol Obstet* 2009; **279**: 493–7.

43. Wang Q, Li TC, Wu YP, Cocksedge KA *et al.* Reappraisal of peripheral NK cells in women with recurrent miscarriage. *Reprod Biomed Online* 2008; **17**(6): 814–19.

44. Turner MW. Mannose-binding lectin: the pluripotent molecule of the innate immune system. *Immunol Today* 1998; **17**: 532–40.

45. Kruse C, Rosgaard A, Steffensen R *et al.* Low serum level of mannan-binding lectin is a determinant for pregnancy outcome in women with recurrent spontaneous abortion. *Am J Ob Gynecol* 2002; **187**(5): 1313–20.

46. Kilpatrick DC, Starrs L, Moore S *et al.* Mannan binding lectin concentration and risk of miscarriage. *Hum Reprod* 1999; **14**(9): 2379–80.

47. Christiansen OB, Henriette S, Neilsen ML *et al.* Mannose-biding lectin -2 genotypes and recurrent late pregnancy losses. *Hum Reprod* 2009; **249**(2): 291–9.

48. Raziel A, Kornberg Y, Friedler S *et al.* Hypercoagulable thrombophilic defects and hyperhomocysteinemia in patients with recurrent pregnancy loss. *Am J Reprod Immunol* 2001; **45**(2): 65–71.

49. Nelen WL, van der Mulen EF, Blom HJ *et al.* Recurrent early pregnancy loss and genetic-related disturbances in folate and homocysteine metabolism. *Br J Hosp Med* 1997; **58**: 511–13.

50. Lissak A, Sharon A, Fruchter O *et al.* Polymorphism for mutation of cytosine to thymine at location 677 in the methylene reductase gene is associated with recurrent early fetal loss. *Am J Obst Gynec* 1999; **181**: 126–30.

51. Holmes ZR, Regan L, Chilcott I, Cohen H. The C677T MTHFR gene mutation is not predictive of risk for recurrent fetal loss. *Br J Haematol* 1999; **105**: 98–101.

52. Suarez MB, Morales MJ, Cadtro V *et al.* A new HLA-Gallele (HLA –G*0105N) and its distribution in the Spanish population. *Immunogenetics* 1997; **45**: 464–5.

53. Aldrich CL, Stephenson MD, Karrison T *et al.* HLA-G genotypes and pregnancy outcome in couples with unexplained recurrent miscarriage. *Mol Hum Reprod* 2001; **7**: 1167–72.

54. Quere I, Mercier E, Bellet H *et al.* Vitamin supplementation and pregnancy outcome in women with recurrent early pregnancy loss and hyperhomocysteinaemia. *Fertil Steril* 2001; **75**: 823–5.

55. Clifford K, Rai R, Regan L. Future pregnancy outcome in unexplained recurrent first trimester miscarriage. *Hum Reprod*; 1997; **12**: 387–9.

# Molar pregnancy

Eric R. M. Jauniaux and Jemma Johns

## Introduction

Molar pregnancy is a term that describes disorders of the villous anatomy which includes pathological anomalies of trophoblast development. The biochemical analysis of the fluid contained in molar vesicles indicates that it is derived from the diffusion of maternal plasma and the accumulation of specific trophoblast proteins. In the case of mole associated with a developing fetus or presenting with fetal remnants the molar vesicle composition is unchanged by any form of fetal metabolism [1]. These biochemical findings suggest that the hydropic (hydatidiform) transformation of the villous mesenchyme results from a lack, maldevelopment or regression of the villous vasculature that makes the drainage of fluid supplied by the trophoblast impossible. The fact that mild to moderate generalized villous edema is often found following the demise of an embryo or early fetus supports this concept and highlights the fact that hydropic villous changes are not synonymous with true molar changes.

The vast majority of molar pregnancies miscarry spontaneously during the first 3–4 months of pregnancy resulting in an incidence of molar placenta of 1 per 41 miscarriages [2,3]. These data suggest that with the development of early pregnancy units (EPU) over the last decade most women with molar pregnancies are likely to be first seen during the first trimester. Gestational trophoblastic disorders (GTD) comprise hydatidiform mole, placental site trophoblastic tumor, choriocarcinoma and gestational trophoblastic neoplasia (GTN). Depending on their origin and anatomical characteristics, GTDs have different fetal and maternal consequences during pregnancy and after delivery. Thus an early and accurate differential diagnosis is important for patient counseling and perinatal management. This chapter reviews the role of ultrasound in early pregnancy in the screening for molar pregnancy.

## True molar pregnancies

Molar pregnancies are characterized by gross waterlogging and villous cistern formation and villous trophoblastic hyperplasia is the microscopic characteristic feature of true molar pregnancies [4–9]. Complete hydatidiform moles (CHM) and partial hydatidiform moles (PHM) are related disorders of human fertilization which constitute the largest group of GTDs. Although both disorders are in themselves benign they both may develop subsequently into GTN and choriocarcinoma [8,9]. To ensure reliable monitoring of human chorionic gonadotropin (hCG) concentrations after a molar pregnancy, all patients in the UK are registered with one of three centers: Ninewells Hospital (Dundee), Weston Park Hospital (Sheffield) and Charing Cross Hospital (London) [9]. Women who present late with clinical GTN have significantly more complications and morbidity, and they are more likely to need surgery and combination chemotherapy than women identified early.

The distinction between CHM and PHM was made in the late 1970s on the basis of gross morphological, histological and cytogenetic criteria [4,5]. The clinical and pathological picture of the two molar syndromes overlap to a degree [6,7] since both the phenotype and natural history of the PHM seem to represent a mild, bland version of those of the CHM (Table 8.1). Gestational trophoblastic neoplasia occurs in around 10% of women with molar pregnancy. Women diagnosed with hydatidiform mole should therefore be registered with a regional center for regular monitoring of hCG to detect malignancy early [8,9].

Ultrasonographic examination of the placenta should correctly identify vesicular villi by the beginning of the second trimester (Figure 8.1) [7]. Before 13 weeks' gestation some partial moles may present

**Table 8.1** Comparison of historical (H) and modern (M) incidence of the main semiological features in complete hydatidiform mole (CHM) and modern incidence in cases of partial hydatidiform mole (PHM) diagnosed during the second trimester of pregnancy.

| Symptoms | CHM | | PHM |
|---|---|---|---|
| | H (%) | M (%) | M (%) |
| Uterine enlargement | 50 | 25 | 10 |
| Vaginal bleeding | 95 | 60 | 4 |
| Hyperemesis | 30 | 10 | Rare |
| Multicystic ovaries | 30 | 1–2 | Rare |
| Pre-eclampsia | 20 | 1–2 | 2.5 |
| Anemia | 55 | 5 | Exceptional |
| High serum hCG | 10–200 MoM | | 10–60 MoM |

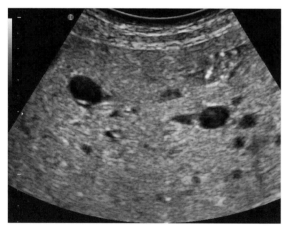

**Figure 8.1** Typical ultrasound appearances of villous molar transformation in an early second-trimester partial mole.

as an enlarged placenta with or without only a few vesicular changes and the classification of some molar pregnancies has become more difficult because they are often evacuated earlier and before the stage of development at which they have the classical morphological features.

## Complete hydatidiform mole (CHM)

Complete hydatidiform moles are characterized by a generalized swelling of the villous tissue, diffuse trophoblastic hyperplasia and no embryonic or fetal tissue. Complete moles are almost always diploid with their chromosomes totally derived from the paternal genome resulting from endoreduplication (duplication without cell cytokinesis) after monospermic fertilization or more rarely dispermic fertilization of an anucleate oocyte (devoid of the maternal X) [10]. This totally androgenic conceptus is characterized by generalized trophoblastic hyperplasia and rapidly developing villous edema with central cistern formation, giving the macroscopic appearance of a "bunch of grapes." The fluid, at first uniformly distributed in the core of the villi, collects in several loculi to coalesce into a central cistern [4–7].

The incidence of CHM varies geographically between 1 in 200 in China and 1 per 1500 pregnancies in Europe and North America [11–13]. Maternal age of less than 20 and over 35 years of age are the best established risk factors for CHM [14]. Complete hydatidiform moles can also develop rarely as part of a multiple pregnancy [15] and exceptionally in postmenopausal women [16]. Following uterine evacuation around 15% of women with a CHM develop a GTN [9], including persistent GTD (pGTD) in 10–20% and choriocarcinoma in 1–2%.

Classically, women with CHM present with vaginal bleeding, uterine enlargement greater than expected for gestational age and abnormally high levels of serum hCG. Medical complications include pregnancy-induced hypertension (PIH), hyperthyroidism, hyperemesis, anemia and the development of ovarian theca lutein cysts in patients with marked hCG elevations as a result of ovarian hyperstimulation (Table 8.1). Historically, 54% of patients presented with hemoglobin levels less than 10 g/dL; now that earlier diagnosis is more common, only 5% of current patients present with anemia. Similarly, theca lutein cysts over 5 cm in diameter were historically present in 46% of patients with CHM, growing sometimes to 20 cm leading to ovarian torsion or rupture of theca lutein cysts. Overall, with the routine use of transvaginal high-resolution ultrasound in the first trimester of pregnancy, the incidence of all of these complications has decreased over the last 20 years [7,8,17–19].

The prenatal ultrasound diagnosis of CHM usually poses little problem from the third month of pregnancy (8–10 weeks) onwards and it can be made antenatally in around 80% of the cases (Table 8.2) [18–26]. Molar changes can now even be detected from the second month of pregnancy by ultrasound which typically reveals a uterine cavity filled with

**Table 8.2** Comparison of ultrasound mean gestational age (MGA) at diagnosis and detection rate (DR) in complete hydatidiform mole (CHM) and partial hydatidiform mole (PHM) in retrospective studies.

| Author(s) | CHM | | | PHM | | |
|---|---|---|---|---|---|---|
| (Year) | n | MGA (weeks) | DR (%) | n | MGA (weeks) | DR (%) |
| Lazarus et al. [21] | 21 | 10.5 | 57 | | | |
| Lindholm & Flam [20] | 75 | 12.4 | 84 | 60 | 14.3 | 30 |
| Benson et al. [22] | 24 | 8.7 | 71 | | | |
| Fowler et al. [23] | 200 | 10.0 | 79 | 178 | 10.0 | 29 |
| Kirk et al. [24] | 20 | | 95 | 41 | | 20 |

**Table 8.3** Ultrasound differential diagnosis of molar pregnancies in early pregnancy.

| Category | Ultrasound features |
|---|---|
| Complete hydatidiform mole (CHM) | |
| Single CHM | Avascular Snowstorm appearance<br>No fetus/multicystic ovaries |
| Twin/Triplet CHM | Avascular Snowstorm appearance<br>Multicystic ovaries<br>Normal fetus with normal placenta |
| Partial hydatidiform mole (PHM) | |
| On-going pregnancy | Swiss Cheese appearance/placentomegaly<br>Small CRL (<10th centile)<br>Fetal malformation (rare <12 weeks) |
| Miscarriages | Increased gestational sac diameter ratios<br>Cystic changes in the placenta<br>Increased placental echogenicity |

multiple sonolucent areas of varying size and shape ("snow storm appearance") without any associated embryonic or fetal structures (Table 8.3). Large sonolucent areas or maternal lakes due to stasis of maternal blood inbetween the molar villi are often found [18–19]. Theca lutein cysts secondary to the very high hCG levels may be diagnosed in up to 30% of the cases, producing enlarged ovaries with either a "soap bubble" or "spoke wheel" appearance [19]. The role of Doppler is limited, although it almost always demonstrates high velocities and low resistance to flow in the uterine arterial circulation and will only be of clinical interest in the diagnosis of an invasive mole [19].

Usually, the ultrasonographic description of CHM applies to pregnancies between 9 and 12 weeks of amenorrhea (Table 8.2). Prior to this, demonstrating villous hydatidiform changes using ultrasound

may be very difficult and inaccurate [19]. Uterine dysgerminomas, which are the most frequent malignant germ cell tumor in women, may appear as an heterogeneous intrauterine mass with multiple echolucent spaces. Other uterine tumors such as sarcomas or lymphomas may also have features similar to those of a CHM on ultrasound and should theoretically be considered in the differential diagnosis [19–27]. These tumors do not usually produce hormonal tumor markers such as hCG or alpha-fetoprotein (AFP). Within the context of an early pregnancy failure, previous ultrasound data [7–11] and our recent series comparing ultrasound and histological features [12] indicate that at least 80% of CHM should be diagnosed at the time of the first ultrasound examination. As ongoing CHM are associated with hCG levels of 10–200 MoM (multiples of the median), and PHM with levels of 10–60 MoM [7,11], pre-evacuation hCG levels may be a useful adjunct to histology in first-trimester spontaneous miscarriages. This is particularly so in cases with unusual ultrasound appearances.

A classical mole coexisting with a normal fetus and placenta in cases of molar transformation of one ovum in a dizygotic twin pregnancy have been most frequently diagnosed at around 15–20 weeks at a later gestational age than would be expected with a complete mole. We have found that as a complete mole produces a characteristic vesicular sonographic pattern, their association with a normal gestational sac can be accurately determined at around 12–14 weeks [15,18,19]. An early ultrasound diagnosis may be difficult because the molar placenta may partially cover the normal placenta. The incidence of this GTD in the first trimester of pregnancy is unknown but as vaginal bleeding is the most common presenting symptom in >95% of cases the first ultrasound

**Table 8.4** Perinatal data of 176 pregnancies combining a normal fetus and placenta with a complete hydatidiform mole (CHM) (modified from Wee & Jauniaux, 2005 [15]).

| Variables | Sebire et al. [42] | Bristow et al. [43] | Steller et al. [44], Fishman et al. [45] | Jauniaux et al. [32] & UCLH (1996–2008)[a] | Single case reports (Wee & Jauniaux) [15] | Total |
|---|---|---|---|---|---|---|
| No of cases | 77 | 26 | 29 | 10 | 34 | 176 |
| Mean gestational age in weeks at diagnosis (range) | NA | 21 (±5) | 21 (±7) | 14 (±3) | 17 (±7) | 18 (±5) |
| Pregnancy complications | | | | | | |
| Vaginal bleeding | NA | 24 (92%) | 25 (86%) | 10 | 17 (47%) | 77% (76/99) |
| PET | 3 (4%) | 7 (26%) | 7 (24%) | 2 | 7 (19%) | 14% (25/176) |
| Theca lutein cyst | NA | 6 (23%) | 6 (21%) | 4 | NA | 25% (16/65) |
| Hyperthyroidism | NA | NA | 1 (11%) | 0 | 3 (5%) | 5% (4/73) |
| Outcome | | | | | | |
| Termination of pregnancy | 26[b] (34%) | 19 (73%) | 17 (59%) | 1 | 19 (56%) | 47% (82/176) |
| Pre-term delivery | 28 (36%) | NA | 7 (24%) | 3 | 4 (12%) | 29% (44/150) |
| Fetal loss[c] | 31 (40%) | NA | 3 (10%) | 3 | 5 (15%) | 27% (41/150) |
| Term livebirth | 20 (26%) | 7 (27%) | 2 (7%) | 3 | 8 (24%) | 23% (40/176) |
| Chemotherapy for PTD | 15 (20%) | 15 (58%) | 16 (55%) | 4 | 12 (35%) | 35% (62/176) |

NA = not available; PET = Pre-eclampsia; PTD = persistent trophoblastic disease.
[a] UCLH Prospective series.
[b] Includes two cases of termination of pregnancy for pre-clampsia.
[c] Includes spontaneous miscarriage, intrauterine death and neonatal death.

examination for these women is likely to take place in the early pregnancy unit. The ultrasound diagnosis becomes easier as pregnancy advances as the marked generalized swelling of the molar tissue with large hemorrhagic areas can be more easily identified on ultrasound [18,19]. The mother must be informed that if she wishes to continue the pregnancy she will be at high risk of developing severe medical complications classically described in CHM before the development of high-resolution ultrasound examination [15]. Overall she only has a one in four chance of a live birth and around 35% chance of developing persistent trophoblastic disease (PTD) after delivery. In ongoing pregnancies there is a greater than 15% risk of early onset of pre-eclampsia (PET) and a 30% risk of fetal loss due to late miscarriage, intrauterine death and neonatal death (Table 8.4). This type of GTD is associated with very high maternal hCG levels [15] which can be used to monitor the growth of the molar mass in women deciding to continue with the pregnancy until fetal viability is reached.

## Partial hydatidiform moles

The term partial hydatidiform mole (PHM) refers to the combination of a fetus with localized placental molar degeneration. Histologically it is characterized by focal swelling of the villous tissue, focal trophoblastic hyperplasia and embryonic or fetal tissue [4–7]. The abnormal villi are scattered within macroscopically normal placental tissue that tends to retain its shape. Theoretically, the histopathological definition should only be applied when villous hydatiform changes are associated with trophoblastic hyperplasia, which cannot be demonstrated by ultrasound. The hydatidiform changes are also focal resulting in an irregular patchwork of seemingly normal and affected areas. Women with PHM generally present with signs and symptoms consistent with missed or incomplete miscarriage. Most often, in fact, the diagnosis of PHM is made upon histological review of curettage specimens [28]. The classical presentation described for complete molar pregnancy is rare in PHM (Table 8.1).

The estimated incidence of partial mole is 1 per 700 pregnancies and does not seem to vary around the world [2,4–7]. Partial moles are triploid in 90% of cases, having inherited two sets of chromosomes from the father and one from the mother [6,7]. Two fetal phenotypes have been delineated: type I (paternally derived, i.e. diandric triploidy) fetuses are relatively well-grown, have a proportionate head size and are associated with placental partial molar changes; in type II (maternally derived, i.e. digynic triploidy) fetuses present with severe asymmetrical growth restriction and an apparently normal placenta [6,7].

Following uterine evacuation between 0.5 and 5.6% of women with a PHM develop pGTD [7–9,29]. True choriocarcinomas are rare after PHM but have been recently reported [30]. Older maternal age and a history of previous molar pregnancy are associated with development of pGTD [29]. Wide variation in the incidence of pGTD after PHM is probably due to the absence of epidemiological data on large unselected populations. Some of this variation is also a result of differences between population-based versus hospital-based pregnancy data.

Triploidies are highly lethal chromosomal abnormalities and most embryos affected by this defect will die within a few weeks following conception [31]. Within this context, paternally inherited or dyandric triploidies are more likely to survive until the second trimester but in PHM, the hydatidiform transformation is slower than in CHM and before 12 weeks' gestation many present simply as an enlarged placenta (Table 8.3) without obvious macroscopic vesicular changes [7,25,26,32,33]. It is therefore not surprising that the ultrasound diagnosis of PHM is less accurate than that of CHM at the same gestational age and that around 70% of those cases will be missed antenatally (Table 8.2). Until recently up to 50% of women with complete moles miscarried spontaneously before the diagnosis was made. Several ultrasound features have been proposed that might increase the ultrasound detection of molar change in missed miscarriages in the first trimester. These include gestational sac diameter ratios, cystic changes in the placenta and the increased echogenicity of placental tissue [7,18,34,35].

Pre-evacuation hCG levels may be a useful adjunct to histology in first-trimester spontaneous miscarriages, in particular in cases with unusual ultrasound appearances [26,33]. In our prospective preliminary study, nine of our 13 molar pregnancies in which a pre-operative hCG was available demonstrated an hCG of 2 to 10.8 MoM. Karyotype or ploidy determination could also be useful in the diagnosis of difficult cases, but are not useful as first-line diagnostic tools as they are expensive and time consuming. DNA ploidy can be useful in problem cases to discriminate between PHM and CHM and is cheaper and faster than karyotyping [3,36,37], but can also be associated with misclassification, particularly if maternal tissue is present. In addition, ploidy analysis cannot distinguish between a diploid molar pregnancy and hydropic abortion [38]. Differences in expression of imprinted genes between complete and partial molar pregnancies have been shown to be useful in differential diagnosis. Using immunohistochemical techniques, the expression of a known imprinted gene can be used to indicate the presence of a functional maternal copy of that gene in partial molar gestations, and absence of the maternal copy in complete moles [39].

We have proposed a combined approach using hCG and ultrasound features in order to screen out those cases that require histology, follow-up and referral [26]. As most women in Europe and North America now have access to an ultrasound examination in early pregnancy, women presenting with ultrasound features suggesting an hydatidiform mole should be fully investigated including cytogenetic or ploidy analysis and detailed histopathology. Women could be further selected for this investigation before a uterine evacuation on the basis of their hCG level but this screening strategy needs to be tested prospectively in a large population.

## Rare causes of true partial hydatidiform mole

Villous hydatidiform transformation can be found in association with tetraploidy and other chromosomal abnormalities [7]. As the vast majority of tetraplodies miscarry spontaneously during the first weeks of pregnancy, tetraploidies resulting from a double or triple paternal contribution and presenting with a partial "molar" placenta have been rarely described in ongoing pregnancies. Confined placental diploid or triploid mosaicism may appear as triploid partial mole on scan but in these cases, the fetus is anatomically normal and has a diploid karyotype [7]. Ultrasound and pathological examination may in rare cases be complicated by the fact that the molar placental tissue comes from a resorbed twin. In these cases, the mother remains at risk for the complications of triploid PHM and in particular she may subsequently develop early pre-eclampsia. In most of these cases, the maternal serum hCG is high [7] and the mother can be at risk of pGTD.

## Pseudo-molar pregnancies

Although there is a well-established clinical association between molar changes of the villi and trophoblastic hyperplasia, hydropic villous changes can be found in conditions unrelated to GTD such as mesenchymal dysplasia [7].

In early pregnancy and in particular in missed miscarriage, independently of the presence of a chromosomal abnormality, the progressive disappearance of the villous vasculature after embryonic death (before 7–8 weeks menstrual age) leads to villous hydrops, which does not however herald a true PHM [28,37,38]. Focal villous hydropic changes may also be found in pregnancies presenting with trisomy or monosomy and are probably related to insufficient development of the villous vasculature in some placental areas as part of a larger vascular maldevelopment involving the fetal circulation or to villous degeneration in cases of placental retention following embryonic/fetal demise [1,40]. Hydrops of the stem villi with placentomegaly but a normal trophoblast have also been observed in cases of Beckwith–Wiedemann syndrome and with a phenotypically normal fetus. This anomaly appears to be a limited malformation of the extraembryonic mesoderm involving the mesenchyme and the vessels of the stem villi of several cotyledons and it has, therefore, been referred to as mesenchymal dysplasia. Beside a partial mole appearance and increased thickness, the placenta show no vascular abnormalities until midgestation. Overall, the risk of pGTD developing from a histologically confirmed non-molar hydropic miscarriage is considered to be less than 1 in 50 000 [41].

## References

1. Jauniaux E, Gulbis B, Hyett J, Nicolaides KH. Biochemical analyses of mesenchymal fluid in early pregnancy. *Am J Obstet Gynecol* 1998; **178**: 765–9.
2. Jeffers MD, O'Dwyer P, Curran B, Leader M, Gillan JE. Partial hydatidiform mole: a common but underdiagnosed condition. *Int J Gynecol Pathol* 1993; **12**: 315–23.
3. Fukunaga M. Early partial hydatidiform mole: prevalence, histopathology, DNA ploidy and persistence rate. *Virchows Arch* 2000; **437**: 180–4.
4. Szulman AE, Surti U. The syndromes of hydatidiform mole. I. Cytogenetic and morphologic correlations. *Am J Obstet Gynecol* 1978; **131**: 665–71.
5. Szulman AE, Surti U. The syndromes of hydatidiform mole. II. Morphologic evolution of complete and partial mole. *Am J Obstet Gynecol* 1978; **132**: 20–7.
6. Szulman AE, Surti U. The clinicopathologic profile of the partial hydatidiform mole. *Obstet Gynecol* 1982; **59**: 597–602.
7. Jauniaux E. Partial moles: from postnatal to prenatal diagnosis. *Placenta* 1999; **20**: 379–88.
8. Berkowitz RS, Goldstein DP. Chorionic tumors. *New Engl J Med* 1996; **335**: 1740–8.
9. Sebire NJ, Seckl MJ. Gestational trophoblastic disease: current management of hydatidiform mole. *Br Med J* 2008; **337**: a1193.
10. Devrientd K. Hydatidiform mole and triploidy: the role of genomic imprinting in placental development. *Hum Reprod Update* 2005; **11**: 137–42.
11. Palmer JR. Advances in the epidemiology of gestational trophoblastic tumors. *J Reprod Med* 1994; **39**: 155–62.
12. Kim S. Epidemiology. In BW Hancock, ES Newlands, RS Berkowitz (eds.), *Gestational Trophoblastic Disease*. London: Chapman & Hall, 1997, pp. 27–42.
13. Shi YF, Li JQ, Zheng W et al. Survey of gestational trophoblastic disease incidence among 3.6 million pregnancies in China. *Zhonghua Fu Chan Ke Za Zhi* 2005; **40**: 76–8.
14. Altman AD, Bentley B, Murray S, Bentley JR. Maternal age-related rates of gestational trophoblastic disease. *Obstet Gynecol* 2008; **112**: 244–50.
15. Wee L, Jauniaux E. Prenatal diagnosis and management of twin pregnancies complicated by a co-existing molar pregnancy. *Prenat Diagn* 2005; **25**: 772–6.
16. Abike F, Temizkan, Payasli A et al. Postmenopausal complete hydatidiform mole: a case report. *Maturitas* 2008; **59**: 95–8.
17. Mangili G, Garavaglia E, Cavoretto P et al. Clinical presentation of hydatidiform mole in northern Italy: has it changed in the last 20 years? *Am J Obstet Gynecol* 2008; **198**: 302.e1–4.

18. Jauniaux E, Nicolaides KH. Early ultrasound diagnosis and follow-up of molar pregnancies. *Ultrasound Obstet Gynecol* 1997; **9**: 17–21.

19. Jauniaux E. Ultrasound diagnosis and follow-up of gestational trophoblastic disease. *Ultrasound Obstet Gynecol* 1998; **11**: 367–77.

20. Lindholm H, Flam F. The diagnosis of molar pregnancy by sonography and gross morphology. *Acta Obstet Gynecol Scand* 1999; **78**: 6–9.

21. Lazarus E, Hulka CA, Siewert B, Levine D. Sonographic appearance of early complete molar pregnancies. *J Ultrasound Med* 1999; **18**: 589–93.

22. Benson CB, Genest DR, Bernstein MR *et al.* Sonographic appearance of first trimester complete hydatidiform moles. *Ultrasound Obstet Gynecol* 2000; **16**: 188–91.

23. Fowler DJ, Lindsay I, Seckl MJ, Sebire NJ. Routine pre-evacuation ultrasound diagnosis of hydatidiform mole: experience of more than 1000 cases from a regional referral center. *Ultrasound Obstet Gynecol* 2006; **27**: 56–60.

24. Kirk E, Papageorghiou AT, Condous G, Bottomley C, Bourne T. The accuracy of first trimester ultrasound in the diagnosis of hydatidiform mole. *Ultrasound Obstet Gynecol* 2007; **29**: 70–5.

25. Fowler DJ, Lindsay I, Seckl MJ, Sebire NJ. Histomorphometric features of hydatidiform moles in early pregnancy: relationship to detectability by ultrasound examination. *Ultrasound Obstet Gynecol* 2007; **29**: 76–80.

26. Johns J, Greenwold N, Buckley S, Jauniaux E. Ultrasound in the screening and diagnosis of molar pregnancies in miscarriages. *Ultrasound Obstet Gynecol* 2005; **25**: 493–7.

27. Jauniaux E, Sebire N. Placental and fetal malignancies. In S Kehoe, E Jauniaux, P Martin-Hirsch, P Savage (eds.), *Cancer and Reproductive Health*. London: RCOG Press, 2008, pp. 187–204.

28. Jauniaux E, Kadri R, Hustin J. Partial mole and triploidy: screening patients with first trimester spontaneous abortion. *Obstet Gynecol* 1996; **88**: 616–19.

29. Feltmate CM, Growdon WB, Wolfberg AJ *et al.* Clinical characteristics of persistent gestational trophoblastic neoplasia after partial hydatidiform molar pregnancy. *J Reprod Med* 2006; **51**: 902–6.

30. Seckl MJ, Fisher RA, Salerno G *et al.* Choriocarcinoma and partial hydatidiform moles. *Lancet* 2000; **1**: 36–9.

31. Zaragoza MV, Surti U, Redline RW *et al.* Parental origin and phenotype of triploidy in spontaneous abortions: Predominance of diandry and association with the partial hydatidiform mole. *Am J Hum Genet* 2000; **66**: 1807–20.

32. Jauniaux E, Brown R, Snijders RJM, Noble P, Nicolaides K. Early prenatal diagnosis of triploidy. *Am J Obstet Gynecol* 1997; **176**: 550–4.

33. Jauniaux E, Bersinger NA, Gulbis B, Meuris S. The contribution of maternal serum markers in the early prenatal diagnosis of molar pregnancies. *Hum Reprod* 1999; **14**: 842.

34. Naumoff P, Szulman AE, Weinstein B, Mazer J, Surti U. Ultrasonography of partial hydatidiform mole. *Radiology* 1981; **140**: 467–70.

35. Fine C, Bundy AL, Berkowitz RS *et al.* Sonographic diagnosis of partial hydatidiform mole. *Obstet Gynecol* 1989; **73**: 414–18.

36. Genest DR. Partial hydatidiform mole: clinicopathological features, differential diagnosis, ploidy, molecular studies and gold standards for diagnosis. *Int J Gynecol Pathol* 2001; **20**: 315–22.

37. Deavers MT, Kalhor N, Silva EG. Diagnostic problems with trophoblastic lesions. *Arch Pathol Lab Med* 2008; **132**: 168–74.

38. Bell KA, Van Deerlin V, Addya K *et al.* Molecular genetic testing from paraffin embedded tissue distinguishes nonmolar hydropic abortion from hydatidiform mole. *Mol Diagn* 1999; **4**: 11–19.

39. Thaker HM, Berlin A, Tycko B *et al.* Immunohistochemistry for the imprinted gene product IPL/PHLDA2 for facilitating the differential diagnosis of complete hydatidiform mole. *J Reprod Med* 2004; **49**: 630–6.

40. Jauniaux E, Hadler A, Partington C. A case of partial mole associated with trisomy 13. *Ultrasound Obstet Gynecol* 1998; **11**: 62–4.

41. Sebire NJ, Foskett M, Fisher RA, Lindsay I, Seckl MJ. Persistent gestational trophoblastic disease is rarely, if ever, derived from non-molar first-trimester miscarriage. *Med Hypotheses* 2005; **64**: 689–93.

42. Sebire NJ, Foskett M, Paradinas FJ *et al.* Outcome of twin pregnancies with complete hydatidiform mole and healthy co-twin. *Lancet* 2002; **359**: 2165–6.

43. Bristow RE, Shumway JB, Khouzami AN, Witter FR. Complete hydatidiform mole and surviving coexistent twin. *Obstet Gynecol Surv* 1996; **51**: 705–9.

44. Steller MA, Genest DR, Bernstein MR *et al.* Clinical features of multiple conception with partial or complete molar pregnancy and coexisting fetuses. *J Reprod Med* 1994; **39**: 147–54.

45. Fishman DA, Padilla LA, Keh P *et al.* Management of twin pregnancies consisting of a complete hydatidiform mole and normal fetus. *Obstet Gynecol* 1998; **91**: 546–50.

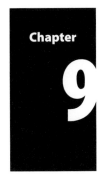

# Uterine natural killer cells and reproduction

Siobhan Quenby and Ai-Wei Tang

## Introduction

Reproductive failure has been thought to have an immune etiology for many years. More recently there has been a focus on the innate immune system in which natural killer (NK) cells play a major role. A particular type of natural killer cell, the uterine natural killer (uNK) cell has been associated with both recurrent miscarriage (three or more consecutive miscarriages) and recurrent implantation failure (failure of pregnancy after three or more cycles of embryo transfer of good-quality embryos). These uNK cells comprise about 20% of human endometrial cells in the luteal phase and have been extensively studied and found to be different from leukocyte populations in peripheral blood [1]. In human endometrium, the population of leukocytes consists mainly of T cells, macrophages and uNK cells [2]. These cells change in proportion and numbers throughout the menstrual cycle and pregnancy with the most predominant of these being uNK cells [1].

In recent years, with greater understanding of the interaction between fetal and maternal cells that occur during placentation in the uterus, the role of uNK cells as a significant factor of reproductive failure has been a subject of discussion. Much of the information on uNK cell biology and function comes from studying mouse endometrium due to difficulty in obtaining human tissue in pregnancy for research purposes. However, work on animals has given much insight into uNK function in humans. While the exact function and origin of uNK cells are still being investigated, there is increasing interest in uNK cells as endometrial causes of reproductive failure have not yet been elucidated.

## Uterine natural killer cells

Uterine natural killer cells are characterized by their cytoplasmic granules and previously had many names,
including "granular endometrial stromal cell," "endometrial granulocytes," "K cells," and "large granulated lymphocyte" [3]. The name "uterine natural killer" has recently been adopted as these cells share similar properties with natural killer (NK) cells in the blood, part of the innate immune system, but are unique with their own distinct antigenic features (Table 9.1) [3].

Both uterine and peripheral blood NK cells express the CD56 antigen [4,5]. It is the intensity of CD56 and the lack of CD16 and CD57 antigens, typical NK cell markers, that differentiate uterine from peripheral NK cells. The density of CD56 on uNK cells is 20 times that of the majority of peripheral blood NK cells. Eighty percent of uNK cells are CD56$^{bright}$ and CD16$^-$ whereas 90% of peripheral NK cells are CD56$^{dim}$ and CD16$^+$ [4,5]. Although about 10% of peripheral NK cells are CD56$^{bright}$ and CD16$^-$, they differ from the uNK subtype as their intensity of CD56 is less and they are agranular [4].

There is also no correlation between the numbers of peripheral NK cells and uNK cells and they both express different functional markers (Table 9.1). All uNK cells express CD94/NKG2 receptors compared with only 50% of peripheral blood NK cells. Although peripheral CD56$^{bright}$ NK cells do not express the killer-cell immunoglobin-like receptors (KIR), this is expressed by both uterine CD56$^{bright}$CD16$^-$ and peripheral CD56$^{dim}$CD16$^+$ NK cells [6]. Despite their name, uNK cells display only weak cytotoxic capabilities against target cells compared to their peripheral NK equivalent [7]. Uterine natural killer cells exert their function by production of high levels of cytokines such as granulocyte-macrophage colony stimulating factor (GM-CSF), colony stimulating factor-1 (CSF-1), tumor necrosis factor-alpha (TNF-α), interferon-gamma (IFN-γ), transforming growth factor-beta (TGF-β), leukemia-inhibitory factor (LIF) and interleukin-2 (IL-2) [8]. No relationship

**Table 9.1** The difference between subsets of natural killer (NK) cells.

| Phenotype and function | Peripheral blood | | Endometrium |
| --- | --- | --- | --- |
| | CD56^dim | CD56^bright | CD56^bright |
| Proportion of NK cells | 90% | 10% | 80% |
| CD56 | + | ++ | ++++ |
| CD16 | ++ | +/− | − |
| CD3 | − | − | − |
| NK activity | High | Low | Low |
| Morphology | Large and granular | Small and agranular | Large and granular |
| Cytokine production | − | + | ++++ |

has been found between specific cytokine production and cytotoxic function between different NK cell phenotypes [7].

Uterine natural killer cells form the largest group of leukocytes in the endometrium but they vary in proportion to other leukocyte populations significantly throughout the menstrual cycle (Figures 9.1 and 9.2). In the proliferative phase, both T cells and uNK cells are of equal proportion, about 40% each of all leukocytes. However, uNK cell numbers increase to encompass about 60% of leukocytes by the mid-luteal phase and continue to peak to >75% of leukocytes in early pregnancy when implantation occurs [1]. Analysis of uNK cells during pregnancy is difficult due to the problems in obtaining tissue for research and thus the level of uNK cells in the second trimester of pregnancy is not certain. In the third trimester, uNK cell numbers generally decrease drastically in the decidua attached to placental membranes and delivered placenta but substantial numbers are still found in placental bed biopsies (3). Uterine natural killer cells tend to also accumulate in large numbers around blood vessels and glands which could implicate either function or origin (Figure 9.3) [1]. The fluctuation of numbers according to the menstrual cycle suggests that their existence depends on hormonal regulation [6].

## The source of uNK cells

The process of how uNK cells arrive in large numbers into the endometrium during the late secretory phase of the menstrual cycle is still questioned but two main theories exist. One is in-utero proliferation and differentiation of stem cells or indigenous NK cells in the endometrium, and the other is recruitment of

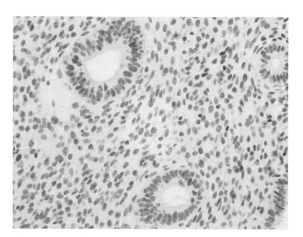

**Figure 9.1** Proliferative phase endometrium showing low levels of uterine natural killer (uNK cells) (stained brown). A color reproduction of this figure can be found in the color plate section.

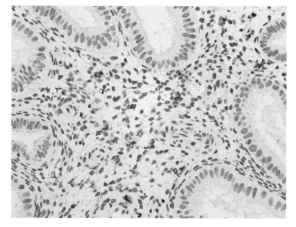

**Figure 9.2** Mid-luteal phase endometrium showing higher numbers of uterine natural killer (uNK) cells (stained brown). A color reproduction of this figure can be found in the color plate section.

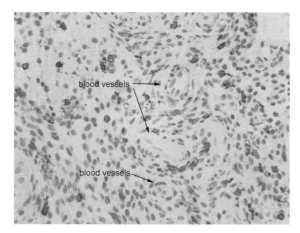

**Figure 9.3** Uterine natural killer (uNK) cells (stained brown) forming aggregates around blood vessels. A color reproduction of this figure can be found in the color plate section.

hematopoietic stem cells or CD56$^{bright}$ cells from peripheral blood which subsequently differentiate in the uterine microenvironment into the uNK cell phenotype.

## In-utero proliferation and differentiation

Although there are only few CD56$^{bright}$ cells in the proliferative phase, they are still present. Therefore, there could be local proliferation of residual uNK cells present in the stratum basalis that is not shed during menstruation [3]. Furthermore, there is an increase in expression of Ki-67, a proliferative marker on uNK cells in both secretory phase endometrium and decidua of early pregnancy which supports this theory. When comparing both tissue types, maximum proliferation was seen in secretory phase endometrium and there was a downward trend of proliferation in the decidua as gestation proceeded [4]. Similarly, the concentration of IL-15, a cytokine uniquely expressed in the endometrium that helps in stimulating proliferation, also peaks during the secretory phase [9].

Another theoretical mechanism arises from the fact that the endometrium sheds every month and is highly regenerative. Hence, the idea of endometrial stem cells and their potential functional capacity has been supported recently [10]. Although the exact markers and function of these stem cells are yet unknown, they could potentially differentiate and proliferate into these special uNK cells in the uterus [6].

## Trafficking from peripheral blood

The alternative theory proposes the recruitment of peripheral blood cells into the endometrium through hormonally regulated methods via chemokines and cytokines [6]. This is because the uNK cell population varies with the menstrual cycle, and immunohisto-chemistry staining for CD56$^{bright}$ cells show that they commonly form aggregates around the spiral arteries and glands [1]. Once these cells are recruited, they could then differentiate into uNK cells.

Progesterone is the main hormone found during the secretory phase of the menstrual cycle and is thus thought to regulate uNK cells. However, these cells express estrogen receptor-β (ER-β) and glucocorticoid receptors but not progesterone receptors [11]. As the precise mechanism of recruitment of cells from the peripheral blood is still unknown, it could either be mediated directly through actions of estrogen via the existing ER-β receptor, directly through action of progesterone via an unidentified receptor, or through progesterone action on endometrial T cells and stromal cells via prolactin, IL-15, macrophage inflammatory protein-1β (MIP-1β) or vascular endothelial growth factor (VEGF) in attracting peripheral NK cells [12].

Two cytokines of interest are IL-15 and MIP-1β. Both are secreted by endometrial stromal cells and believed to be chemo-attractants for recruitment of peripheral cells as they are distinctly expressed in the vascular and perivascular areas in the secretory phase endometrium at a higher concentration compared with the proliferative phase [9,13]. There is also a strong correlation between cytokine levels and the number of uNK cells. Once recruited, IL-15 can continue to assist in its proliferation and differentiation into unique uNK cells [9].

## Regulation of menstruation

The time period between implantation and menstruation (7–14 days after ovulation) is crucial as the endometrium has to either decidualize to prepare for pregnancy or initiate menstruation. If implantation does not occur, then the functional layer of the endometrium is shed. Prior to menstruation, a fall in progesterone levels is synonymous with characteristic nuclear changes similar to apoptosis occurring in uNK cells [6]. These changes are only seen in late-secretory endometrium and not in normal decidua. They also occur before any other features of menstrual breakdown such as neutrophil infiltration, clumping of stromal cells and interstitial hemorrhage are present. Therefore the death of uNK cells could be the initial triggering event for mucosal breakdown and menstruation [6].

# The functions of uNK cells

## Regulation of trophoblast invasion and growth

Despite extensive studies into uNK cells, their exact roles remain unknown. One of their functions could be in the establishment and maintenance of early pregnancy as their presence peaks at a time when implantation should occur. Human species have the most invasive placenta. When implantation occurs, there needs to be adequate invasion of the trophoblast to allow for good maternal blood supply but at the same time invasion should not be so deep that it causes pathology such as placenta accreta or gestational trophoblastic disease [6]. There is evidence to imply that uNK cells play an important role in initiating decidualization and regulating trophoblast invasion as these cells are hormonally dependent and accumulate as a dense infiltrate at the implantation site near stromal cells, glands, blood vessels and trophoblast cells in early pregnancy [4]. In-vitro studies have also shown that extravillous trophoblast and uNK cell interaction can occur and may regulate the maternal immune response to the fetal allograft [14].

## Regulation via extravillous trophoblast and uNK cell interaction

Trophoblast cells constitute the fetal side of the interface between fetal and maternal tissue. Trophoblast mediates the implantation of embryo into the endometrium and has specialized immunological features. Neither syncytiotrophoblast nor cytotrophoblast cells express classical class I human leukocyte antigen-A (HLA-A) or HLA-B or class II HLA-DP, HLA-DQ or HLA-DR major histocompatibility complex (MHC) alloantigens involved in graft rejection. Instead, the invasive, extravillous trophoblast (EVT) cells express an unusual combination of non-classical class I MHC molecules, HLA-E and HLA-G with low expression of HLA-C [14]. Uterine natural killer cells are found to express receptors such as killer-cell immunoglobulin-like receptors (KIR), immunoglobin-like transcripts (ILT) and CD94/NKG2 proteins which recognize all these non-classical MHC molecules [14]. Thus, there are potential molecular interactions for maternal recognition

of trophoblast which results in either activating or inhibitory mechanisms.

The receptors on uNK cells for HLA-C are members of the KIR multigene family. All women express KIRs for HLA-C alleles and because HLA-C is polymorphic, maternal uNK cells can encounter non-self paternal HLA-C alleles on trophoblast and each pregnancy may present a different combination of KIRs and HLA-C [15]. The percentage of KIR expressed and density of receptor expression also differ between individuals. This interaction plays a physiological role related to immune regulation and placental development. Obvious differences were observed with different combinations of polymorphic ligand-receptor pairs and have been associated with pre-eclampsia, a condition that is known to be secondary to poor trophoblast invasion [16]. These specific fetal HLA-C/maternal KIR genotype combinations have also been identified in recurrent miscarriage [17].

HLA-E has a high affinity for CD94/NKG2 dimers on uNK cells. The overall effect is inhibition of cytolysis of either maternal or fetal tissues by uNK cells [18]. However, uNK cells are unable to kill trophoblast even when these receptors are blocked by antibodies which suggests that this interaction may regulate other functions besides cytolysis during implantation. It could be that other inhibitory pathways exist or trophoblast lacks specific surface molecules to initiate killing [18].

Specific receptors for HLA-G, which is expressed only by EVT are yet to be defined [14]. HLA-G is recognized by CD94/NKG2 via co-expression with HLA-E or by ILT-2 leading to decreased sensitivity to NK cell-mediated cytotoxicity [6]. HLA-G interaction has also been shown to stimulate proliferation of uNK cells and increased production of IFN-γ and vascular endothelial growth factor (VEGF) [19]. Although there is evidence for uNK and EVT interaction through these MHC molecules and receptors, the final consequences of these interactions are still unclear.

## Regulation via cytokine production

Control of trophoblast invasion was initially thought to be via cell-mediated cytotoxicity as uNK cells were capable of cytolysis although less than their peripheral equivalent [7]. However, as mentioned before, trophoblast cells are resistant to lysis by uNK cells as they express non-classical HLA class I antigen, unless stimulated by IL-2, which is not present in the endometrium in large amounts in normal pregnancy.

Thus, a different mechanism had been proposed, that uNK cells and EVT interactions altered the profile of cytokine production, ultimately resulting in a change in the invasive behavior of trophoblast [6].

Uterine natural killer cells are known to produce many cytokines such as GM-CSF, CSF-1, TNF-α, IFN-γ, TGF-β, LIF, IL-2 and IL-10, some of which trophoblast has receptors for [8,20]. Thus, there could be a role for these uNK cell-derived cytokines on trophoblast growth and differentiation or apoptosis and defective invasion of the endometrium. For example, GM-CSF has been shown to stimulate DNA synthesis in culture of murine trophoblast and CSF-1 increases production of hCG and human placental lactogen (hPL) by trophoblast. Both these cytokines have also been shown to cause placental cell proliferation in mouse models [12]. Similarly, IL-4, IL-6 and LIF stimulate hCG secretion by trophoblast cells [21]. Another cytokine, macrophage migration inhibitory factor (MIF), produced by uNK cells and expressed highly in endometrium and human placenta, reduces the cytolytic capabilities of uNK cells [22].

On the other hand, IFN-γ has been shown to inhibit EVT invasion within early human pregnancy decidua both by increased EVT apoptosis and reduced levels of active proteases [23]. Similarly, TNF-α impairs trophoblast invasion through elevation of plasminogen activator inhibitor-1 (PAI-1) [24]. Transforming growth factor-beta (TGF-β) is also known to affect growth and differentiation of first-trimester trophoblast by inhibiting intergrin expression, HPL and hCG secretion [21]. Some of these cytokines also regulate production of matrix metalloproteinases (MMP) -2 and MMP-9 that plays a role in trophoblast invasion [21]. A recent study demonstrated that granulysin, a cytotoxic granule protein produced by uNK cells causes apoptosis of EVT and granulysin-positive uNK cells can attack EVT [25]. Therefore, any alternations in the production of cytokines could contribute to the imbalance of this unique fetal–maternal interface immune phenomena leading to abnormal implantation and the clinical presentation of a miscarriage.

## Regulation of vascular remodeling

These uNK cells are found in high numbers around blood vessels. Whether their location is a reflection of trafficking cells from peripheral circulation or due to the possible function of uNK cells in development and remodeling of uterine spiral arteries is still not known. However, early structural changes including dilatation and medical disorganization that occurs in decidual spiral arteries happen at the time when uNK cells are present. These cells also reduce in number after 20 weeks' gestation when vascular changes are generally complete. The variation in numbers and timeline implicate its function in vascular remodeling [3].

Apart from cytokines, uNK cells are also found to secrete high levels of angiogenic growth factors such as VEGF-C, placental growth factor, angiopoietin-1 (Ang-1), Ang-2 and TGF-β in both non-pregnant endometrium and early pregnancy decidua [26,27]. Their levels decrease with increasing gestation which suggests their role in modulating vascular growth in early pregnancy could be regulated by other cytokines, such as IL-2 and IL-15, that are secreted by uNK cells [26]. For example, Ang-2 may be an important mediator for spiral artery transformation and destabilization of vessel structure and is only expressed in tissues associated with vessels undergoing remodeling [26]. Another cytokine thought to play a role is IFN-γ secreted by uNK cells. Studies in mice models, from which a lot of evidence for uNK cells' involvement in spiral artery transformation has come, show that mice deficient in uNK cells or IFN-γ signaling have implantation site abnormalities and failure of decidual artery remodeling [28].

A recent study has also showed that uNK cell density was positively correlated with the formation of blood vessels, lymphatics, spiral arterial smooth muscle differentiation and endometrial edema [29]. Clinically, increased uNK cell density was associated with reduced uterine artery resistance to blood flow. Hence it was proposed that the mechanism by which high uNK cell density was associated with reproductive failure was one of increased angiogenic cytokine production leading to increased angiogenesis and inappropriate blood flow to the developing fetal–placental unit, cause oxidative stress and subsequent miscarriage.

## Uterine NK cells and recurrent miscarriage

Recurrent miscarriage (RM) is a stressful condition for both patients and clinicians. There is no cause found in up to 50% of cases for the repeated losses despite numerous investigations [30]. Many clinicians believe that there is an underlying endometrial factor contributing to these recurrent pregnancy losses [31]. As uNK cells are the most predominant leukocyte in the endometrium in early pregnancy, they could play a major role in recurrent miscarriage. Moreover, studies comparing normal and miscarried early pregnancy decidua have implicated uNK cells in the etiology of RM by being phenotypically different in these two patient groups [32,33]. This relationship could be explained in two ways. These cells are either hostile to the invading trophoblast, or they may facilitate implantation of abnormal blastocysts, both leading to the clinical presentation of miscarriage [34].

Although the association between uNK cells and RM has been repeatedly reported, there are differences in the methods of analysis of uNK cells in pre-implantation endometrium, leading to differing results. A study using flow cytometry found decreased numbers of CD56$^{bright}$CD16$^-$ NK cells and increased CD56$^{dim}$CD16$^+$ NK cells in mid-luteal endometrium [35]. Conversely, studies using immunochemistry staining have found increased numbers of CD56$^{bright}$CD16$^-$ NK cells in patients with RM [36–38] (Figure 9.4). However, numbers of uNK cells may not correlate directly with function and the significance of these observations is still not known. We know that in mice, uNK cells are needed for decidualization and appropriate vascularization of the implantation site to occur [39]. Thus, there is doubt if high numbers of uNK cells are harmful to the trophoblast.

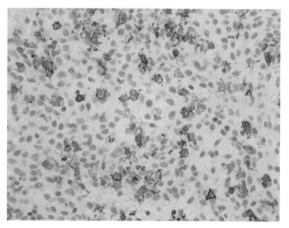

**Figure 9.4** Immunochemistry staining on patient with RM showing high levels of uterine natural killer uNK cells (stained brown) in mid-luteal phase endometrium. A color reproduction of this figure can be found in the color plate section.

There is also an association between high numbers of uNK cells and women with RM of severe phenotype [40]. It has been suggested that the significantly decreased number of uNK cells in controls who all have had previous births were due to the effect of a previous term pregnancy as pregnancy and birth involve extensive changes in size and vascularization of the uterus. However, a study showed that five women who had a previous birth had >5% of uNK cells, excluding the possibility that a live birth reduces uNK cells to <5% in all women [40]. Whether high numbers of uNK cells in the mid-luteal phase predict subsequent miscarriage is controversial. One study suggested that they do [36] but a more recent slightly larger study refuted this [38]. However, both these studies are inadequately powered and did not undergo rigorous methodology to assess if uNK cell population predicted reproductive failure.

The other explanation of uNK cells facilitating implantation of abnormal blastocyts including those with abnormal karyotype is supported by findings of differences in uNK cell populations in decidua of RM patients with normal and abnormal karyotype [32]. Additionally, uNK cells are more numerous in the decidua of chromosomally abnormal miscarriages compared with chromosomally normal miscarriages [33].

The use of steroids in an attempt to improve pregnancy outcomes by pharmacological manipulation has been suggested as uNK cells express glucocorticoid receptors and ER-β [11]. There are also case reports of success with its use. Although there was no uNK cells measurement, a patient with ten previous miscarriages had a live birth after receiving preconceptual steroids [41]. More recently, a patient with excessive uNK cells with 19 previous miscarriages had a successful pregnancy outcome after receiving preconceptual steroids [42]. Furthermore, a prospective study using 20 mg prednisolone from day 1 to day 21 of the cycle demonstrated a reduction in uNK cells in the pre-implantation endometrium of patients with RM [40]. Although the number or density of uNK cells may not reflect their function, the profound difference in numbers seen in women with reproductive failure is likely to implicate a functional endometrial change.

As uNK cells share many similar properties with peripheral blood NK cells, their population in the blood has also been reported to be associated with RM. A higher level of peripheral NK cells and higher activity pre-conceptionally were found in patients with RM and to be predictive of further miscarriages in this group of women [43]. However, the value of testing peripheral blood for NK cells to gauge the state of the endometrium is questioned [44]. Moreover, any tests for NK cells, either in the peripheral blood or in endometrium biopsies to guide potential treatment are controversial and should not be routinely offered [44]. Apart from steroids, other immunomodulation therapies such as intravenous immunoglobulin (IvIg), third-party donor cell immunization, paternal cell immunization and trophoblast membrane infusion have been proposed. However, there is conflicting evidence as to their efficacies and a meta-analysis of trials comparing these immunotherapies has found no evidence of a beneficial effect over placebo in preventing further miscarriages [45].

## Uterine natural killer cells and recurrent implantation failure

Some couples have recurrent implantation failure despite producing high-quality embryos. Although it is known that there may be other causes contributing to their infertility, it is logical to assume that this group of women have an endometrial pathology that is contributing to these pregnancy failures. There is also a similar relationship between uNK cells and uterine artery Doppler in women with RM and in women with recurrent implantation failure (RIF) which suggests a similar underlying endometrial pathology in these two conditions [29]. However, high uNK cells are only part of a complex array of immune and vascular abnormalities in the endometrium of patients with RIF and more research is needed to understand the immunology of inadequate uterine receptivity [46].

There are also controversies regarding the association of NK cells in the endometrium and blood of patients with RIF. Immunochemistry staining has found increased numbers of $CD56^{bright}CD16^-$ NK cells in secretory endometrium of patients with RIF [46]. However, when flow cytometry was used, no difference in uNK cell populations was detected in patients with RIF compared with those reported in normal human endometrium [47]. Peripheral blood analysis for NK cells have found that a higher number of $CD56^{dim}CD16^+$ NK cells which are more cytotoxic when activated were associated with poorer pregnancy outcomes due to a harmful role in successful implantation [48]. However, the debate of associating peripheral

NK cell counts which are phenotypically and functionally different to uNK cell activity in the endometrium has not been resolved [44].

Steroids have been used as anti-inflammatory agents to try to improve success of implantation, as aside from the immunology of pregnancy, there could be other inflammatory processes in the practice of in-vitro fertilization (IVF) such as stimulation from the intrauterine catheter during embryo transfer [49]. Additionally, a study using 10 mg prednisolone a day for 5 weeks prior to IVF and embryo transfer found a significantly increased implantation rate in women with a possible autoimmune cause to their infertility [50]. It was suggested that since the dose was too low to reduce auto-antibody titers, it was the action on reducing NK cells that contributed to the improved rates. However, there are also studies which showed that prednisolone did not make a significant difference [51,52], but these studies did not assess the endometrium for any possible endometrial factors for the infertility. In the recent study that showed a trend towards lower miscarriage rate with prednisolone, it was suggested that steroids may be useful in raising a low pregnancy and implantation rate rather than increasing the standards of clinical results and thus could be useful in recurrent implantation failure [52].

As with RM, immunomodulation therapies such as IvIg and anti-TNF-α agents have been tried to suppress NK cell activity. A recent meta-analysis of three trials has shown that IvIg treatment significantly increases the live-birth rate in patients who fail IVF [53]. There were, however, variables in the patient selection and treatment process of IvIg. As it has potentially severe side effects and is very expensive, it should not be routinely recommended until more evidence is available.

## Conclusion

A successful pregnancy is the result of a delicate immunological balance of the maternal immune system in preventing rejection of the fetal allograft and at the same time recognizing it adequately to promote satisfactory trophoblast invasion and placental growth. There still remains considerable controversy over the exact role and function of uNK cells in this immunological phenomenon. However, there is increasing evidence that uNK cells, the most predominant leukocytes in early pregnancy, are associated with reproductive failure although the mechanisms of this association are not clear. Therefore, more investigations into the relationship between uNK cells and reproductive failure are needed before any tests, either peripheral blood sampling or endometrium biopsies for NK cells level are routinely advised. At the present moment, although patients may be disappointed at the lack of a proven intervention and treatment, it is not in their best interest to recommend any immunomodulation therapy with the lack of strong evidence. Instead, patients should be encouraged to participate in research involving NK cells to generate more information of their function in reproduction and subsequently attempt to offer treatment to improve pregnancy outcomes.

# References

1. Bulmer JN, Morrison L, Longfellow M et al. Granulated lymphocytes in human endometrium: histochemical and immunohistochemical studies. *Hum Reprod* 1991; **6**(6): 791–8.

2. Bulmer JN. Cellular constituents of human endometrium in the menstrual cycle and early pregnancy. In RA Bronson, NJ Alexander, D Anderson et al. (eds.), *Reproductive Immunology*. Oxford: Blackwell Science, 1996, pp. 212–39.

3. Bulmer JN, Lash GE. Human uterine natural killer cells: a reappraisal. *Mol Immunol* 2005; **42**: 511–21.

4. King A, Balendran N, Woodling P et al. CD3-leukocytes present in the human uterus during early placentation: phenotypic and morphologic characterization of the CD56++ population. *Dev Immunol* 1991; **1**(33): 169–90.

5. Nagler A, Lanier LL, Cwiria S et al. Comparative studies of human FcRIII-positive and negative natural killer cells. *J Immunol* 1989; **143**(10): 3183–91.

6. Trundley A, Moffet A. Human uterine leukocytes and pregnancy. *Tissue Antigens* 2004; **63**(1): 1–12.

7. Christmas SE, Bulmer JN, Meager A et al. Phenotypic and functional analysis of human CD3- decidual leukocyte clones. *Immunology* 1990; **71**(2): 182–9.

8. Jokhi PP, King A, Sharkey AM et al. Screening for cytokine messenger ribonucleic acids in purified human decidual lymphocyte populations by the reverse-transcriptase polymerase chain reaction. *J Immunol* 1994; **153**(10): 4427–35.

9. Kitaya K, Yamaguchi T, Honjo H. Central role of interleukin-15 in postovulatory recruitment of peripheral blood CD16(–) natural killer cells into human endometrium. *J Clin Endocrinol Metab* 2005; **90**(5): 2932–40.

10. Garget CE, Chan RW, Schwab KE. Endometrial stem cells. *Curr Opin Obstet Gynecol* 2007; **19**(14): 377–83.

11. Henderson TA, Saunders PT, Moffett-King A. Steroid receptor expression in uterine natural killer cells. *J Clin Endocrinol Metab* 2003; **88**(1): 440–9.

12. Dosiou C, Giudice LC. Natural killer cells in pregnancy and recurrent pregnancy loss: endocrine and immunologic perspectives. *Endocr Rev* 2005; **26** (1): 44–62.

13. Kitaya K, Nakayama T, Okubo T et al. Expression of macrophage inflammatory protein-1beta in human endometrium: its role in endometrial recruitment of natural killer cells. *J Clin Endocrinol Metab* 2003; **88**(4): 1809–14.

14. Moffet-King A. Natural killer cells and pregnancy. Nature reviews. *Immunology* 2002; **2**: 656–63.

15. Verma S, King A, Loke YW. Expression of killer cell inhibitory receptors on human uterine natural killer cells. *Eur J Immunol* 1997; **27**(4): 979–83.

16. Hiby SE, Walker JJ, O'shaughnessy KM et al. Combinations of maternal KIR and fetal HLA-C genes influence the risk of preeclampsia and reproductive success. *J Exp Med* 2004; **200**(8): 957–65.

17. Hiby SE, Regan L, Lo W et al. Association of maternal killer-cell immunoglobulin-like receptors and parental HLA-C genotypes with recurrent miscarriage. *Hum Reprod* 2008; **23**(4): 972–6.

18. King A, Allan DS, Bowen M et al. HLA-E is expressed on trophoblast and interacts with CD94/NKG2 receptors on decidual NK cells. *Eur J Immunol* 2000; **30**(6): 1623–31.

19. van der Meer A, Lukassen HG, van Lierop MJ et al. Membrane-bound HLA-G activates proliferation and interferon-gamma production by uterine natural killer cells. *Mol Hum Reprod* 2004; **10**(3): 189–95.

20. Saito S, Nishikawa K, Morii T et al. Cytokine production by CD16-CD56[bright] natural killer cells in the human early pregnancy decidua. *Int Immunol* 1993; **5**(5): 559–63.

21. Laird SM, Tuckerman EM, Cork BA et al. A review of immune cells and molecules in women with recurrent miscarriage. *Hum Reprod Update* 2003; **9**(2): 163–74.

22. Arcuri F, Cintorino M, Carducci A et al. Human decidual natural killer cells as a source and target of macrophage migration inhibitory factor. *Reproduction* 2006; **131**(1): 175–82.

23. Lash GE, Otun HA, Innes BA et al. Interferon-gamma inhibits extravillous trophoblast cell invasion by a mechanism that involves both changes in apoptosis and protease levels. *FASEB J* 2006; **20**(14): 2512–18.

24. Bauer S, Pollheimer J, Hartmann J et al. Tumor necrosis factor-alpha inhibits trophoblast migration through elevation of plasminogen activator inhibitor-1 in first-trimester villous explant cultures. *J Clin Endocrinol Metab* 2004; **89**(2): 812–22.

25. Nakashima A, Shiozaki A, Myojo S et al. Granulysin produced by uterine natural killer cells induces apoptosis of extravillous trophoblasts in spontaneous abortion. Am J Pathol 2008; 173(3): 653–64.

26. Li XF, Charnock-Jones DS, Zhang E et al. Angiogenic growth factor messenger ribonucleic acids in uterine natural killer cells. J Clin Endocrinol Metab 2001; 86(4): 1823–34.

27. Lash GE, Schiessl B, Kirkley M et al. Expression of angiogenic growth factors by uterine natural killer cells during early pregnancy. J Leukoc Biol 2006; 80(3): 572–80.

28. Ashkar AA, Di Santo JP, Croy BA. Interferon gamma contributes to initiation of uterine vascular modification, decidual integrity, and uterine natural killer cell maturation during normal murine pregnancy. J Exp Med 2000; 192(2): 259–70.

29. Quenby S, Nik H, Innes B et al. Uterine natural killer cells and angiogenesis in recurrent reproductive failure. Hum Reprod 2009; 24(1): 45–54.

30. Quenby SM, Farquharson RG. Predicting recurring miscarriage: what is important? Obstet Gynecol 1993; 82(1): 132–8.

31. Li TC, Tuckerman EM, Laird SM. Endometrial factors in recurrent miscarriage. Hum Reprod 2002; 8(1): 43–52.

32. Quack KC, Vassiliadou N, Pudney J et al. Leukocyte activation in the decidua of chromosomally normal and abnormal fetuses from women with recurrent abortion. Hum Reprod 2001; 16(5): 949–55.

33. Yamamoto T, Takahashi Y, Kase N et al. Role of decidual natural killer (NK) cells in patients with missed abortion: differences between cases with normal and abnormal chromosome. Clin Exp Immunol 1999; 116(3): 449–52.

34. Quenby S, Vince G, Farquharson R et al. Recurrent miscarriage: a defect in nature's quality control? Hum Reprod 2002; 17: 1959–63.

35. Lachapelle MH, Miron P, Hemmings R et al. Endometrial T, B and NK cells in patients with recurrent spontaneous abortion. Altered profile and pregnancy outcome. J Immunol 1996; 156(10): 4027–34.

36. Quenby S, Bates M, Doig T et al. Pre-implantation endometrial leukocytes in woman with recurrent miscarriage. Hum Reprod 1999; 14(9): 2386–91.

37. Clifford K, Flanagan AM, Regan L. Endometrial CD56+ natural killer cells in women with recurrent miscarriage: a histomorphometric study. Hum Reprod 1999; 14: 2727–30.

38. Tuckerman E, Laird SM, Prakash A et al. Prognostic value of the measurement of uterine natural killer cells in the endometrium of women with recurrent miscarriage. Hum Reprod 2007; 22(8): 2208–13.

39. Guimond MJ, Wang B, Croy BA. Engraftment of bone marrow from severe combined immunodeficient (SCID) mice reverses the reproductive deficits in natural killer cell-deficient tg epsilon 26 mice. J Exp Med 1998; 187(2): 217–23.

40. Quenby S, Kalumbi C, Bates M et al. Prednisolone reduces preconceptual endometrial natural killer cells in women with recurrent miscarriage. Fertil Steril 2005; 84(4): 980–4.

41. Ogasawara M, Aoki K. Successful uterine steroid therapy in a case with a history of ten miscarriages. Am J Reprod Immunol 2000; 44(4): 253–5.

42. Quenby S, Farquharson R, Young M et al. Successful pregnancy outcome following 19 consecutive miscarriages: case report. Hum Reprod 2003; 18(12): 2562–4.

43. Yamada H, Morikawa M, Kato Eh et al. Preconceptual natural killer cell activity and percentage as predictors of biochemical pregnancy and spontaneous abortion with normal chromosome karyotype. Am J Reprod Immunol 2003; 50(4): 351–4.

44. Moffett A, Regan L, Braude P. Natural killer cells, miscarriage, and infertility. Br Med J 2004; 329: 1283–5.

45. Scott JR. Immunotherapy for recurrent miscarriage. Cochrane Database Syst Rev 2003; (1): CD000112.

46. Ledee-Bataille N, Bonet-Chea K, Hosny G et al. Role of the endometrial tripod interleukin-18, -15 and -12 in inadequate uterine receptivity in patients with a history of repeated in-vitro fertilisation-embryo transfer failure. Fertil Steril 2005; 83(3): 598–605.

47. Matteo MG, Greco P, Rosenberg P. Normal percentage of CD56[bright] natural killer cells in young patients with a history of repeated unexplained implantation failure after in vitro fertilization cycles. Fertil Steril 2007; 88(4): 990–3.

48. Thum MY, Bhaskaran S, Abdalla HI et al. An increase in the absolute count of CD56[dim]CD16[+]CD69[+] NK cells in the peripheral blood is associated with a poorer IVF treatment and pregnancy outcome. Hum Reprod 2004; 19(10): 2395–400.

49. Hill JA. Immunological mechanisms of pregnancy maintenance and failure: a critique of theories and therapy. Am J Reprod Immunol 1990; 22(1–2): 33–41.

50. Hasegawa I, Yamanoto Y, Suzuki M et al. Prednisolone plus low-dose aspirin improves the implantation rate in women with autoimmune conditions who are

undergoing in vitro fertilization. *Fertil Steril* 1998; **70**(6): 1044–8.

51. Moffitt D, Queenan JT Jr, Veeck LL. Low-dose glucocorticoids after in vitro fertilization and embryo transfer have no significant effect on pregnancy rate. *Fertil Steril* 1995; **63**(3): 571–7.

52. Ubaldi F, Rienzi L, Ferrero S *et al.* Low dose prednisolone administration in routine ICSI patients

does not improve pregnancy and implantation. *Hum Reprod* 2002; **17**(6): 1544–7.

53. Clark DA, Coulam CB, Stricker RB. Is intravenous immunoglobulins (IVIG) efficacious in early pregnancy failure? A critical review and meta-analysis for patients who fail in vitro fertilization and embryo transfer (IVF). *J Assist Reprod Genet* 2006; **23**(1): 1–13.

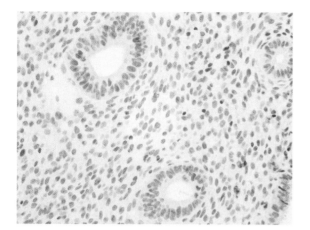

**Figure 9.1** Proliferative phase endometrium showing low levels of uterine natural killer (uNK cells) (stained brown).

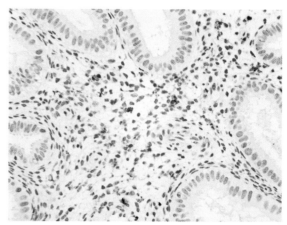

**Figure 9.2** Mid-luteal phase endometrium showing higher numbers of uterine natural killer (uNK) cells (stained brown).

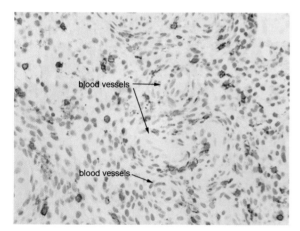

**Figure 9.3** Uterine natural killer (uNK) cells (stained brown) forming aggregates around blood vessels.

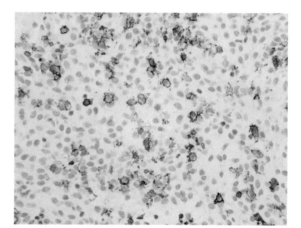

**Figure 9.4** Immunochemistry staining on patient with RM showing high levels of uterine natural killer uNK cells (stained brown) in mid-luteal phase endometrium.

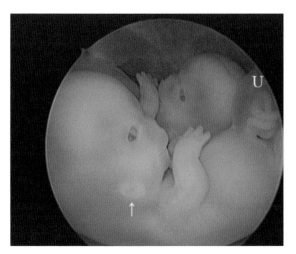

**Figure 12.1b** Embryoscopic lateral view of the two embryos. Note the developing eye lids. The arrow marks the external ear. The elbow is bent .The fingers are separated. Herniation of the midgut into the umbilical cord (U) is still physiological at this developmental stage. A normal karyotype (46,XX) was diagnosed cytogenetically.

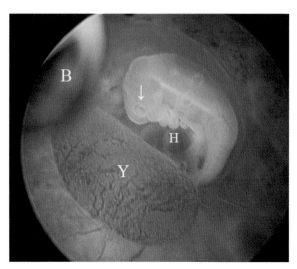

**Figure 12.2b** Four branchial arches an the lens plakode (arrow) are clearly discernible. The head is close contact to the heart prominence (H). Note the yolk (Y) sac with fetal blood islands. (M) marks a micro-bubble. Chromosome analysis revealed a normal (46,XX) karyotype.

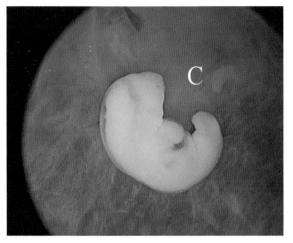

**Figure 12.3b** Embryoscopic examination revealed a GD 3 embryo measuring 6 mm crown–rump length. A short body stalk connected the GD3 embryo to the chorionic plate (C). Cytogenetically trisomy 7 (47, XY, +7) was diagnosed.

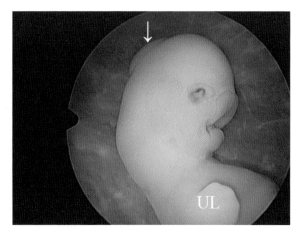

**Figure 12.4b** Close up, lateral view of the upper portion of the trisomy 15(47,XY,+15) embryo with a parietal encephalocele (arrow). The embryo showed on embryoscopic examination abnormal lip development and a dysplastic face. Based on the crown–rump length, the head is too small and the upper limbs (UL) are retarded in their development.

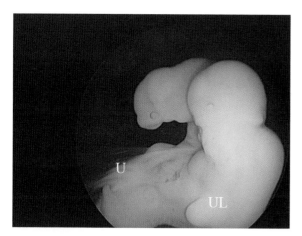

**Figure 12.5b** Embryoscopic examination from a lateral view
**(b)** showed dicephalus conjoined twins. The microcephalic
conjoined twins showed dysplastic faces and shared a body from the
upper chest downwards. Two upper (UL) and no lower limbs and a
single umbilical cord (U) were seen by embryoscopy. A normal
karyotype (46,XY) was diagnosed cytogenetically.

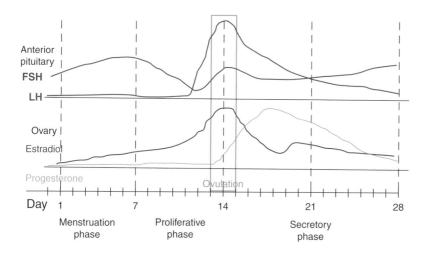

**Figure 17.1** Profile of expression of the
hormones during the menstrual cycle.

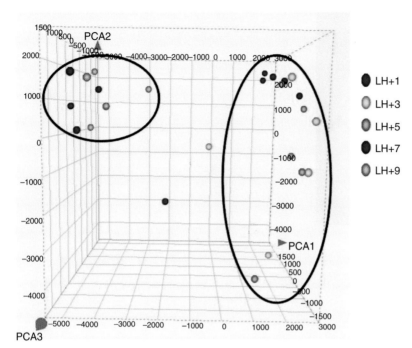

**Figure 17.3** Principal component analysis of human endometrium throughout the development of the secretory phase (after the endogenous pick of LH) in natural cycle (adapted from Horcajadas *et al.* [30]).

● LH+1
○ LH+3
◐ LH+5
● LH+7
◑ LH+9

# Cytogenetic factors in recurrent early pregnancy loss

Sony Sierra and Mary D. Stephenson

Longitudinal studies in reproductive-aged couples have demonstrated the inefficiencies in human reproduction. In any given cycle, there is only an estimated one in five chance of conception, and before clinical recognition or development of embryonic heart activity; almost 50% of all pregnancies end in miscarriage [1,2]. Whether this is due to errors in fertilization or the result of a high-functioning quality control process remains unclear. In either case, observations on chances to reproduce successfully initiated early efforts to assess the risk of miscarriage.

In 1975, Boue *et al.* reported that 60% of miscarriages were due to numeric cytogenetic abnormalities, specifically, aneuploidies or polyploidies, based on the cytogenetic results of 1500 miscarriages [3]. The authors hypothesized that pregnancies with numeric cytogenetic abnormalities were generally not compatible with life, and therefore ended in miscarriage. Further data found that the frequency of cytogenetic abnormalities changes as gestational age advances.

Edmonds *et al.* [1] and Wilcox *et al.* [2] reported that prior to 6 weeks' gestation, the risk of miscarriage is 30–50%. Ohno *et al.* reported that 70% of pre-clinical miscarriages, defined as demise of less than 6 weeks' gestation, are due to numeric cytogenetic abnormalities [4]. Between 6 and 10 weeks' gestation, approximately 15% of such pregnancies end in demise, of which 50% are due to numeric cytogenetic abnormalities [5]. After 10 weeks' gestation, the risk of pregnancy loss is much less, estimated at approximately 2–3%, of which approximately 5–6% are due to numeric cytogenetic abnormalities [6]. A small percentage of term deliveries, estimated at 0.6%, will have a numeric cytogenetic abnormality, most commonly trisomy 21, 18 or 13, or a sex chromosome aneuploidy [7].

This chapter will discuss the cytogenetic factors involved in miscarriage in the general population and in couples with recurrent pregnancy loss. The process of meiosis in gametogenesis will be reviewed, as well as the errors of meiosis which lead to aneuploidy. The importance and limitations of cytogenetic analyses of miscarriage tissue is highlighted. Finally, the management of cytogenetic factors in miscarriage will be summarized.

## Cytogenetics in human reproduction

Meiosis is a specialized cell division process occurring in human reproduction generating gametes with the haploid (23n) chromosome number from diploid (46n) germ cells. Germ cells undergo one round of DNA replication initially, followed by two cell divisions producing four daughter cells. The first division, termed meiosis I, involves the segregation of homologous chromosomes to opposite poles of the cell. Meiosis II involves segregation of the sister chromatids, producing four cells each with a haploid chromosome number (23n). During the meiotic prophase, the homologous chromosomes synapse and undergo recombination. This unique and intricate phenomenon accounts for genetic variation among species.

In females, germ cells increase by mitotic proliferation during early embryogenesis, and reach a maximum of 8 million by the end of the first trimester. This active period of cell division is followed by entry into meiotic prophase. Numerous germ cells undergo apoptosis, or programmed cell death, at this time, reducing the pool of potential oocytes at birth to approximately 800 000. At birth, oocytes are surrounded by somatic cells forming primordial follicles. At this time they enter a period of extended meiotic arrest. Resumption of meiosis and the completion of the first cell division occurs after the onset of puberty. Completion of meiosis I occurs just prior to ovulation. The oocyte arrests briefly at the

**Table 10.1** Aneuploidy at various stages of reproduction and development. Adapted from Hassold & Hunt (2001) [8].

|  | Sperm | Oocytes | Pre-implantation embryos | Pre-clinical miscarriage | Early miscarriage | Fetal demise | Livebirths |
|---|---|---|---|---|---|---|---|
| Incidence of aneuploidy | 1–2% | 20% | ~20% | ~50–70%* | 35% | 4% | 0.3% |
| Most common aneuploidies | Various | Various | Various | Not known | 45X;+16; +21; +22 | +13; +18; +21 | +13; +18; +21; XXX; XXY; XYY |

metaphase of meiosis II, with the completion of the second cell division after fertilization [8].

In males, the process follows a slightly different timeline. Meiosis begins with puberty; germ cells progress from prophase to metaphase I to metaphase II without delay, producing four haploid gametes. In comparison, in females, each cell that enters meiosis produces only one functional haploid oocyte and three polar bodies which degenerate.

Normal meiosis I (MI) division results in the segregation of homologous chromosomes. Abnormal MI segregation can result from true non-disjunction, where homologs travel to the same spindle pole, rather than opposing. Achiasmatic non-disjunction occurs when homologous chromosomes fail to pair and/or undergo recombination and travel independently to the same spindle pole. Premature separation of sister chromatids occurs when chromatids, rather than homologous chromosomes, segregate from one another [8].

Normal meiosis II (MII) division results in the segregation of sister chromatids. MII non-disjunction occurs when sister chromatids do not separate. The final result from these erroneous cell divisions is aneuploidy, defined as the addition (trisomy) or absence (monosomy) of individual chromosomes (Table 10.1). Such numeric chromosome errors are frequently found in miscarriages.

It is recognized that trisomy is the most frequent type of numeric chromosome error in miscarriage. Hassold & Chiu [9] showed the frequency of trisomy increases with advancing maternal age, notably after the maternal age of 35 years. Maternally derived trisomy occurs more frequently in meiosis I, than in meiosis II. This holds true for trisomy of chromosome numbers 2, 15, 16, 21, 22 and sex chromosomes resulting in XXY and XXX [10].

Non-disjunction errors occur much less frequently in sperm, although paternal errors account for the majority of monosomy X (45 X) [11] and sex trisomies

XXY, XYY [12]. Fluorescent in situ hybridization (FISH) analyses of sperm collected from couples with a history of recurrent miscarriage revealed an increase of sex chromosome disomy (0.45% vs 0.37%, $P < 0.01$) [13]. Despite this finding, miscarriages from couples with recurrent miscarriage have equivalent frequencies of sex chromosome aneuploidies compared with the general reproductive population [14] suggesting that sperm with such numeric chromosome abnormalities may be selected against during fertilization.

A case–control study published in 2003 reported evidence of an association between elevated sperm chromosome aneuploidy and apoptosis in couples with recurrent miscarriage. Carrell *et al.* [15] evaluated semen quality parameters and sperm chromosome aneuploidy for chromosomes X, Y, 13, 18 and 21 in patients with unexplained recurrent miscarriage (n = 24), fertile controls (n = 42) and a control group of men from the general population (n = 26). The mean aneuploidy rate in the recurrent miscarriage group was 2.77% ± 0.22, significantly higher ($P < 0.005$) than the control groups (1.19% and 1.48%, respectively). This study, while small in size, supports the findings of other smaller studies documenting increased sperm aneuploidy in couples with unexplained recurrent miscarriage [13,16]. While these studies are limited by their power, further research may clarify the contribution of sperm aneuploidy in recurrent miscarriage.

Recently, "recurrent aneuploidy" has been suggested as a factor associated with a history of recurrent pregnancy loss. This theory has led to the empiric use of in-vitro fertilization with pre-implantation genetic screening (IVF/PGS) in patients with unexplained recurrent miscarriage. On the basis of the cytogenetic data of 420 miscarriages in 285 patients with a history of recurrent miscarriage, Stephenson *et al.* [14] did not find any difference in the distribution of aneuploidies, when stratified for maternal age and compared with data of the general reproductive population [10]. The most frequent trisomies in the recurrent miscarriage cohort were of chromosomes 15, 16, 22, 21, 14 and 13.This study did not find evidence of recurrent aneuploidy in couples with recurrent miscarriage. Therefore, "recurrent aneuploidy" remains theoretical and further studies are warranted before IVF/PGS is considered evidence-based.

## Evaluation of the miscarriage

Identification of numeric or unbalanced cytogenetic abnormalities in miscarriages is paramount for counseling and developing a management plan for subsequent pregnancies in couples with a history of recurrent pregnancy loss. Unfortunately, cytogenetic analyses of miscarriages is not routinely performed, despite a favorable cost–benefit analysis [17].

Cytogenetic analyses can be performed on miscarriage tissue using several techniques, including cell culture followed by chromosome banding, microsatellite testing and comparative genomic hybridization. Correlation of cytogenetic results with embryopathology, either by sending the specimen for evaluation or imaging of the miscarriage in utero by hysteroscopic visualization prior to dilation and curettage, is the optimal way of evaluating the miscarriage for cytogenetic and/or congenital abnormalities.

The classic method of cytogenetic analysis of miscarriage tissue is through cell culture of the isolated pregnancy tissue followed by Giemsa banding analysis of metaphase chromosomes. This method of analysis has well-described limitations because it relies on the timely collection of viable pregnancy tissue, preferably embryo proper or amnion. Unfortunately, it is usually the chorionic villi that are isolated, with maternal decidual cells attached. Either due to a lack of chorionic villi, or to robust decidual cell overgrowth in culture, often a disproportionately high percentage of 46,XX results are reported [18]. The rate of maternal contamination for an individual laboratory can be estimated by comparing the number of 46,XX to 46, XY results. Microsatellite testing, which compares highly polymorphic DNA loci in miscarriage DNA to maternal DNA, can be used to determine whether a 46,XX result is a true result or due to maternal cell contamination.

In addition, culture failure can occur, usually when there has been a prolonged period of time from demise to the collection of the miscarriage tissue [18].

Comparative genomic hybridization (CGH) with flow cytometry (FCM) is an innovative improvement for cytogenetic analysis of miscarriage specimens, although it has its own inherent limitations. This technique involves the simultaneous hybridization of DNA extracted from miscarriage cells and reference DNA, each labeled fluoroscopically and matched to a set of normal metaphase chromosomes. Comparison of the fluorochrome intensities for each of the target chromosomes allows for the detection of trisomies and monosomies. Comparative genomic hybridization cannot assess for ploidy, therefore, flow cytometry is required. A comparison of CGH/ FCM technology to conventional Giemsa banding revealed that CGH/FCM has a higher success rate (99.7%) and less maternal contamination, therefore more accurate results [19]. Unfortunately, balanced structural chromosome rearrangements cannot be assessed with CGH and visualization with conventional cytogenetic analysis is necessary.

Comparative genomic hybridization is not yet widely available, however, it can be applied to stored miscarriage tissue, usually as paraffin blocks. Bell et al. [20] reported their results from an academic center with retrospective analysis of stored miscarriage tissue as paraffin blocks following fixation with formalin. DNA was extracted from nine paraffin blocks with known aneuploidy, followed by whole genome amplification by degenerate oligonucleotide-primed PCR. Comparative genomic hybridization was able to detect aneuploidy in 7 of the 9 cases. Comparative genomic hybridization followed by flow cytometry may prove a powerful technique to provide chromosome results on paraffin-stored miscarriage tissue.

## Investigation and management of genetic factors in recurrent pregnancy loss

Inherited genetic factors as a potential causative factor in the investigation and management of patients with recurrent pregnancy is recognized by the American College of Obstetrics and Gynecology and the Royal College of Obstetrics and Gynecology, UK [21,22]. Chromosome analyses of miscarriage specimens are recommended in both guidelines to assess for numeric errors (such as trisomy, monosomy or polyploidy) or structural chromosome rearrangements. The results of such studies are useful in determining whether additional factors of maternal or paternal origin are required. In couples with a history of recurrent pregnancy loss, if cytogenetic analysis of miscarriage tissue confirms a diagnosis of aneuploidy, that same couple can be counseled to try to conceive again without further evaluation. If the second miscarriage is found to be associated with a numeric chromosome error, the couple can be counseled that this miscarriage was a random event and that the risk of miscarriage in the subsequent pregnancy is not increased since such chromosome errors have been shown to be random events, although the frequency of such events are highly dependent on maternal age. Without such information, an extensive evaluation is often performed, which is both costly and time-consuming. Furthermore, with chromosome results of prior miscarriages, the couple is often left without answers, which can lead to heightened anxiety and feelings of hopelessness.

## Pre-implantation genetic screening and recurrent pregnancy loss

The possibility of recurring chromosome errors as etiologic for recurring pregnancy loss, has led to the recent application of pre-implantation genetic screening (PGS) for management of idiopathic recurrent miscarriage. In the mid 1990s, PGS was developed in conjunction with in-vitro fertilization (IVF) to optimize embryo selection by screening for aneuploidy and reducing the number of embryos for transfer [23]. The first successful embryo biopsy was performed in 1968 [24]. Embryo biopsy involves a polar body biopsy or aspiration of 1–2 blastomeres from the six-to eight-celled embryos, followed by fluorescent in-situ hybridization (FISH) of a limited number of chromosomes. Unfortunately there is a high rate of mosaicism (>25%) in day 2–3 blastomeres, thus limiting the accuracy of this technique [25,26].

There have been two studies assessing the utility of this procedure in unexplained recurrent miscarriage.

The first study was retrospective in design, including 58 women with three or more miscarriages from various IVF centers [27]. It is unclear what investigations were done prior to IVF/PGS other than to rule out parental genetic factors. Nine PGD cycles were not included due to low numbers of embryos. A single day 3 blastomere was biopsied and fewer than 5 embryos transferred on day 4 or 5. FISH screening from chromosomes X, Y, 13, 15, 16, 17, 18, 21 and 22 was done. In women aged less than 35 years, a total of 25 cycles were completed, and 8% (2/21) did not have a transfer. FISH results were abnormal in 12/21 (57%) of cases. The pregnancy rate was 52% (13/21) and the take-home baby rate was 40% (10/25). In women over age 35, a total of 44 cycles were completed with 16% (6/37) not having embryos to transfer. FISH results were abnormal in 30/44 (67%) of cycles.The pregnancy rate was 39% (17/37) and the take-home baby rate was 34% (15/44).

A second study by Platteau in 2005 [28] was prospective in design, based on the same hypothesis that repeated chromosome errors may be causative in idiopathic recurrent miscarriage. To examine the role of IVF/PGD, patients were divided into two groups by age. A total of 35 cycles were done in 25 patients less than 37 years of age and a total of 34 cycles in 24 patients over age 37. All patients had a history of three or more unexplained miscarriages, with parental genetic factors, anatomical factors and antiphospholipid syndrome ruled out. Two blastomeres were biopsied and FISH for chromosomes X, Y, 13, 16, 18, 21 and 22 were done. Two embryos were transferred on day 5. In the younger group, 4/35 cycles (11%) resulted in no transfer; FISH results were abnormal in 44% of embryos. The pregnancy rate was 10/35 or 29%, with a take-home baby rate of 9/35 or 26%. In the older group, 47% (16/34) of cycles resulted in no transfer and 67% of the embryos were abnormal by FISH analysis. The pregnancy rate was 18% (5/34), and the take-home baby rate was 3% (1/34).

Both of these studies used FISH techniques to screen for aneuploidy, however neither was fully inclusive of the most frequent trisomies found in miscarriages from couples with a history of recurrent miscarriage [13,14,15,16,21,22]. Comparison of the pregnancy rates in these two studies to a historic control group of patients with idiopathic recurrent miscarriage managed conservatively is shown in Table 10.2.

It has been demonstrated that in the management of idiopathic recurrent miscarriage, conservative treatment consisting of early pregnancy monitoring by ultrasound every 2 weeks in a dedicated miscarriage clinic led to a pregnancy rate of 70% and successful take-home baby in 75% of cases [29]. In the studies discussed above where assisted reproductive techniques were applied with PGS the live-birth rate is similar, however, the pregnancy rates are much lower than expected with a natural cycle.

**Table 10.2** Pregnancy outcome in idiopathic recurrent miscarriage: IVF/PGS vs. control group.

| | Intervention | Pregnancies | Pregnancy rate | Successful outcome/pregnancy |
|---|---|---|---|---|
| Munne *et al.* [27] | IVF/PGS | 30/78 completed cycles | 38%** | 83%** |
| Platteau *et al.* [28] | IVF/ICSI$^a$/PGS | 15/69 cycles started | 22%* | 67%* |
| Brigham *et al.* [29] | Conservative | 226/302 patients | 70% | 75% |

* not significant.
** $P < 0.001$.
$^a$ ICSI, Intracytoplasmic sperm injection.

The American Society for Reproductive Medicine (ASRM) has released the committee opinion stating that the available evidence does not support the use of IVF/PGS to improve the live-birth outcome in patients with recurrent pregnancy loss [30]. The evidence indicates that instead of providing benefit, these techniques may actually lower the take-home baby rate in these already vulnerable, anxious couples in addition to subjecting them to the costs and invasiveness of assisted reproductive therapies designed for infertility. A better approach is to encourage these couples with evidence from studies indicating that treatment consisting of supportive care and early pregnancy monitoring leads to a much higher success rate of a good pregnancy outcome [31,32].

## Summary

Human reproduction appears to be a very inefficient process, primarily because of a high frequency of chromosome errors in gametes and the resultant embryos. New techniques for the diagnosis of chromosome errors in miscarriages are being offered for couples facing the burden of recurrent pregnancy loss. Conventional cytogenetic analyses have a proven role but complementary techniques are required in specific cases, for example, with culture failure, when maternal cell contamination is suspected or when fresh tissue was not sent for analysis.

Although initially promising, pre-implantation genetic screening does not appear to be effective for couples with recurrent pregnancy loss. An evidence-based evaluation followed by close, supportive monitoring in subsequent pregnancies appears to be effective in improving the pregnancy outcome. If unfortunately another miscarriage occurs, chromosome testing is paramount to determine whether the miscarriage is "explained," due to a numeric chromosome error, or "unexplained" and perhaps a treatment failure.

## References

1. Edmonds DK, Lindsay KS, Miller JF, Williamson E, Wood PJ. Early embryonic mortality in women. *Fertil Steril* 1982; **38**(4): 447–53.

2. Wilcox AJ, Weinberg CR, O'Connor JF *et al.* Incidence of early loss of pregnancy. *New Engl J Med* 1988; **319**: 189–94.

3. Boue J, Boue A, Lazar P. Retrospective and prospective epidemiological studies of 1500 karyotyped spontaneous human abortions. *Teratology* 1975; **12**: 11–26.

4. Ohno M, Maeda T, Matsunobu A. A cytogenetic study of spontaneous abortions with direct analysis of chorionic villi. *Obstet Gynecol* 1991; **77**(3): 394–8.

5. Jacobs PA, Hassold T. Chromosome abnormalities: origin and etiology in abortions and livebirths. In F Vogel, K Sperling (eds), *Human Genetics*. Berlin: Springer-Verlag, 1987, pp. 233–44.

6. Simpson JL. Incidence and timing of pregnancy losses: relevance to evaluating safety of early prenatal diagnosis. *Am J Med Genet* 1990; **35**(2): 165–73.

7. Neilson JP, Wohort M. Chromosome abnormalities found among 34,910 newborn children: results from a 13-year incidence study in Arhus, Denmark. *Hum Genet* 1991; **22**: 81–3.

8. Hassold T, Hunt P. To err (meiotically) is human: the genesis of human aneuploidy. *Nature Rev Genet* 2001; **1**: 280–91.

9. Hassold T, Chiu D. Maternal age-specific rates of numerical chromosome abnormalities with special reference to trisomy. *Hum Genet* 1985; **70**: 11–17.

10. Hassold T, Abruzzo M, Adkins K *et al.* Human aneuploidy:incidence, origin, and etiology. *Environ Mol Mutagen* 1996; **28**: 167–75.

11. Chamley LW, McKay EJ, Pattison NS. Inhibition of heparin/antithrombin III cofactor activity by anticardiolipin antibodies: a mechanism for thrombosis. *Thromb Res* 1993 15; **71**(2): 103–11.

12. Hawley R, Frazier J, Rasooly R. Separation anxiety: the etiology of nondisjunction in flies and people. *Hum Mol Genet* 1994; **3**: 1521–8.

13. Rubio C, Gil-Salom M, Simon C *et al.* Incidence of sperm chromosomal abnormalities in a risk population: relationship with sperm quality and ICSI outcome. *Hum Reprod* 2001; **16**(10): 2084–92.

14. Stephenson MD, Awartani KA, Robinson WP. Cytogenetic analysis of miscarriages from couples with recurrent miscarriage: a case-control study. *Hum Reprod* 2002; **17**(2): 446–51.

15. Carrell D, Wilcox A, Lowy L *et al.* Elevated sperm chromsome aneuploidy and apoptosis in patients with unexplained recurrent pregnancy loss. *Obstet Gynecol* 2003; **101**: 1229–35.

16. Rubio C, Simon C, Blanco V *et al.* Implications of sperm chromosome abnormalities in recurrent miscarriage. *J Assist Reprod Genet* 1999; **16**: 253–8.

17. Wolf GC, Horger E. O. Indications for examination of spontaneous abortion specimens: a reassessment. *Am J Obstet Gynecol* 1995; **173**: 1364–8.

18. Bell KA, Van Deerlin PG, Haddad BR, Feinberg RF. Cytogenetic diagnosis of "normal 46, XX" karyotypes in spontaneous abortions frequently may be misleading. *Fertil Steril* 1999; **71**(2): 334–41.

19. Lomax B, Tang S, Separovic E *et al.* Comparative genomic hybridization in combination with flow cytometry improves results of cytogenetic analysis of spontaneous abortions. *Am J Hum Genet* 2000; **66**(5): 1516–21.

20. Bell KA, Van Deerlin PG, Feinber RF, du Manoir S, Haddad BR. Diagnosis of aneuploidy in archival, parafffin-embedded pregnancy-loss tissues by comparative genomic hybridization. *Fertil Steril* 2001; **75**(2): 374–9.

21. American College of Obstetricians and Gynecologists. ACOG Practice Bulletin. Management of recurrent pregnancy loss. Number 24, February 2001 (replaces Technical Bulletin Number 212, September 1995). *Int J Gynaecol Obstet* 2002; **78**(2): 179–90.

22. Royal College of Obstetricians and Gynaecologists. The Investigation and Treatment of Couples with Recurrent Miscarriage. RCOG Guideline No. 17. 2003.

23. Harper JC, Coonen E, Ramaekers FC *et al.* Identification of the sex of human preimplantation embryos in two hours using an improved spreading method and fluorescent in-situ hybridization (FISH) using directly labelled probes. *Hum Reprod* 1994; **9**(4): 721–4.

24. Edwards RG, Gardner RL. Choosing sex before birth. *New Scientist* 1968; **38**: 218–20.

25. Munne S, Magli C, Cohen J *et al.* Positive outcome after preimplantation diagnosis of aneuploidy in human embryos. *Hum Reprod* 1999; **14**(9): 2191–9.

26. Delhanty JD. Chromosome analysis by FISH in human preimplantation genetics. *Hum Reprod* 1997;**12** (11 Suppl): 153–5.

27. Munne S, Chen S, Fischer J *et al.* Preimplantation genetic diagnosis reduces pregnancy loss in women aged 35 years and older with a history of recurrent miscarriages. *Fertil Steril* 2005; **84**, 331–5.

28. Platteau P, Staessen C, Michiels A *et al.* Preimplantation genetic diagnosis for aneuploidy screening in patients with unexplained recurrent miscarriages. *Fertil Steril* 2005; **83**(2): 393–7.

29. Brigham SA, Conlan C, Farquharson R. A longitudinal study of pregnancy outcome following idiopathic recurrent miscarriage. *Hum Reprod* 1999; **11**: 2868–71.

30. The Practice Committee of the American Society of Reproductive Technology, The Practice Committee of the American Society of Reproductive Medicine. Preimplantation genetic testing: A practice committee opinion. *Fertil Steril* 2008; **90**: S136–43.

31. Stray-Pederson B, Stray-Pederson S. Etiologic factors and subsequent reproductive performance in 195 couples with a prior history of habitual abortion. *Am J Obstet Gynec* 1984; **148**: 140–6.

32. Clifford K, Rai R, Regan L. Future pregnancy outcome in unexplained recurrent first trimester miscarriage. *Hum Reprod* 1997; **12**: 387–9.

# Parental chromosome testing

M. Goddijn and Nico J. Leschot

## Background

Couples with recurrent miscarriage are offered a diagnostic work-up to show or rule out an underlying cause known to be associated with recurrent miscarriage. These factors are antiphospholipid syndrome, uterine abnormalities, parental structural chromosome abnormalities and hyperhomocysteinemia. In this chapter parental chromosome testing is addressed.

Parental chromosome patterns are most frequently investigated, in routine care, by conventional chromosome techniques (G-banding or Q-banding technique). See Figure 11.1 as an example of trypsin-G-banding technique. The aim is to detect a balanced structural chromosome abnormality in the male or female partner. Structural chromosome abnormalities can be subdivided into translocations, inversions, deletions and duplications, but only translocations and inversions are known to be associated with recurrent miscarriage. This is a result of translocations and inversions sharing the ability to be inherited also in a balanced form. Structural chromosome abnormalities other than translocations and inversions, which are potentially associated with recurrent miscarriage, like sex chromosomal mosaicism and uniparental disomy are discussed. Another genetic mechanism, skewed sex chromosome inactivation, potentially related to recurrent miscarriage is discussed as well.

Structural chromosome abnormalities involve the rearrangement of chromosome segments. Within chromosome translocations and inversions in their balanced form there is no overall loss or gain of genetic material.

The incidence of carrier status for balanced chromosome translocations has been reported to increase from approximately 0.7% in the general population to 2.2% after one miscarriage, 4.8% after two miscarriages and 5.2% after three miscarriages [1,2].

Women appear more likely to be carriers than men and translocations are more frequent than inversions [1]. More recent studies report an overall incidence of approximately 3% in couples with a history of recurrent miscarriage, probably due to the use of more restrictive criteria for structural chromosome abnormalities, this way excluding normal variant chromosome patterns [3,4].

If a balanced structural chromosome abnormality is found this should be communicated to the patient by explaining to him or her that he or she is a healthy carrier. The test result will have no medical consequences for him or her, with the exception of the increased risk of another miscarriage and of abnormal offspring. In the genetic counseling of patients who are carriers of a balanced chromosome translocation, it is important to stress the absence of medical consequences for the carriers themselves as couples not infrequently have the perception that they carry a severe disease. The products of conception in carriers can have a normal karyotype, the same karyotype as the carrier parent, or an unbalanced karyotype. The latter can lead to miscarriage, stillbirth or the birth of a child with major congenital impairments. The expected chances of adverse pregnancy outcome in a carrier of a specific chromosome abnormality should be shared with the patient if available.

For many years it has been good clinical practice to offer chromosome testing to women with recurrent miscarriage. Recurrent miscarriage is most frequently interpreted as two or three miscarriages, and varies between different guidelines. In actual practice we are of the opinion that gynecologists take a different view of the pros and cons of the parental chromosome test in couples with recurrent miscarriage than geneticists. Gynecologists mostly share the opinion that a possible unbalanced combination in a subsequent pregnancy would end in another miscarriage. Geneticists

---

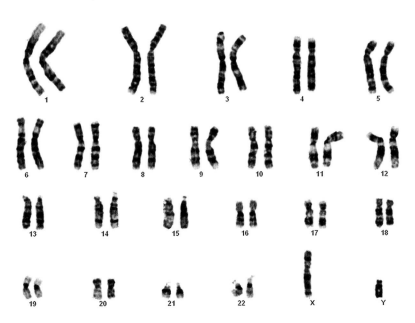

**Figure 11.1** A normal male karyotype with 46 chromosomes. The chromosomes are ordered from large to small and have a trypsin-Giemsa banding pattern, which is specific to each chromosome.

however are more focused on unbalanced combinations that might survive pregnancy and result in a newborn with severe malformations and a mental handicap. Their view is based on the knowledge that in a reciprocal translocation two abnormal, but different, combinations in the gametes are possible. Theoretically, a pregnancy could end in miscarriage in the majority of cases, while the other combination could be viable and result in a live-born severely handicapped child. We will address the theoretical and empirical chances of unbalanced outcomes in subsequent pregnancies. Cytogenetic and clinical information on rare chromosomal disorders can be found on internet facilities for professionals (www. ecaruca.net, www.ncbi.nlm.nih.gov/omim) and for patients (chromosomehelpstation.com).

The chance of viable unbalanced offspring resulting from carrier status is the most important reason to offer parental chromosome testing. Other reasons might be to find an explanation for the recurrence of the miscarriages, prognostic reasons, i.e. to investigate the chances of delivering a healthy child and the risk of a future miscarriage, and furthermore to reduce anxiety and distress by identifying or excluding carrier status as a likely cause of the recurrent miscarriages.

It should be realized that the majority of unbalanced structural chromosome abnormalities are inherited from either one of the parents while a smaller proportion arise *de novo*. It is, however, hard to establish the incidence of *de novo* translocations, especially for the category ascertained by recurrent

miscarriage. In general, the incidence of *de novo* translocations might be up to one third of unbalanced cases detected prenatally [5], or 23% at birth [6]. Furthermore, most viable unbalanced offspring are ascertained through the previous birth of a child with an unbalanced karyotype, rather than through recurrent miscarriage. Some viable unbalanced offspring will not be detected antenatally because parents deliberately decide to refrain from prenatal diagnosis or from termination of a pregnancy.

In this chapter, couples carrying a structural chromosome abnormality ascertained through recurrent miscarriage work-up are described. Their accompanying epidemiological figures and subsequent results of pregnancy outcome should not be confused with those in couples which carry a structural chromosome abnormality ascertained through a preceding live-born child with major congenital abnormalities or a preceding late stillbirth, for which other subsequent pregnancy outcomes might apply. Chapter 10 of this book deals with fetal chromosome abnormalities which might account for RM as well.

## Biological basis of chromosome abnormalities

### Reciprocal translocations

During meiosis in a carrier of a balanced chromosome translocation, theoretically three possible types of gametes are produced. In the case of the example

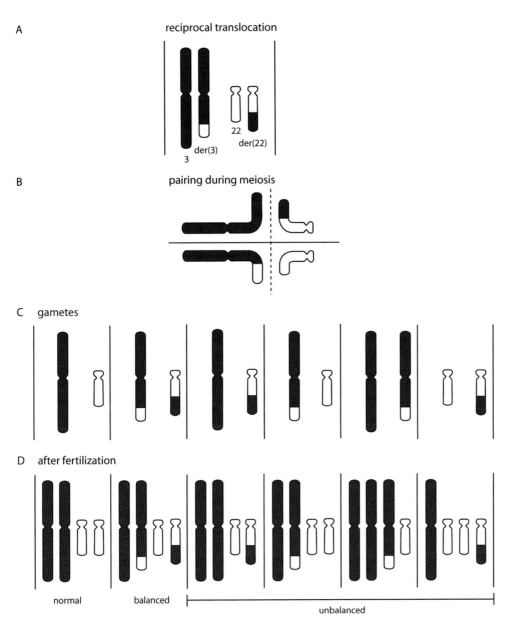

**Figure 11.2** In this diagram the theoretically possible gametes in a balanced carrier of a translocation between chromosome 3 and chromosome 22 is depicted. Of the six possible combinations, four of these will, after fertilization, result in an unbalanced combination. One in six will have a normal karyotype and the sixth combination will result in a balanced chromosome translocation. From Heineman *et al.* 2007 [38].

below (3/22 chromosome translocation) there is a theoretical chance of one in six for a gamete to have a normal chromosome 3 and a normal chromosome 22. There is also a chance of one in six for a gamete to have a balanced chromosome translocation. But there is a chance of four in six of a gamete having either too much genetic material of chromosome 3 (partial trisomy 3) and too little of chromosome 22 (partial monosomy 22), or the other way round: too much genetic material of chromosome 22 (partial trisomy 22) and too little of chromosome 3 (partial monosomy 3) (see Figure 11.2).

Assuming that the partner has a normal chromosome complement, the situation directly after fertilization might be as follows: statistically only two out of six early-stage embryos will have a normal or balanced

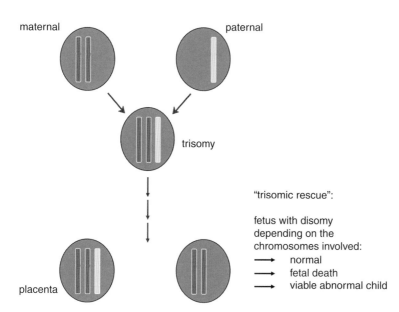

**Figure 11.3** One of the possible mechanisms that can explain an uniparental disomy: "trisomic rescue."

maternal

paternal

trisomy

"trisomic rescue":

fetus with disomy depending on the chromosomes involved:
→ normal
→ fetal death
→ viable abnormal child

placenta

karyotype, but four out of six embryos will have an unbalanced translocation. During further development a strong selection against the unbalanced embryos will occur. One of the possibilities is early death, after mitosis, resulting in failure to implant or a sub-clinical biochemical pregnancy, unnoticed by the woman herself. A further possibility is that the development of an unbalanced combination stops in the first trimester of gestation and the pregnancy ends in a miscarriage; furthermore, there is a small chance of a live-born child with, in the majority of cases, various congenital malformations and a severe mental handicap in later life.

A special type of chromosome translocation is the *Robertsonian translocation* (or centric fusion translocation). This translocation is restricted to the so-called acrocentric chromosomes, namely chromosomes 13, 14, 15, 21 and 22.

This type of translocation can be responsible for viable unbalanced offspring i.e. Down's syndrome or non-viable offspring. For instance in the most frequently occurring Robertsonian translocation between chromosome 14 and 21, trisomy 14, monosomy 14 and monosomy 21 are all non-viable. This type of chromosome translocation is responsible for the so-called "hereditary form of Down's syndrome" (about 1% of all patients with Down's syndrome).

Within this group of Robertsonian chromosome translocations there is a subgroup of homologous translocations. Someone can be a balanced carrier of a 14/14 translocation, t(14;14)(q10;q10) or a

t(15;15)(q10;q10) chromosome translocation. Such carriers of Robertsonian translocations have a risk of a child with (non-viable) trisomy 14 of almost 100%. However there is a chance of uniparental disomy (UPD).

*Uniparental disomy* (UPD) is an epigenetic phenomenon in which the total number of chromosomes is normal, but for a particular chromosome pair, both chromosomes originate from one parent only. One of the mechanisms is shown in Figure 11.3.

For chromosome regions that are imprinted (chromosome regions: 1p, 6q, 7q, 11p, 14q, 15q, 18q, 19q and 20q), there is a chance of a specific syndrome. Imprinted means that the DNA is methylated and that the genes in that region cannot be expressed. Paternal UPD of chromosome 14 is associated with a polyhydramnion, dysmorphic symptoms and a severe mental handicap. Maternal UPD 14 is associated with growth retardation and only a mild mental retardation. Maternal UPD 15 is associated with Prader–Willi syndrome, while paternal UPD 15 results in Angelman syndrome. In the meiosis of the healthy carrier mentioned above of a (14;14)(q10;q10) chromosome translocation, the translocation chromosome will be present in every early-stage embryo, while a normal chromosome 14 from the other parent results in a (non-viable) trisomy 14. However such a combination is sometimes "saved" by a mechanism that is called "trisomic rescue." The normal chromosome 14 is lost and the result is a carrier of the translocation chromosome only, however, he or she will have uniparental disomy for chromosome 14. For this particular chromosome, there is no chance of the result being normal offspring [7].

It is important to realize that uniparental disomy can only be confirmed by DNA analysis of the father, the mother and the fetus or child.

The second structural chromosome abnormality associated with recurrent miscarriage is a *chromosome inversion*. A segment of a particular chromosome is turned 180 degrees. For carriers of an inverted chromosome it is important to know whether the inversion is restricted to one chromosome arm (paracentric inversion) or whether both breakpoints of the inversion are on both chromosome arms (pericentric inversion). For carriers of paracentric inversions the chances of viable unbalanced offspring are very small, and reported at a maximum percentage of 3.8% [8,9]. In these older studies patients with recurrent miscarriage as well as other indications were included, this way explaining the relatively high percentage of unbalanced offspring. For carriers of a pericentric inversion the situation concerning the offspring is complicated. During meiosis a loop structure is formed, in order to try and achieve homolog pairing of both chromatides. If, however, a crossover in that loop occurs, the result is duplication of a part of the chromosome and deficiency of another segment of the same chromosome. These combinations can therefore result in miscarriages or abnormal viable offspring.

(*Sex*) *chromosomal mosaicism*, mostly hyperploidy in the mother has been reported as a cause for couples with RM [10,11]. However no control groups have been included in these studies and the weight of the association with recurrent miscarriage therefore remains unknown. An increased miscarriage rate has been found in couples with X-chromosome mosaicism and diminished ovarian reserve when compared with the same couples without diminished ovarian reserve [12].

# Technique of conventional chromosome studies

Chromosome studies of a blood sample are done by culturing lymphocytes for 72 hours, using a mitotic stimulant. Then cell division is blocked by a mitotic inhibitor. Hypotonic treatment is applied to let the cells swell, then a fixative is used. Metaphase spreads are studied under the microscope after a banding technique has been applied (mostly trypsin-Giemsa or Q-banding is used). The analysis is done semi-automatically.

# Recently developed laboratory techniques (molecular cytogenetics)

The resolution of conventional chromosome studies is limited. The smallest deletion that can be detected in this way is 5 mb. Therefore additional techniques are used, of which the most well known is fluorescence in situ hybridization (FISH). The principle here is that one or more specific small DNA probes are used, that are labeled with a colored signal that can be seen under a fluorescence microscope. In normal cells such probes should be seen as two signals in a normal diploid cell (either in a metaphase spread or in an interphase nucleus).

In this way submicroscopic translocations can be detected. In actual practice the FISH technique is mostly applied in cases of doubt about the morphological aspect of a particular chromosome in a conventional chromosome test.

Three other techniques that have been developed in the area of molecular cytogenetics are the Quantitative–PCR (QF–PCR) technique, the MLPA approach and the CGH array.

The QF–PCR technique is mostly used as a quick and cheap way to carry out prenatal diagnosis of trisomy 13, 18 and 21, using fluorescent primers for chromosomes 13, 18 and 21, mostly using X and Y and Y-primers as well. Abnormalities concerning other chromosomes are missed in this way. However, simple and multiplex QF–PCR has also been used successfully in studying 160 miscarriages [13].

Multiplex Ligation-dependent Probe Amplification (MLPA) was developed by MRC Holland (see Figure 11.4). It is mostly used for frequently investigated genes, where probe sets are commercially available. It is also widely used for prenatal diagnosis as in QF–PCR.

One of the standard kits is a (sub) telomere set of probes, which can be used if there is a suspicion about the tip of the long or short arm of one or more of the chromosomes in a conventional chromosome test. A validation study in a diagnostic center was recently published by Ahn *et al.* [14].

Comparative genomic hybridization (CGH) is a technique for detecting sequences anywhere in the genome that are present in an abnormal number of copies (see Figure 11.5).

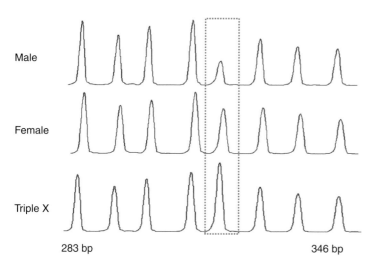

Male

Female

Triple X

283 bp                                                    346 bp

**Figure 11.4** This is an example of the result after application of Multiplex Ligation dependent Probe Amplification (MLPA). The area under the curves in the frame is an indication of the quantity of X-chromosome material in a normal male, normal female and a triple X karyotype. From Heineman *et al.* 2007 [38].

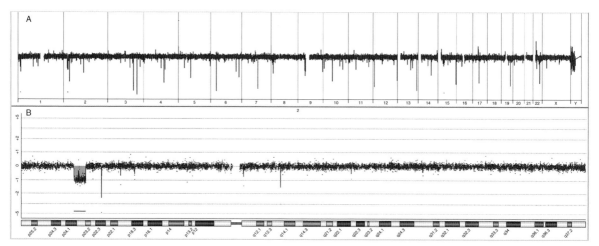

**Figure 11.5** Detection of submicroscopic copy number aberrations using Agilent 105 k oligonucleotide arrays (CGH). Panel A shows the weighted moving average of log2 ratios as a function of chromosomal position using DNA Analytics 4.076 software. Called aberrations are shown by a line on top (gain) or bottom (loss) of the graph. Panel B shows chromosome 2 in detail, where a deletion of 5.15 Mb on 2p24.1 to 2p23.2 was found. The boundaries of the deletion were confirmed using FISH analysis.

One of the latest techniques based on this principle is the CGH array. With this technique it is possible to detect very small deletions and duplications.

However, the three high-resolution techniques, FISH, MLPA and CGH array mentioned above are unable to detect very small *balanced* aberrations in healthy carriers. This can be explained by the fact that however large the chromosome segments that are involved in the translocation may be in a balanced translocation, there is no unbalance at the cell level: a part of the genetic material of two chromosomes has only changed place, with all the potential complications in the meiosis that were mentioned above.

If we want to use high-resolution techniques in the scientific genetic unraveling of recurrent miscarriages,

we should consider focusing primarily on a genetic diagnosis of the spontaneous miscarriage itself in order to find a very small unbalanced abnormality which can then be used to investigate the parents using specific tests, e.g. FISH probes.

Initially this approach might feel like a step backwards, since we are all aware of the small chance of setting up a successful cell culture with material from a stillborn fetus. But with these new approaches it is often not necessary to have living cells for further analyses as a DNA sample might suffice. Benkhalifa *et al.* concluded that CGH is becoming an important clinical assay for unbalanced chromosome abnormalities whether cells grow in culture or not and in cases of one or a few cells [15]. Schaeffer *et al.* reported a similar conclusion in 2004 [16]. The disadvantages are the costs of the technique and the finding of small copy number variances for which the clinical relevance is only applicable if not detected in the parents of the person tested. Thus far, the approach of applying high resolution techniques to fetal samples has not proved to be suitable for implementation in daily routine clinical care.

Finally we would refer to a paper by Kaare *et al.*, who investigated whether *skewed X-chromosome inactivation* (XCI) could be associated with recurrent miscarriage [17]. In a retrospective study in 46 women with recurrent miscarriage and a control group of 95 women with no history of recurrent miscarriage, the frequency of both extremely and mildly skewed XCI proved to be similar.

## Screening strategies

Only very few cases of viable unbalanced offspring will be prevented as the result of an extensive screening procedure for structural chromosome abnormalities in couples with recurrent miscarriage. Recent studies have shown percentages ranging from 0.0 to 1.0% of potentially viable unbalanced chromosome abnormality in pregnancies after ascertainment of carrier status of a structural chromosome abnormality [18–22]. Screening *all* couples with recurrent miscarriage for structural chromosome abnormalities therefore is not an effective strategy.

In an ideal screening setting only few couples are tested (low costs and little effort) and no undesired preventable abnormalities are missed (high preventive potential). In the search for an ideal screening strategy there has been a great deal of debate as to whether parental chromosome testing should be offered after two or three miscarriages. On this subject, up until now, no consensus has been reached as evidenced by the guidelines from different countries. To date, the American College of Obstetrics and Gynecology (ACOG) defines RM as two or three or more consecutive pregnancy losses, the Royal College of Obstetricians and Gynaecologists (RCOG) as three or more miscarriages, the European Society of Obstetrics and Gynaecology (ESHRE) defines RM as three or more consecutive miscarriages and the Dutch Society of Obstetrics and Gynaecology as two or more miscarriages [23–26].

Recent evidence shows an independent influence of the number of miscarriages on the probability of carrier status; three or more miscarriages is a stronger predictor of carrier status than two miscarriages [4].

However, there are other factors which influence the probability of carrier status. In fact, maternal age at second miscarriage is by far the most influential predictive factor. The higher the maternal age, the lower the probability of carrier status. This could be explained by the fact that the risk of repeat aneuploid conceptions steeply increases at advanced maternal age which would explain the higher risk of (recurrent) miscarriage at higher maternal age [27,28]. Other factors influencing the risk of carrier status are a family history of recurrent miscarriage in either the couple's parents or in siblings. A model based on these four factors was developed to calculate the probability of carrier status more accurately (Table 11.1).

When applying the selective karyotyping strategy, chromosome testing is withheld below a 2.2% risk of carrier status. After one miscarriage, in which the reported incidence of carrier status is 2.2%, parental chromosome testing is not recommended. As a probability of 2.2% is apparently considered acceptable, it is reasonable to withhold chromosome testing from couples with an even lower chance of carrier status. This screening advice has been adopted by ESHRE [25].

It is widely recognized that implementing a complicated model into clinical practice does not improve the advice being followed [29,30]. But if, for practical reasons, only one parameter could be used to select couples with the highest probability of carrier status, maternal age at second miscarriage would provide more information than the number of miscarriages. The number of previous miscarriages alone is not sufficient information on which to base the decision as to whether or not to offer parental chromosome testing to couples. Couples with a history of only two miscarriages may well have a high probability of carrier status if concomitant factors exist like low maternal age at second miscarriage and a positive family history of recurrent miscarriage. Couples with a history of three or more miscarriages may be at low risk in the absence of these factors.

Screening family members of carriers ascertained after recurrent miscarriage – in our opinion – does not have a role in routine care. It could be considered only in specific rare abnormal chromosome test results.

It is acknowledged among both patients and physicians that there are subjective arguments to retaining parental chromosome testing in couples with recurrent miscarriage such as fear of under-diagnosing viable unbalanced offspring, the wish to find or exclude a

**Table 11.1** Probability of carrier status in couples with two or more miscarriages according to the multivariable logistic regression model [4].

| Maternal age at *second* miscarriage | | $(RM_{parents})$ + | | $(RM_{parents})$ – | |
|---|---|---|---|---|---|
| | | ≥3 misc. | 2 misc. | ≥3 misc. | 2 misc. |
| <23 years | $(RM_{bs})$ + | 10.2% | 7.3% | 7.3% | 5.2% |
| | $(RM_{bs})$ – | 5.7% | 4.0% | 4.1% | 2.8% |
| 23–34 years | $(RM_{bs})$ + | 10.0% | 7.2% | 7.2% | 5.1% |
| | $(RM_{bs})$ – | 5.7% | 4.0% | 4.0% | 2.8% |
| 34–37 years | $(RM_{bs})$ + | 5.8% | 4.1% | 4.1% | 2.9% |
| | $(RM_{bs})$ – | 3.2% | 2.2% | 2.2% | 1.6% |
| 37–39 years | $(RM_{bs})$ + | 4.0% | 2.8% | 2.8% | 2.0% |
| | $(RM_{bs})$ – | 2.2% | 1.5% | 1.5% | 1.1% |
| ≥39 years | $(RM_{bs})$ + | 1.8% | 1.2% | 1.3% | 0.9% |
| | $(RM_{bs})$ – | 1.0% | 0.7% | 0.7% | 0.5% |

Shaded area shows a probability of carrier status <2.2%. In these couples karyotyping can be withheld.
$RM_{bs}$ = a history of ≥2 miscarriages in a brother or sister of either partner; $RM_{parents}$ = a history of ≥2 miscarriages in parents of either partner; ≥3 misc. = a history of ≥3 miscarriages in the couple; 2 misc. = a history of ≥2 miscarriages in the couple.
Multivariable regression analysis was limited to 528 couples in whom the data collection was complete.
Intercept based on the total population = −5.388.

(possible) cause of the recurrent miscarriage, or the possibility of predicting the chance of a healthy child.

Further research is needed into existing facilitating factors or barriers in implementing the selective karyotyping strategy. To abandon an ineffective screening strategy will probably present a big problem. It is therefore vital that care providers involved in the field of recurrent miscarriage, in particular geneticists and gynecologists, consider this matter carefully and decide on future management.

## Pregnancy outcome in carriers

Conventional parental chromosome testing is offered to couples after they have experienced recurrent miscarriage. Carrier status was formerly regarded as a serious condition or problem, with negative consequences for reproductive outcome. Nowadays, we know that although there is an increased risk of another miscarriage the cumulative chance of a healthy live-born child is generally high.

In a large study, reproductive outcomes of carrier couples and non-carrier couples, referred for parental chromosome testing after two or more miscarriages before 20 weeks were collected. Data were obtained from medical records, questionnaires and interviews. All pregnancy outcomes were recorded for a period of at least 2 years after testing. A total of 278 carrier couples and 427 non-carrier couples were included. The mean follow-up period after testing was 5.8 years. Forty-nine percent of the carrier couples experienced one or more miscarriages after PCA compared with 29% of the non-carrier couples ($P < 0.001$). The percentage of couples with at least one healthy child, born after testing was not significantly different between carrier couples (83%) and non-carrier couples (84%). Amongst 550 pregnancies after chromosome testing in carrier couples the combined incidence of viable unbalanced chromosome abnormalities detected at prenatal diagnosis and live-born children with an unbalanced karyotype was 0.7%. The interpretation of this study is that the risk of viable unbalanced offspring is very low in couples with structural chromosome abnormalities ascertained through two or more miscarriages. Their chances of having a healthy child are as high as in non-carrier couples, despite a higher risk of a subsequent miscarriage [21].

Other research reporting on smaller study groups confirm the low percentages of potentially viable unbalanced chromosome abnormality in pregnancies after ascertainment of carrier status: these percentages ranged from 0.0 to 1.0% [19–20,22]. Altogether outcomes of over 800 subsequent pregnancies in carriers are described and the conclusion can be drawn that a theoretical risk of a viable unbalanced outcome, as described earlier in this chapter, drops from 66% (4/6) to a maximum of 1.0% empirical risk by means of natural selection.

From the point of view of prenatal diagnosis, it was confirmed that viable unbalanced offspring at prenatal diagnosis is mainly ascertained through the previous birth of a child with an unbalanced karyotype rather than through recurrent miscarriage [31].

It has been demonstrated that carrier couples are at higher risk of future miscarriage than non-carrier couples. The long-term chance of a miscarriage in carriers is 49% compared with 30% in non-carriers ($P < 0.01$) [21].

Couples carrying a structural chromosome abnormality with a history of recurrent miscarriage have an excellent prognosis of delivering a healthy child in future pregnancies. The live-birth rate in the first pregnancy after chromosome testing has been reported to range from 32% to 60% [18–21]. In the long term, the cumulative live-birth rate rises to as high as nearly 85% [19–21]. A longer time horizon to establish a successful pregnancy seems to be an an important factor.

## Counseling and therapeutic options (PND vs PGD)

In the case of detected carrier status, couples will be advised to consult a clinical geneticist with whom the options in subsequent pregnancies can be discussed, e.g. prenatal diagnosis (PND). There are no causal therapeutic options with regard to carrier status. As an alternative to prenatal diagnosis, couples can proceed to pre-implantation genetic diagnosis (PGD).

## Prenatal diagnosis

Despite the relatively low risk mentioned above for carrier women with RM to have a viable child with an unbalanced translocation, there is, in our opinion, an indication to counsel carriers for prenatal chromosome testing. The pros and cons of chorion villi sampling versus amniotic fluid cell culture should be discussed with the future parents. Guidelines also emphasize the importance of referral to a clinical geneticist in order to counsel carriers on PND [23–26]. In cases of an unbalanced fetal karyotype, detected at PND, termination of the pregnancy may be considered after careful and thorough counseling.

Contrary to our a priori expectations, many couples with an established structural chromosome abnormality refrained from an invasive PND procedure (CVS or amniocentesis) in subsequent pregnancies. Thus, although all of these couples underwent proper genetic counseling in which the need for PND was stressed, many couples disregarded this advice. Overall, almost half of the carrier couples in our study group underwent no invasive PND procedures in any subsequent ongoing pregnancies. In the subgroup of carrier couples with advanced maternal age (≥36 years) more than 60% decided against any type of invasive PND [32]. The motivations of carrier couples to opt for or refrain from invasive PND-procedures should be a topic for further research to optimize clinical care and informed decision making.

## Pre-implantation genetic diagnosis

Pre-implantation genetic diagnosis can be used as an alternative to invasive prenatal diagnosis to avoid termination of pregnancy in the case of an unbalanced fetal karyotype. The technique is restricted to couples at high risk of transmitting genetic disorders such as X-linked diseases, various monogenic diseases and also for structural chromosome abnormalities. In these cases, IVF/ICSI treatment is required. A single cell from each embryo is aspirated, its nucleus isolated and the nuclear DNA investigated for the specific translocation or inversion. An embryo or embryos without abnormal test results can then be transferred to the uterus.

Pre-implantation genetic diagnosis is used increasingly frequently for these patients as an alternative to prenatal diagnosis. With the results of the large multicenter cohort in mind that showed the combined incidence of fetal karyotypes at prenatal diagnosis and live-born children with an unbalanced karyotype was 0.7% in couples with two or more miscarriages carrying a structural chromosome abnormality [21], and additional smaller studies it can be asked whether it is necessary to perform prenatal or pre-implantation diagnosis to further reduce this already low chance of unbalanced offspring.

Apart from preventing the birth of unbalanced offspring, PGD has also been claimed by some investigators to increase a woman's chance of achieving a live birth [33] or to decrease the miscarriage rate [34]. In clinical practice, patients are easily tempted to use this relatively new technique as its rationale speaks for itself and patients wish to avoid going through another miscarriage. However, there is currently some controversy about the efficacy of PGD in terms of live-birth and miscarriage rates for this particular group of patients.

No randomized controlled trials or non-randomized comparative studies comparing the effects of PGD with natural conception are available. The published literature of results after PGD consists only of case series or case reports with the exception of two larger studies [34,35]. These two studies report a successful clinical outcome of respectively 28.6% (14/49) live births/carrier couple and 54.5% (18/33) ongoing pregnancies/carrier couple after PGD in respectively 64 and 41 embryo-transfer cycles. At present, there is no evidence of a high live-birth rate or ongoing pregnancy rate when performing PGD in couples with a history of recurrent miscarriage and carrying a structural chromosome abnormality [36]. Unfortunately, the most recent ESHRE PGD Consortium data do not report details of obstetric history, causing these results not to be eligible for interpretation with regard to recurrent miscarriage couples [37].

The combined data of studies reporting on live-birth rates after natural conception in couples carrying a structural chromosome abnormality and with a history of recurrent miscarriage were mentioned in the previous section.

We are of the opinion that there are insufficient data to recommend PGD in these couples over spontaneous conception. Considering the good prognosis of achieving a live birth after spontaneous conception, PGD should not be used in routine care of these couples until convincing data shows otherwise. Preimplantation genetic diagnosis could only be chosen if the aim is to prevent the very low chance at all costs of viable unbalanced offspring in couples with recurrent miscarriage.

## Summary, conclusions and focus of future research

Couples with recurrent miscarriage are at an increased risk of either of the partners carrying a structural chromosome abnormality. Structural chromosome abnormalities involve the rearrangement of chromosome segments. In their balanced form there is no overall gain or loss of genetic material, but in the unbalanced form segments of chromosomes are added ((partial) trisomies) or deleted ((partial) monosomies) during the second meiotic division. The most common types are translocations and inversions. The incidence of carrier status of a structural chromosome abnormality rises from approximately 0.7% in the general population to 2.2% after one miscarriage, 4.8% after two miscarriages and 5.2% after three miscarriages.

It has been shown that it is possible to distinguish between couples with recurrent miscarriage with a high chance of carrying a structural chromosome abnormality and couples with a low chance. Besides the number of miscarriages, there are other factors which affect the probability of carrier status, maternal age at the second miscarriage being the most influential factor. Another important finding is that the prognosis of delivering a healthy child is good or comparable to non-carrier couples with a history of recurrent miscarriage and the chances of viable unbalanced offspring due to the chromosome abnormality is very low. To date the accepted advice is to use the model based on four influential risk factors to assess the risk of carrier status and subsequently offer parental chromosome testing only to couples at high risk of carrier status.

If one of the partners carries a structural chromosome abnormality, products of conception can have a normal karyotype, the same karyotype as the carrier parent, or an unbalanced karyotype. The latter can lead to miscarriage, stillbirth or the birth of a child with major congenital impairments.

(Conventional) parental chromosome testing is offered to couples who have experienced recurrent miscarriage. In the past carrier status was regarded as a serious condition/problem, with negative consequences for reproductive outcome. Nowadays, we know that although there is an increased risk of another miscarriage the cumulative chances of having a healthy live-born child are generally high. The chances of a severely handicapped child on the contrary are very low, and thus couples can be encouraged to conceive again.

In the case of detected carrier status, couples will be advised to consult a clinical geneticist with whom the options in subsequent pregnancies should be discussed, i.e. prenatal diagnosis. There are no causal therapeutic options with regard to carrier status. As an alternative to prenatal diagnosis, couples can proceed to pre-implantation genetic diagnosis. For PGD, IVF treatment is required. It has been shown that data with regard to live birth and miscarriage rates after PGD are scarce and prove low percentages of live births or ongoing pregnancies per carrier couple.

The question might even arise whether to refrain from parental chromosome testing in all couples with recurrent miscarriage, based on the low risk of unbalanced viable offspring. Further discussion on this topic should be encouraged. In current clinical practice, evidence-based medicine may conflict with patients' (or physicians') desire for diagnostic testing and treatment.

Molecular cytogenetic techniques (e.g. FISH, QF-PCR, MLPA, CGH) are improving all the time and could play a role in the future in establishing submicroscopic chromosome abnormalities, resulting in another way of assessing abnormalities which play a role in couples with RM. Until now, not enough evidence has been available for the role of genetic mechanisms, like (sex chromosome) mosaicism, uniparental disomy or skewed X chromosome inactivation with regard to their association with recurrent miscarriage. Other potentially interesting fields of research are patient preferences with regard to parental chromosome testing and reproductive choices putatively influenced by abnormal parental chromosome test results.

## Acknowledgments

The authors wish to thank E. Roos and A. Mul for producing the Figures 11.1–11.5.

## References

1. Braekeleer M de, Dao TN. Cytogenetic studies in couples experiencing repeated pregnancy losses. *Hum Reprod* 1990; **5**: 518–28.

2. Tharapel AT, Tharapel SA, Bannerman RM. Recurrent pregnancy losses and parental chromosome abnormalities: a review. *BJOG* 1985; **92**: 899–914.

3. Clifford K, Rai R, Regan L. An informative protocol for the investigation of recurrent miscarriage: preliminary experience of 500 consecutive cases. *Hum Reprod* 1994; **9**: 1328–32.

4. Franssen MTM, Korevaar JC, Leschot NJ *et al.* Selective chromosome analysis in couples with two or more miscarriages: a case-control study. *Br Med J* 2005; **331**: 137–41.

5. Hume RF, Kilmer-Ernst P, Wolfe HM *et al.* Prenatal cytogenetic abnormalities: correlations of structural rearrangements and ultrasonographically detected fetal anomalies. *Am J Obstet Gynecol* 1995; **173**: 1334–6.

6. Forrester MB, Merz RD. Patterns of chromosomal translocations identified by a birth defects registry, Hawaii, 1986–2000. *Genetic Testing* 2004; **8**: 204–8.

7. Kotzot D. Review and meta-analysis of systematic searches for uniparental disomy (UPD) other than UPD 15. *Am J Med Genet* 2002; **111**: 366–75.

8. Madan K. Paracentric inversions: a review. *Hum Genet* 1995; **96**: 503–15.

9. Pettenati MJ, Rao PN, Phelan MC *et al.* Paracentric inversions in humans: a review of 446 paracentric inversions with presentation of 120 new cases. *Am J Med Genet* 1995; **55**: 171–87.

10. Holzgreve W, Schonberg SA, Douglas RG *et al.* X-Chromosome hyperploidy in couples with multiple spontaneous abortions. *Obstet Gynecol* 1984; **63**: 237–40.

11. Sachs ES, Jahoda MGJ, van Hemel JO *et al.* Chromosome studies of 500 couples with two or more abortions. *Obstet Gynecol* 1985; **63**: 375–8.

12. Kuo P, Guo HR. Mechanism of recurrent spontaneous abortions in women with mosaicism of X-chromosome aneuploidies. *Fertil Steril* 2004; **82**: 1594–601.

13. Diego-Alvarez D, Garcia-Hoyos M, Trujillo MJ *et al.* Application of quantitative fluorescent PCR with short tandem repeat markers to the study of aneuploidies in spontaneous miscarriages. *Hum Reprod* 2005; **20**: 1235–43.

14. Ahn JW, Ogilvie CM, Welch A. Detection of subtelomere imbalance using MLPA: validation, development of an analysis protocol, and application in a diagnostic centre. *BMC Med Genet* 2007; **8**: 1–13.

15. Benkhalifa M, Kasakyan S, Clement P *et al.* Array comparative genomic hybridization profiling of first-trimester spontaneous abortions that fail to grow in vitro. *Prenatal Diagnosis* 2005; **25**: 894–900.

16. Schaeffer AJ, Chung J, Heretis K *et al.* Comparative Genomic Hybridization-Array analysis enhances the detection of aneuploidies and submicroscopic imbalances in spontaneous miscarriages. *Am J Hum Genet* 2004; **74**: 1168–74.

17. Kaare M, Painter JN, Ulander VM *et al.* Sex chromosome characteristics and recurrent miscarriage. *Fertil Steril* 2008; **90**: 2328–33.

18. Carp H, Feldman B, Oelsner *et al.* Parental karyotype and subsequent live births in recurrent miscarriage. *Fertil Steril* 2004; **81**: 1296–301.

19. Sugiura-Ogasawara M. Ozaki Y, Sato T *et al.* Poor prognosis of recurrent aborters with either maternal or

paternal reciprocal translocations. *Fertil Steril* 2004; **81**: 367–73.

20. Stephenson MD, Sierra S. Reproductive outcomes in recurrent pregnancy loss associated with a parental carrier of a structural chromosome arrangement. *Hum Reprod* 2006; **21**: 1076–82.

21. Franssen MT, Korevaar JC, van der Veen F *et al.* Reproductive outcome after chromosome analysis in couples with two or more miscarriages: an index-control study. *Br Med J* 2006; **332**: 759–63.

22. Sugiura-Ogasawara M, Aoki K, Fujii T *et al.* Subsequent pregnancy outcomes in recurrent miscarriage patients with a paternal or maternal carrier of a structural chromosome rearrangement. *J Hum Genet* 2008; **53**: 622–8.

23. American College of Obstetricians and Gynecologists. Practice Bulletin. Management of recurrent early pregnancy loss. *Int J Gynaecol Obstet* 2002; **78**: 179–90.

24. Royal College of Obstetricians and Gynaecologists. *The Investigation and Treatment of Couples with Recurrent Miscarriage.* Guideline No. 17. 2003.

25. Jauniaux E, Farquharson RG, Christiansen OB *et al.* Evidence-based guidelines for the investigation and medical treatment of recurrent miscarriage. *Hum Reprod* 2006; **21**: 2216–22.

26. Dutch Society of Obstetricians and Gynaecologists. *Guideline: Recurrent Miscarriage.* Utrecht, the Netherlands, 2007 (in Dutch).

27. Hassold T, Chiu D. Maternal age-specific rates of numerical chromosome abnormalities with special reference to trisomy. *Hum Genet* 1985; **70**: 11–17.

28. Nybo-Andersen AM, Wohlfahrt J, Christens P *et al.* Maternal age and fetal loss: population based register linkage study. *Br Med J* 2000; **320**: 1708–12.

29. Foy R, Penney GC, Grimshaw JM *et al.* A randomised controlled trial of a tailored multifaceted strategy to promote implementation of a clinical guideline on induced abortion care. *BJOG* 2004; **111**: 726–33.

30. Bero LA, Grilli R, Grimshaw JM *et al.* Closing the gap between research and practice: an overview of systematic reviews of interventions to promote the implementation of research findings. The Cochrane Effective Practice and Organization of Care Review Group. *Br Med J* 1998; **317**: 465–8.

31. Franssen MTM, Korevaar JC, Tjoa WM *et al.* Inherited unbalanced structural chromosome abnormalities at prenatal diagnosis are rarely ascertained through recurrent miscarriage. *Prenatal Diagn* 2008; **28**: 408–11.

32. Vansenne F, de Borgie AJM, Korevaar JC *et al.* Low uptake of prenatal diagnosis after established carrier status of a balanced structural chromosome abnormality in couples with recurrent miscarriage. *Fertil Steril* 2010; in press.

33. Otani T, Roche M, Mizuike M *et al.* Preimplantation genetic diagnosis significantly improves the pregnancy outcome of translocation carriers with a history of recurrent miscarriage and unsuccessful pregnancies. *Reprod Biomed Online* 2006; **13**: 869–74.

34. Munne S, Sandalinas M, Escudero T *et al.* Outcome of preimplantation genetic diagnosis of translocations. *Fertil Steril* 2000; **73**: 1209–18.

35. Lim CK, Jun JH, Min DM *et al.* Efficacy and clinical outcome of preimplantation genetic diagnosis using FISH for couples of reciprocal and Robertsonian translocations: the Korean experience. *Prenat Diagn* 2004; **24**: 556–61.

36. Sugiura-Ogasawara M, Suzumori K. Can preimplantation genetic diagnosis improve success rates in recurrent aborters with translocations? *Hum Reprod* 2005; **20**: 3267–70.

37. Goossens V, Harton G, Moutou C *et al.* ESHRE PGD Consortium data collection VIII: cycles from January to December 2005 with pregnancy follow-up to October 2006; *Hum Reprod* 2008; **23**: 2629–45.

38. Heineman MJ, Bleker OP, Evers LH, Heintz APH. *Obstetrie en Gynaecologie.* Maarssen: Elsevier Press, 2007.

# Chapter 2

# Embryoscopy

Thomas Philipp

## Introduction

It is thought that 15–20% of all clinically recognized pregnancies are miscarried. The incidence of clinical pregnancy losses after in-vitro fertilization (IVF) is equally high and approximately 1–3 % of fertile couples experience recurrent early pregnancy losses [1]. The vast majority of these early intrauterine deaths are embryos. A failed pregnancy is a highly emotional event. Parents demand answers to their questions concerning the likely cause of the event and the risk of recurrence in future pregnancies.

To answer these questions as well as to initiate appropriate treatment, the gynecologist has to make an accurate diagnosis of the cause. Investigation protocols for the examination of recurrent early pregnancy loss focus on maternal factors such as maternal thrombophilic disorders, structural uterine anomalies, maternal immune dysfunction, endocrine abnormalities and parental chromosomal anomalies, as described in other chapters of this book. Despite major advances in this field, more than 50% of couples with recurrent miscarriage are assigned to the category of unexplained or idiopathic recurrent miscarriage [2–4]. Whether embryonic causes of recurrent early pregnancy loss exist is currently unknown. For practical reasons the demised embryo or early fetus is rarely subjected to a detailed cytogenetic or morphologic evaluation.

At the end of development the embryo measures 30 mm. Ultrasound resolution does not permit precise viewing of this entity. Due to its minute size and fragility the demised embryo is usually destroyed by instrumental evacuation or spontaneous passage and cannot be subjected to a detailed pathological investigation [5].

The only method which permits visualization of the embryo in utero is embryoscopy. Using the transcervical approach prior to curettage in cases of early pregnancy loss, the outer aspect can be accurately assessed and a variety of developmental defects diagnosed without causing artificial damage [6].

In this chapter we will describe the technique and various embryoscopic findings in cases of early intrauterine death and discuss whether a detailed morphologic and cytogenetic evaluation of the conceptus helps in accurately diagnosing embryonic and early fetal reasons for loss of pregnancies.

## Technique of transcervical embryoscopy

Transcervical embryoscopy is performed in patients who have experienced a first-trimester fetal loss and are scheduled to undergo instrumental evacuation of the uterus under general anesthesia. An early fetal loss (missed abortion) on ultrasound is defined as an embryo or early fetus without heart action, whose crown–rump length can be measured by transvaginal ultrasound. The CRL must be precisely measured. It is one of the criteria to establish the developmental age and prerequisite to assess the embryo morphologically. Embryoscopy is performed before curettage using a rigid hysteroscope (12-degree angle of view with both the biopsy and the irrigation working channel, Circon Ch 25–8 mm). Continuous normal saline flow is used throughout the procedure (pressure, 40–120 mm Hg) to help distend and clean, and thus provide a clear view.

Embryoscopy is a stepwise investigation. The steps have to be performed cautiously in order to avoid bleeding that would obscure the examiner's vision.

### Dilatation of the cervical canal

Before the embryoscope is inserted transcervically into the uterine cavity the cervical canal is gently dilated.

Care must be taken to avoid injury to the uterine cavity.

## Localization of the gestational sac and assessment of the uterine cavity

The uterine cavity is obliterated mid-trimester by fusion of the decidua capsularis and the decidua parietalis. In first-trimester pregnancies, the decidua capsularis and parietalis are not yet fused. After dilation of

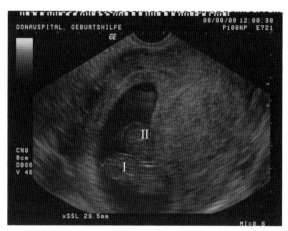

**Figure 12.1a** Ultrasonogram before embryoscopy examination showed monochorionic monoamniotic twin pregnancy with two embryos (I+II), each measuring 29 mm in crown–rump length.

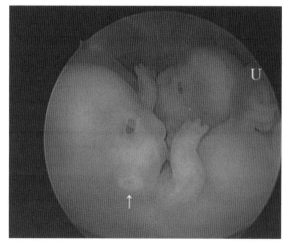

**Figure 12.1b** Embryoscopic lateral view of the two embryos. Note the developing eye lids. The arrow marks the external ear. The elbow is bent .The fingers are separated. Herniation of the midgut into the umbilical cord (U) is still physiological at this developmental stage. A normal karyotype (46,XX) was diagnosed cytogenetically. A color reproduction of this figure can be found in the color plate section.

the cervical canal the hysteroscope is thus inserted into the uterine cavity and congenital and acquired uterine defects can be diagnosed.

After inspection of the uterine cavity the gestational sac is localized.

## Incision of the chorion and the amnion

The gestational sac is seen on embryoscopy as a white and opaque protuberance. Its greater part is in contact with the decidua capsularis. Over this portion the chorionic villi undergo atrophy later on and form the chorion laeve. The future chorion laeve can be opened next to the site of implantation using microscissors, without causing hemorrhage.

In early pregnancy the chorion is separated from the amnion by a fluid-filled space known as the extra-embryonic coelom. The embryo is thus viewed through the amnion. In early intrauterine deaths the cloudy amniotic sac tends to obscure vision by reflecting light.

The small size of the embryo requires a very high image resolution. At the end of the 8th week it measures 30 mm but already possesses a variety of minute structures. The embryoscope should be advanced close to the embryo in order to identify delicate developing structures (Figures 12.1 and 12.2). In failed pregnancies there is no need to avoid amniotic rupture. The hysteroscope can be inserted into the amniotic cavity after opening this membrane with microscissors.

The investigation can be performed satisfactorily by adjusting the pressure of the distension medium if

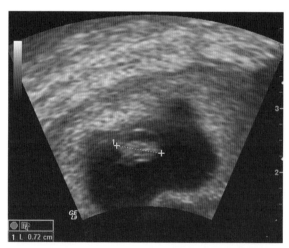

**Figure 12.2a** Ultrasonogram before embryoscopy examination showed an embryo without heart action measuring 7 mm in crown–rump length.

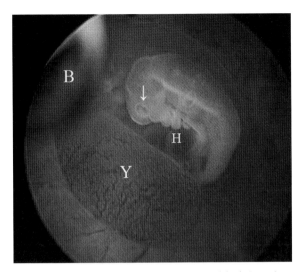

**Figure 12.2b** Four branchial arches an the lens plakode (arrow) are clearly discernible. The head is close contact to the heart prominence (H). Note the yolk (Y) sac with fetal blood islands. (M) marks a micro-bubble. Chromosome analysis revealed a normal (46,XX) karyotype. A color reproduction of this figure can be found in the color plate section.

necessary and opening the membranes (chorion and amnion) using microscissors. The distension medium should be set to low pressure in order to prevent the membrane from collapsing. The chorion and amnion should be opened with microscissors to avoid tenting of these structures.

## Morphological evaluation of the embryo

A comprehensive examination of the conceptus includes visualization of the head, face, dorsal and ventral walls, limbs and umbilical cord. Embryos – especially macerated specimens – are extremely fragile and should not be touched by the tip of the scope or the micro instruments. A gentle drift achieved by adjusting the flow of the hysteroscope usually permits full assessment of the embryo.

To evaluate embryonic development accurately it is essential to take photographs of the embryo from the anterior, posterior and lateral aspect. After the procedure has been concluded these photographs may be compared with illustrations of normal embryos of each developmental stage.

## Tissue sampling

Cytogenetic assessment of early intrauterine deaths is hampered by maternal contamination. An apparently normal 46,XX karyotype in the curettage material of

early miscarriage specimens is not always a reliable result. Transcervical embryoscopy permits selective and reliable sampling of chorionic tissues with minimal potential for maternal contamination [7]. Direct chorion biopsies can be taken by embryoscopy at the end of the morphological examination [8]. At our hospital, chorionic villus sampling is performed under direct vision through the hysteroscope. A microforceps (CH 7–2 mm) is used to sample the chorionic villi from the implantation site (the future chorion frondosum) of the gestational sac. The villi are then dissected in normal saline, placed in culture medium, and immediately sent to the cytogenetic laboratory for further processing. The tissue is subsequently cultured and analyzed cytogenetically, using standard G-banding cytogenetic techniques.

## Instrumental evacuation of the uterus

At the end of the procedure the curettage is performed.

## Embryonic malformations

The developing human is considered to be an *embryo* from conception to the end of the 8th week. From the beginning of the 9th week until birth the developing infant is known as a *fetus*. The distinction between an embryo and a fetus is more than a matter of terminology. The prevalence of developmental defects and the rate of chromosomal abnormalities are particularly high in embryonic specimens.

The embryonic period is a highly dynamic process during which the appearance of the conceptus is constantly changing. At the end of the 8th week it measures 30 mm but already possesses a variety of named structures. In order to diagnose developmental defects accurately the clinician must be aware of the embryo's developmental age. The developmental age or conceptional age of an embryo or fetus extends from the day of fertilization to the day of intrauterine death or expulsion. The developmental age is established by the CRL, measured on ultrasound and by developmental hallmarks, established by embryoscopy. Any discrepancy between embryonic length and specific developmental hallmarks points to the existence of an embryonic developmental defect.

In miscarriage specimens, on the other hand, gestational or menstrual age extends from the first day of the last menstrual period to the expulsion or removal of the conceptus.

This term used in clinical terminology and ultrasound is not helpful when studying early miscarriage specimens because early pregnancy losses are usually retained in utero for several days or weeks.

Abnormal embryonic development may be local or general. General abnormal embryonic development is named embryonic growth disorganization.

## Embryonic growth disorganization

General maldevelopment is a typical malformation of the embryo. It suggests a severe disturbance in early human development that is incompatible with normal fetal development. The embryos are marked by an abnormal, slow growth pattern before cessation of their heart action on ultrasound investigation.

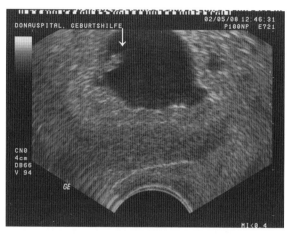

**Figure 12.3a** Sonography before the embryoscopic examination showed embryonic structure (arrow) in a disproportionately large chorionic sac.

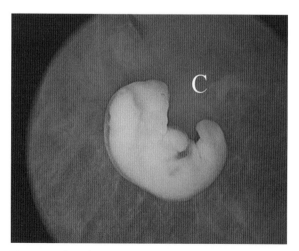

**Figure 12.3b** Embryoscopic examination revealed a GD 3 embryo measuring 6 mm crown–rump length. A short body stalk connected the GD3 embryo to the chorionic plate (C). Cytogenetically trisomy 7 (47, XY, +7) was diagnosed. A color reproduction of this figure can be found in the color plate section.

Based on the degree of abnormal embryonic development, a distinction is made between four types: GD 1 to GD 4 [9].

- GD 1 is marked by an *empty sac* or anembryonic sac. The amnion, if present, is often fused to the chorion. Fusion of the amnion to the chorion prior to 10 weeks' gestation is abnormal.
- GD 2 conceptuses are characterized by 3–5 mm of embryonic tissue with no identifiable external embryonic landmarks and no retinal pigment. It is not possible to delineate a caudal or cephalic pole. Often the embryo is directly attached to the chorionic plate.
- GD 3 embryos are up to 10 mm long. They lack limb buds but frequently possess retinal pigment (Figure 12.3).
- GD 4 embryos have a crown–rump length of more than 10 mm, a discernible head, trunk and limb buds. The limb buds are significantly retarded and the development of the facial structures tends to be very abnormal.

## Localized developmental defects

Localized developmental defects may be isolated or combined. They are similar to the malformations seen in fetuses and newborns. The following local defects have been diagnosed on embryoscopy.

### Head defects

Some of the head defects seen on embryoscopy are microcephaly, anencephaly, faciocranioschisis, encephalocele (Figure 12.4), inencephaly, facial dysplasia, lateral and median cleft lip, cleft palate, fusions of the

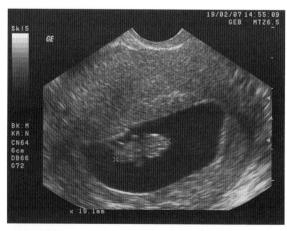

**Figure 12.4a** Sonographic and (b) embryoscopic examination of a missed abortion measuring 19 mm crown–rump length.

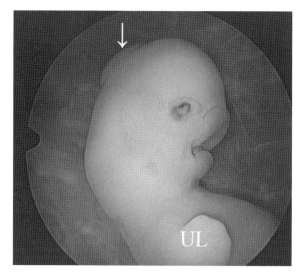

**Figure 12.4b** Close up, lateral view of the upper portion of the trisomiy 15(47,XY,+15) embryo with a parietal encephalocele (arrow). The embryo showed on embryoscopic examination abnormal lip development and a dysplastic face. Based on the crown–rump length, the head is too small and the upper limbs (UL) are retarded in their development. A color reproduction of this figure can be found in the color plate section.

face to the chest, absence of eyes, unfused eye globes and proboscis.

Microcephaly and facial dysplasia are common defects in embryos and are usually observed in combination. *Microcephaly* is seen on embryoscopy as an embryo with a poorly developed cranium with loss of normal vascular markings. The bulge of the frontal area, which is common in embryos of this size, is absent.

Embryos with a *dysplastic face* show poorly developed branchial arches and midface structures on embryoscopic examination.

A *cleft lip* occurs when the maxillary prominence and the united medial nasal prominences do not fuse. In the embryo a cleft lip cannot be diagnosed until after 7 weeks of development because fusion does not occur until this time.

A *cleft palate* occurs when the primary anterior palate, the lateral palatine processes and the nasal septum fail to unite. A cleft palate can only be diagnosed in the fetal period because fusion is completed after the 10th week of development.

### Trunk defects

Trunk defects include spina bifida, omphalocele and gastroschisis. The phenotype of *spina bifida* in the early developmental stages differs from its well-known appearance in the fetus or neonate. In the embryo, a

spina bifida is frequently seen as a plaque-like protrusion of neural tissue over the caudal spine [10].

Herniation of the midgut is still physiological at 8 developmental weeks. Therefore, an *omphalocele* can only be diagnosed in the fetal period.

### Limb defects

Preaxial and postaxial hexadactyly, syndactyly, split-hand malformation, and transverse limb reduction defects are the most commonly observed limb malformations.

In the embryo *syndactyly* cannot be diagnosed until after the end of the 8th week of development because the fingers are not separated before this time.

### Umbilical cord defects

*Umbilical cord cysts* and *abnormal thin* and/or *short cords* are usually found in chromosomally abnormal embryos. *Umbilical cord torsion and stricture* are rarely observed on embryoscopy and are usually postmortem artifacts.

### Duplication abnormalities

Chorangiopagus parasiticus (CAPP) or acardiac conjoined twins, and other conjoined twins (Figure 12.5) have been identified on embryoscopy [11].

### Amnion rupture sequence

Amnion rupture sequence (ARS) may cause abnormalities that are detectable on embryoscopy, such as encephaloceles, cleft lip and amputations. In early abortion specimens the amniotic bands are often much finer than they are in the later fetal period [12].

## Prevalence of embryonic developmental defects in early intrauterine deaths

As shown in Table 12.1, only 58 (11.3%) of 514 early fetal losses had no external abnormalities whereas 456 (88.7%) were marked by abnormal development. Of the latter cases, embryonic growth disorganization (GD 1–4) was seen in 237 (46.1 %) while 198 cases (38.5%) showed no disorganization of development but did have severe combined localized defects. Twenty-one specimens had isolated local developmental defects.

## Correlation of embryonic morphology and karyotype in early abortion specimens

Correlation of embryonic morphology and karyotype (Table 12.1) in early abortion specimens reveals a high

**Table 12.1** Specimen morphology and karyotype of 514 early intrauterine deaths. From Philipp (2007) [22].

| Morphology | Total specimens | | Total specimens successfully karyotyped | | Specimens with abnormal karyotype | |
|---|---|---|---|---|---|---|
| | No. | %[a] | No. | %[b] | No. | %[c] |
| Normal | 58 | 11.3 | 56 | 96.2 | 23 | 41.1 |
| Embryonic growth disorganization | 237 | 46.1 | 225 | 95 | 156 | 69.3 |
| Combined localized defects | 198 | 38.5 | 193 | 97.3 | 166 | 86.0 |
| Isolated localized defects | 21 | 4.1 | 21 | 100 | 14 | 66.7 |
| Total | 514 | 100 | 495 | 96.3 | 359 | 72.5 |

[a] Percentage of total number of specimens with that morphology.
[b] Percentage of each morphological category successfully karyotyped.
[c] Percentage of each morphological category with an abnormal karyotype.

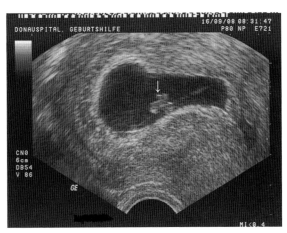

**Figure 12.5a** Ultrasonogram before embryoscopy examination showed an embryo (arrow) without heart action measuring 7 mm in crown–rump length in a disproportionately large chorionic sac. No distinct abnormalities were identified on sonography.

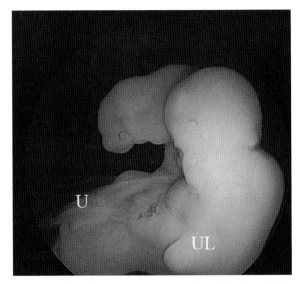

**Figure 12.5b** Embryoscopic examination from a lateral view (b) showed dicephalus conjoined twins. The microcephalic conjoined twins showed dysplastic faces and shared a body from the upper chest downwards. Two upper (UL) and no lower limbs and a single umbilical cord (U) were seen by embryoscopy. A normal karyotype (46,XY) was diagnosed cytogenetically. A color reproduction of this figure can be found in the color plate section.

rate of chromosomal abnormalities in phenotypically abnormal embryos. The highest rate of chromosomal abnormalities (86%) is seen in embryos with combined local developmental defects [13,14]. Of grossly disorganized embryos, about 70% are cytogenetically abnormal. A relatively low frequency of chromosomal abnormalities is seen in embryos of normal phenotype (41%).

The majority (95%) of the observed chromosomal mutations is not hereditary and signify no increased risk for future pregnancies. They originate *de novo* either in gametogenesis (trisomy and monosomy) or may result from polyspermic fertilization or failure of normal cleavage (triploidy and tetraploidy).

Aneuploidy/polyploidy is the major factor affecting normal embryonic development in early intrauterine deaths and may explain why spontaneous abortion is usually a sporadic event in a patient's reproductive history although the prevalence of developmental defects among early intrauterine deaths is high. Therefore, all embryoscopic findings should be supplemented by cytogenetic analysis in order to distinguish between non-chromosomal and chromosomal causes of abnormalities.

# Indications for a detailed embryoscopic evaluation of early intrauterine deaths

Embryoscopy should be offered to a patient when a reliable cytogenetic evaluation of the abortus is indicated. Typical situations would be:

- Patients with a history of infertility who conceived but whose pregnancy failed.
- Patients with a fetal loss and a history of recurrent pregnancy loss.
- Women who were receiving treatment to prevent miscarriage but were diagnosed with a non-viable pregnancy.

# Advantages of a detailed embryoscopic and cytogenetic evaluation of early intrauterine deaths: accurate diagnosis of fetal causes of pregnancy loss

Loss of pregnancy may be due to maternal or fetal factors. Its etiology may be diverse.

In early pregnancy loss, current investigation protocols frequently do not permit a conclusive diagnosis because maternal factors are assessed but fetal causes of pregnancy loss are usually not investigated.

Fetal causes of pregnancy loss include (a) chromosomal aberrations and (b) structural abnormalities of the embryo that are indicative of non-viability or associated with a high rate of intrauterine mortality.

## Reliable cytogenetic evaluation of the conceptus

The value of karyotyping early abortion specimens is limited by false negative results due to maternal contamination. A 46,XX karyotype in the curettage material is not always a reliable finding [15].

Transcervical embryoscopy permits selective and reliable sampling of uncontaminated embryonic tissue prior to dilatation and curettage (D&C). Direct chorion biopsies can be taken embryoscopically at the end of the morphological examination under visual monitoring using a microforceps. This approach ensures minimal maternal contamination.

Seventy percent of all early intrauterine deaths losses are marked by chromosomal abnormalities. The principal categories of chromosomal abnormalities are autosomal trisomies, sex chromosome monosomy and polyploidy. About 2–5% of abnormal karyotypes that occur in early spontaneous losses are structural chromosomal abnormalities. The majority of chromosomal abnormalities observed among early spontaneous losses are incompatible with fetal development. Most (95%) of these chromosomal mutations are not hereditary and signify no additional risk for future pregnancies.

In summary, a reliable cytogenetic evaluation of the conceptus alone will permit investigators to elicit a causal explanation for about 70% of all early pregnancy losses.

# What additional information can be gained from a morphological examination of the embryo with a normal karyotype?

In cases of a normal karyotype the embryonic morphology might yield additional information about the individual cause and the risk of recurrence of early pregnancy loss.

Some of the observed embryonic malformations are either incompatible with fetal development (embryonic growth disorganization) or associated with a high intrauterine mortality rate (CNS defects, amniotic bands, duplication abnormalities, vascular disruptions). This information would be completely lost and the embryonic developmental defect would remain unidentified if embryoscopy were not performed.

The finding of a normal embryo with a normal karyotype (Figure 12.2) might also be valuable in terms of supportive information because the loss of pregnancy is more likely due to maternal factors. A detailed investigation of the mother is indicated in these cases.

To give individual answers to the questions of the parents concerning the probable risk of recurrence of the observed developmental defects in future pregnancies, an accurate description of these specimens is essential. Specific mechanisms leading to the observed developmental defects can be identified by a detailed morphological evaluation of the embryo.

In fetuses or live-born infants, congenital malformations are commonly explained by Mendelian and multifactorial disorders. Isolated localized embryonic developmental defects diagnosed on embryoscopy, similar to those observed among fetuses and live-born infants, might also be heterogeneous in terms of their origin. They may be of multifactorial origin or caused by non-genetic mechanisms (e.g. amniotic bands, duplication anomalies, vascular disruptions). The probability of recurrence of these defects in future pregnancies differs according to their etiology. If the observed defects (e.g. isolated neural tube defects, cleft lip, limb malformations) are multifactorial in origin, the risk of recurrence is estimated to be approximately 2–5%. The recurrence rate may be not significantly increased if a non-genetic mechanism (amniotic bands, duplication anomalies, vascular disruptions) is responsible for abnormal embryonic development.

Multiple localized developmental defects without a chromosomal anomaly are rare (nearly 90% of embryos with combined developmental defects show a chromosomal abnormality) and may indicate a single gene defect [16]. In these cases a high recurrence rate cannot be excluded. Diagnosis of a specific syndrome is usually not possible at these early stages. However, a detailed description of the observed developmental defects might be valuable for first-trimester ultrasound screening in future pregnancies in order to exclude recurrence of the observed developmental defects.

The etiology of embryonic growth disorganization with an apparently normal karyotype is currently unknown. Knowledge about generalized embryonic maldevelopment is scarce because it is a typical malformation of the embryo which could not be investigated morphologically in the past.

Embryonic growth may be affected by maternal factors such as anti-phospholipid antibodies, endocrine factors and immunological causes. However, these factors are known to be non-teratogenic.

Embryonic development is a precisely choreographed event of programmed developmental steps, involving many genes that regulate growth and morphogenesis. Embryonic growth disorganization possibly resulting from an aneuploidy/polyploidy suggests that there may be a genetic cause which cannot be identified by current cytogenetic techniques [17]. Sub-microscopic chromosomal rearrangements containing genes required for embryonic growth and morphogenesis have only recently been considered to be etiologically related to loss of pregnancy [18,19]. The fact of these genetic mechanisms challenges the prevailing assumption that the absence of a genetic disorder on routine laboratory testing is a reason to look for non-genetic causes.

If we are correct in hypothesizing that single gene defects and submicroscopic chromosomal rearrangements (e.g. microdeletions, duplications) exist in chromosomally normal embryos with developmental defects, it might explain why the identification of a normal karyotype in early abortion specimens is usually interpreted as a poor prognostic sign [20,21].

Our present knowledge about these factors is limited. However, correlations of embryoscopic and cytogenetic findings will confront investigators with factors currently not known to be involved in early pregnancy loss. This might serve as an impetus for further detailed genetic studies of abnormal embryos with a normal karyotype, which are needed to achieve a better understanding of embryopathy and as a consequence of early pregnancy loss itself.

# References

1. Goddijn M, Leshot N. Genetic aspects of miscarriage. *Bailliére's Clinical Obstetrics and Gynaecology* 2000; **14** (5): 855–65.

2. Stephenson MD. Frequency of factors associated with habitual abortion in 197 couples. *Fertil Steril* 1996; **66** (1): 24–9.

3. Ansari AH, Kirkpatrick B. Recurrent pregnancy loss. *JReprod Med* 1998; **43**(9): 806–14.

4. Ward KJ. Genetic factors in recurrent pregnancy loss. *Semin Reprod Med* 2000; **18**(4): 425–32.

5. Kalousek DK. Anatomical and chromosomal abnormalties in specimens of early spontaneous abortions: seven years experience. *Birth Defects* 1987; **23**: 153–68.

6. Philipp T, Kalousek DK. Transcervical embryoscopy in missed abortion. *J Assist Reprod Genet* 2001; **18**: 285–90.

7. Ferro J, Martinez MC, Lara C et al. Improved accuracy of hysteroembryoscopic biopsies for karyotyping early missed abortions. *Fertil Steril* 2003; **80**: 1260–4.

8. Philipp T, Feichtinger W, Van Allen M et al. Abnormal embryonic development diagnosed embryoscopically in early intrauterine deaths after in vitro fertilization (IVF): a preliminary report of 23 cases. *Fertil Steril* 2004; **82**: 1337–42.

9. Poland BJ, Miller JR, Harris M et al. Spontaneous abortion: a study of 1961 women and their conceptuses. *Acta Obstet Gynecol Scand* (Suppl.), 1981; **102**: 5–32.

10. Philipp T, Kalousek DK. Neural tube defects in missed abortions – embryoscopic and cytogenetic findings. *Am J Med Genet* 2002; **107**: 52–7.

11. Philipp T, Separovic ER, Philipp K et al. Trancervical fetoscopic diagnosis of structural defects in four first trimester monochorionic twin intrauterine deaths. *Prenat Diagn* 2003; **12**: 964–9.

12. Philipp T, Kalousek DK. Amnion rupture sequence in a first trimester missed abortion. *Prenat Diagn* 2001; **21**: 835–8.

13. Philipp T, Philipp K, Reiner A, Beer F, Kalousek DK. Embryoscopic and cytogenetic analysis of 233 missed abortions: factors involved in the pathogenesis of developmental defects of early failed pregnancies. *Hum Reprod* 2003; **18**: 1724–32.

14. Kalousek DK, Pantzar T, Tsai M *et al*. Early spontaneous abortion: morphologic and karyotypic findings in 3912 cases. *Birth Defects* 1993; **29**: 53–61.

15. Bell KA, Van Deerlin PG, Haddad BR *et al*. Cytogenetic diagnosis of "normal 46, XX" karyotypes in spontaneous abortions frequently may be misleading. *Fertil Steril* 1999; **71**: 334–41.

16. Dimmick JE, Kalousek DK. *Developmental Pathology of the Embryo & Fetus*. Philadelphia, PA: JB Lippincott Co., 1992.

17. Philipp T, Kalousek DK. Generalized abnormal embryonic development in missed abortion: embryoscopic and cytogenetic findings. *Am J Med Genet*. 2002; **111**: 41–7.

18. Schaeffer AJ, Chung J, Heretis K *et al*. Comparative genomic hybridization-array analysis enhances the detection of aneuploidies and submicroscopic imbalances in spontaneous miscarriages. *Am J Med Gen* 2004; **6**: 1168–74.

19. Le Caignec C, Boceno M, Saugier-Veber P *et al*. Detection of genomic imbalances by array based comparative genomic hybridisation in fetuses with multiple malformations. *J Med Genet* 2005; **2**: 121–8.

20. Osagawara M, Aoki K, Okada S *et al*. Embryonic karyotype of abortuses in relation to the number of previous miscarriages. *Fertil Steril* 2000; **73**: 300–4.

21. Stephenson M, Awartani KA, Robinson WP. Cytogenetic analysis of miscarriages from couples with recurrent miscarriage: a case control study. *Hum Reprod* 2002; **17**: 446–51.

22. Philipp T. Fetal structural malformations – embryoscopy. In JAH Carp (ed.), *Recurrent Pregnancy Loss. Causes, Controversies and Treatment*. London: Informa Healthcare Ltd, 2007, pp. 67–78.

# Acquired thrombophilia and recurrent early pregnancy loss

Aisha Hameed and Lesley Regan

## Acquired thrombophilia and recurrent early pregnancy loss

Miscarriage is the commonest complication of pregnancy. Only one in four conceptions results in a live birth; some 30% of fertilized eggs fail to implant, a similar number are lost at the early embryonic stage and about 15% of clinically recognized pregnancies end in miscarriage at the fetal stage. In summary, the vast majority of miscarriages occur early in pregnancy, well before 10–12 weeks' gestation and the incidence of late or second-trimester pregnancy loss between 12 and 24 weeks' gestation is no more than 2% [1,2].

Recurrent miscarriage, defined as three or more consecutive pregnancy losses before the fetus has reached the age of viability, affects 1% of couples [3]. If two or more pregnancy losses are included in the definition, the scale of the problem increases from 1% to 5% of all couples trying to achieve a successful pregnancy outcome. By contrast, at least 25% and probably as many as 50% of all women experience one or more sporadic miscarriages. In the majority of cases, the pregnancy loss is due to a random fetal chromosomal abnormality [4], the risk of which rises with increasing maternal age [5].

Recurrent miscarriage is a heterogeneous condition and no single abnormality will account for all cases. Historically the causes have been grouped into genetic, anatomical, infective, endocrine, immune, environmental and unexplained categories. However, the numerical contributions that these individual categories make to the overall problem are variably reported, reflecting the referral and ascertainment bias introduced by clinicians with specialist interests and expertise and the misleading conclusions that may be drawn from studies that only include small patient numbers [1,6].

Amongst 500 women with a history of recurrent miscarriage attending a specialist clinic at St Mary's Hospital, London, 3% had a parental chromosomal abnormality, 15% had an acquired thrombophilic disorder and in approximately 50% of these women no underlying cause was detected [7]. This contrasts with the percentages reported from a US thrombosis clinic asked to investigate 350 women with a history of recurrent miscarriage (mean 2.8; range 2–8 losses) – 7% had a parental chromosomal abnormality, approximately 60% were diagnosed with blood coagulation protein/platelet defects and only 6% of cases remained unexplained after investigation [8]. Nevertheless, our recent understanding that thrombophilic disorders play an important part in the etiology of recurrent pregnancy loss at various gestational ages has widened the scope of investigations and management options for this distressing condition.

A thrombophilic defect is an abnormality in the coagulation system that predisposes an individual to thrombosis. Indeed, the term thrombophilia was first coined in 1965 to describe the increased risk of venous thrombosis in a Norwegian family with antithrombin deficiency [9]. Since then, the number of detectable thrombophilic defects has increased dramatically and we now recognize that these defects can be inherited or acquired. In addition to the knowledge that deficiencies in the endogenous anticoagulants protein C, protein S and antithrombin 111 have a heritable basis, three common thrombophilic gene mutations have been identified: Factor V Leiden G1691A [10]; Factor II Prothrombin G20210A [11]; and the methylene tetrahydrofolate reductase (MTHFR) thermolabile variant C677T [12] (which leads to hyperhomocysteinemia). These are now firmly established causes of systemic thrombosis.

These thrombophilic defects do not necessarily cause a thrombosis but may weaken the ability to cope with a further prothrombotic insult, such as pregnancy. Pregnancy is a hypercoagulable state secondary to an increase in the levels of certain co-agulation factors and a decrease in the levels of anti-coagulant proteins and fibrinolysis. The first studies of the prevalence of coagulation abnormalities in women with adverse pregnancy outcomes appeared in the mid 1990s [13,14], the presumed hypothesis being that an exaggerated hemostatic response during pregnancy leads to thrombosis of the uteroplacental vasculature and fetal demise.

Since then, numerous studies of the prevalence of individual coagulation defects have reported very variable findings, with one study suggesting that as many as 66% of women with RM have at least one thrombophilic defect as compared with 28% of controls with normal pregnancy histories [15]. In a comprehensive meta-analysis of 31 studies of thrombophilic disorders and fetal loss, Rey *et al.* concluded that there is an increased prevalence of several acquired and inherited thrombo-philic disorders in women with previously unexplained recurrent miscarriage compared with women with no history of adverse pregnancy outcome [16].

This chapter examines the role that the acquired thrombophilic defects play in the magnitude of early pregnancy loss, with particular reference to Primary Antiphospholipid syndrome, hyperhomocysteinemia and Acquired protein C resistance.

## Antiphospholipid syndrome

Antiphospholipid syndrome (APS) is now recognized to be the most important treatable cause of recurrent miscarriage [3]. When first described, this syndrome referred to the association of antiphospholipid antibodies with recurrent miscarriage, thrombosis or thrombocytopenia [17]. However, it has now become apparent that these three clinical features of APS are too limiting. Revised criteria for the diagnosis of APS recognize the importance of additional obstetric mani-festations of antiphospholipid antibodies(aPL), such as a history of pre-eclampsia, intrauterine growth restriction, intrauterine death, placental abruption and pre-term labor [18,19]. In addition there are a variety of neurological, vascular and dermatological presentations of aPL, which are listed in Table 13.1. Primary APS affects patients with no identifiable underlying systemic connective tissue disease, whereas APS in patients with chronic inflammatory diseases such as systemic lupus erythematosus is referred to as secondary APS.

**Table 13.1** Clinical manifestations of antiphospholipid antibodies.

| Neurological | Dermatological |
|---|---|
| Transient ischemic attacks | Livedo reticularis |
| Cerebrovascular accidents | Cutaneous necrosis |
| Chorea | |
| Peripheral neuropathy | Hematological |
| Migraine | Thrombocytopenia |
| Epilepsy | Prothrombin deficiency |
| Obstetric | Vascular |
| Recurrent miscarriage | Venous thrombosis |
| Intrauterine growth retardation | Arterial thrombosis |
| Intrauterine death | Mitral valve prolapse |
| Pre-eclampsia | Thrombotic endocarditis |
| Chorea gravidarum | |
| Neonatal | |
| Neonatal thrombosis | |
| Congenital heart block | |

## Screening for Antiphospholipid syndrome

Antiphospholipid antibodies are a family of approxi-mately 20 heterogeneous autoantibodies that are directed against phospholipid-binding plasma pro-teins (see list in Table 13.2). In the etiology of early pregnancy loss, the two most clinically important aPLs are the lupus anticoagulant (LA) and anticardiolipin antibodies (aCL) of the immunoglobulin G (IgG) and IgM subclasses.

Antiphospholipid antibodies can be associated with pregnancy loss and morbidity in each of the three trimesters of pregnancy [3]. Women with aPL may have an unusually high proportion of later preg-nancy losses at 10 or more weeks' gestation [20], but since the vast majority of miscarriages occur early in pregnancy before 10 weeks' gestation, numerically the impact of APS is greatest during the pre-embryonic (<6 weeks) and embryonic period (6–9 weeks) [21,22].

The diagnosis of APS is determined by the detec-tion of either the LA or aCL of the same subclass, in blood samples taken on at least 2 occasions more than 6 weeks apart. The detection of aPL is subject to considerable inter-laboratory variation [23], due to temporal fluctuations of aPL titres in individual patients, transient positivity secondary to infection, suboptimal sample collection and preparation and lack of standardization of laboratory tests for their detection. In order to avoid these diagnostic inaccuracies, international guidelines for optimal sample collection and test performance have been introduced. For example, ensuring that samples for LA testing are collected using minimal venous stasis and are double centrifuged within 2 hours of collection in

order to prepare platelet-poor plasma [24]. The dilute Russell's Viper Venom Time (dRVVT) with platelet neutralizing procedure is the most sensitive assay to detect LA [21]. Both IgG and IgM aCL are assayed using a standardized enzyme linked immunosorbent assay (ELISA) [25].

The most recent international consensus statement has further updated the classification criteria for definitive Antiphospholipid syndrome [26]. In this latest revision, anti-$\beta_2$ glycoprotein-I antibodies were added to the laboratory criteria and more precise pregnancy-related complications were described. The revised clinical and laboratory criteria are detailed in Table 13.3. However, it should be noted by clinicians that the recommendation to allow 12 weeks between test samples 1 and 2 will prove difficult to uphold if current UK health service waiting list targets for outpatients are to be met.

**Table 13.2** Common antiphospholipid antibodies.

Anticardiolipin antibodies

Lupus anticoagulant

Anti-phosphatidylserine

Anti-phosphatidylinositol

Anti-phosphatidylcholine

Anti-phosphatidic acid

Anti-phosphatidylethanolamine

Anti-phosphatidic acid

Anti-phosphatidylglycerol

Anti-annexin-v antibody

$\beta_2$ glycoprotein-I

Hexagonal phospholipid

## Prevalence of Antiphospholipid syndrome

It is generally accepted that some 15% of women with recurrent miscarriage have persistently positive tests for aPL, both LA and aCL [21], although this figure may vary depending on the criteria used for the diagnosis of APS. In a review of 16 published studies the prevalence of LA ranged from 0–9% and that of aCL from 5–51% [27]. By comparison, the prevalence of aPL in women with a "low risk" obstetric history is less than 2% [28,29]. Experience gained from our specialist clinic at St Mary's London, emphasizes the importance

**Table 13.3** Current criteria for the diagnosis of Antiphospholipid syndrome.

Antiphospholipid antibody syndrome (APS) is present if at least one of the clinical criteria and one of the following laboratory criteria are met.
Clinical criteria
1. Vascular thrombosis
   One or more clinical episodes of arterial, venous or small vessel thrombosis, in any tissue or organ. Thrombosis must be confirmed by objective validated criteria (i.e. unequivocal findings of appropriate imaging studies or histopathology). For histopathologic confirmation, thrombosis should be present without significant evidence of inflammation in the vessel wall.
2. Pregnancy morbidity
   (a) One or more unexplained deaths of a morphologically normal fetus at or beyond the 10th week of gestation, with normal fetal morphology documented by ultrasound or by direct examination of the foetus, or
   (b) One or more premature births of a morphologically normal neonate before the 34th week of gestation because of: (i) eclampsia or severe pre-eclampsia defined according to standard definitions, or (ii) recognized features of placental insufficiency, or
   (c) Three or more unexplained consecutive spontaneous abortions before the 10th week of gestation, with maternal anatomic or hormonal abnormalities and paternal and maternal chromosomal causes excluded.

Laboratory criteria
1. Lupus anticoagulant (LA) present in plasma, on two or more occasions at least 12 weeks apart, detected according to the guidelines of the International Society on Thrombosis and Haemostasis (Scientific Subcommittee on LAs/phospholipid-dependent antibodies).
2. Anticardiolipin (aCL) antibody of IgG and/or IgM isotype in serum or plasma, present in medium or high titer (i.e. >40 GPL or MPL, or >99th percentile), on two or more occasions, at least 12 weeks apart, measured by a standardized ELISA.
3. Anti-$\beta_2$ glycoprotein-I antibody of IgG and/or IgM isotype in serum or plasma (titer >99th percentile), present on two or more occasions, at least 12 weeks apart, measured by a standardized ELISA, according to recommended procedures.

of testing for both LA and aCL since there is little cross reactivity between them. Furthermore, a previous personal or family history of thrombosis, cardiovascular disease, epilepsy or migraine is strongly predictive of positive aPL status [21]. Testing for aPL other than LA and aCL is of no proven benefit in the investigation of women with recurrent miscarriage [30,31].

## Outcome of pregnancy in women with untreated aPL

The outcome of pregnancy in untreated women with aPL and a history of recurrent miscarriage is invariably poor. The earliest studies were undertaken by physicians and reported that the fetal loss rate in women with APS was in the range of 50–70% [28,32]. It was subsequently realized that these figures underestimated the scale of the problem because recruitment only took place after these women had presented for antenatal care (at approximately 12 weeks) by which time the majority of miscarriages have already occurred. In a prospective observational study which recruited women with APS before pregnancy, the miscarriage rate was 90% with no pharmacological treatment. By contrast, the miscarriage rate amongst a control group of aPL-negative women with recurrent miscarriage was significantly lower – in the region of 40% [33].

## Mechanism of aPL pregnancy loss

The mechanisms by which aPL cause adverse pregnancy outcome are varied, reflecting in part their heterogeneity. A growing body of evidence has implicated thrombophilia in late pregnancy complications such as intrauterine growth restriction, severe pre-eclampsia and placenta abruption ([34,35] and there is also reasonable evidence to suggest that some cases of recurrent miscarriage are associated with thrombosis of placental vessels and infarction [36,37]. Firstly, microthrombi are a common finding in the placental vasculature and decidua of women with recurrent miscarriage [38]. Secondly, placental thrombosis and infarction have been described in association with certain thrombophilic defects [39,40]. Thirdly, thrombophilic defects are significantly more prevalent amongst women with such pregnancy complications [16]. Fourthly, there is an increased incidence of pregnancy loss amongst women carrying thrombophilic defects [38]. However, pathological placental and decidual features are neither specific nor universal

[41,42] and adverse pregnancy outcomes can occur in women with thrombophilic disorders in the absence of placental thrombosis [43].

In summary, additional or alternative non-thrombotic mechanisms must have a part to play in a proportion of women with aPL and recurrent miscarriage. Indeed, more recent advances in our understanding of early pregnancy development and the biology of aPL have provided new insights into the mechanisms of aPL-related pregnancy failure. In vitro studies report that aPL (a) impair signal transduction mechanisms controlling endometrial cell decidualization [44]; (b) increase trophoblast apoptosis [45]; (c) decrease trophoblast fusion [45–47]; and (d) impair trophoblast invasion [42,46]. Interestingly, the effects of aPL on trophoblast function are reversed, at least in vitro, by low molecular weight heparin [45–48].

Elegant experiments in mice have highlighted the pivotal role that complement plays in the pathogenesis of aPL-induced fetal damage. Antiphospholipid antibodies activate the classical complement pathway, generating the potent anaphylatoxin C5a which in turn recruits and activates inflammatory cells leading to tissue damage in the placenta and fetal death or growth restriction [49,50]. Heparin prevents aPL-induced fetal loss by inhibiting complement activation [51] which raises the possibility that complement inhibitory therapies targeted to the placenta may be a useful treatment option for prevention of miscarriage in the future.

## Treatment of Antiphospholipid syndrome in pregnancy

A variety of treatments including corticosteroids, low-dose aspirin, low-dose heparin and immunoglobulins have been tried either singly, or in combination, in an attempt to improve the live-birth rate of women with APS.

Our understanding of this complex syndrome continues to evolve. Having moved away from considering APS to be a systemic connective tissue disease, we went on to recognize that many cases have a thrombotic etiology. However, we now appreciate that APS is an example of an acquired thrombophilic disorder (as opposed to an inherited defect) that leads to fetal loss and later pregnancy complications. Furthermore, evidence is now emerging that aPL can exert adverse effects on the decidual immune response, which may be responsive to immunomodulatory treatments.

Currently, the use of thromboprophylactic agents are the favored treatment options for pregnant aPL-positive women with a history of recurrent miscarriage. A meta-analysis has shown that a combination of aspirin and heparin can significantly improve the live-birth rate in women with recurrent miscarriage and APS [52].

## Corticosteroids and Antiphospholipid syndrome

When Antiphospholipid syndrome was first linked to fetal loss and pregnancy morbidity in the early 1980s, it was considered to be an autoimmune disorder [53]. Hence, glucocorticoid therapy was widely used in an attempt to dampen the so-called excessive maternal immune response that damaged the pregnancy. A recent Cochrane review [54] identified two trials comparing prednisone and aspirin with placebo or aspirin alone and concluded that prednisone and aspirin did not improve the live-birth rate (RR 0.85, 95% CI 0.53 to 1.36) [55,56]. However, the use of corticosteroids was associated with a significant increase in both maternal and fetal morbidity. There was a significant increase in pre-term births and in one study admission to the neonatal intensive care unit was nine times more likely in the prednisone-treated group than the placebo group (95% CI 2.14–37.78) [55]. Amongst the women treated with prednisone the rate of pre-eclampsia and hypertension was higher and a 3.3 times (95% CI 1.53–6.98) greater risk of gestational diabetes was noted when compared with placebo, aspirin alone, heparin and aspirin, or IvIg [55–58]. Neonatal birth weight was significantly less in the prednisone and aspirin-treated groups compared with aspirin (weighted mean difference (WMD) −552.00, 95% CI −1064.79 to −39.21) [56] or IvIg (WMD −351.00, 95% CI −587.94 to −114.06) [57].

## Role of aspirin in Antiphospholipid syndrome

Aspirin is an anti-platelet agent which irreversibly inhibits platelet cyclo-oxygenase and thereby decreases the production of thromboxane A2 (TXA2), a potent vasoconstrictor. Because aspirin reduces the risk of platelet-mediated vascular thrombosis, it has been widely used in an attempt to improve pregnancy outcome for women with aPL and a history of recurrent miscarriage and a variety of auto-immune conditions [59–68]. Aspirin has also been prescribed with increasing frequency before pregnancy in an attempt to improve the success of in-vitro fertilization (IVF), reduce the risk of miscarriage and improve the outcome of pregnancy [61].

It is generally believed that women with APS who use low-dose aspirin (LDA) have improved pregnancy outcomes. There have been three randomized trials of aspirin in combination with heparin for the treatment of APS [59,60,62] but no trials that compare aspirin alone with heparin alone. Furthermore, of the three trials that have studied aspirin versus placebo or supportive care, none has reported that aspirin confers a significant benefit [29,58,63]. Even when the results were combined in a meta-analysis, aspirin compared with placebo or supportive care had no significant effect on any of the outcomes of pregnancy (RR 1.05; 95% CI 0.66–1.68) [64]. It remains unclear as to whether women with APS have improved pregnancy outcomes with LDA therapy.

For women with unexplained recurrent early miscarriage, a large observational prospective study has reported that aspirin taken from the time of a positive pregnancy test does not improve the live-birth rate (OR 1.24; 95% CI 0.93–1.67) [65]. Of interest, the same study did report an improvement in the live-birth rate for women with a history of unexplained late miscarriage treated with LDA.

A population-based observational cohort study has examined aspirin and non-steroidal anti-inflammatory (NSAID) exposure in pregnancy and the risk of sporadic miscarriage [66]. Aspirin users were defined as those women who reported using aspirin or preparations containing aspirin after their last menstrual period. After adjustment for potential confounders, NSAID use was associated with an 80% increased risk of miscarriage. The association was stronger if the initial NSAID use was around the time of conception or if NSAID use lasted more than a week. The use of aspirin in early pregnancy was similarly associated with an increased risk of miscarriage. However, the data from this study should be interpreted with caution, since the reason for taking aspirin and the doses of aspirin taken were not known. It is possible that the aspirin and NSAID users did so because of cramping pain from an inevitable miscarriage or alternatively they may have had conditions like systemic lupus erythematosus (SLE) and APS that placed them at increased risk of miscarriage [61].

Pre-implantation aspirin therapy is a topical and controversial issue. The use of aspirin and other NSAIDs prior to conception has been associated with a high miscarriage rate [66]. In mice, Cyclooxygenase-2 ( COX-2) expression during the phase of blastocyst attachment to the decidua is critical to implantation and since aspirin suppresses COX-2 activity, it has the theoretical potential to interfere with implantation [67]. On the other hand, there are data that suggest that maintenance of pregnancy is dependent on a mechanism that suppresses prostaglandin synthesis throughout gestation. Aspirin, which suppresses COX-2, has the potential to support this mechanism [61].

Aspirin crosses the placenta and although it has not been linked to major congenital anomalies [68] aspirin has been associated with an increased risk of vascular disruptions, particularly gastroschisis [68,69]. Gastroschisis, which complicates approximately one in 5000 births, is an open abdominal wall defect thought to occur at 7 weeks' gestation due to inadequate perfusion of the omphalomesenteric artery. Both a case-controlled study [69] and a meta-analysis of 22 studies published between 1971 and 2002 [68] reported a two- to three-fold increased risk of fetal gastroschisis in mothers taking aspirin during the first trimester of pregnancy. The same meta-analysis also found an increased risk of central nervous system defects (OR 1.68, 95% CI 1.23–2.30) and cleft lip and palate (OR 2.87, 95% CI 2.04–4.02) and there is a potential risk that aspirin could lead to premature closure of the ductus arteriosus [70].

Aspirin ingestion during pregnancy is not without risk and can contribute to maternal and fetal bleeding. Although LDA has been shown to reduce the risk of venous thromboembolism by one third in postoperative patients, in women at high risk for venus thromboembolism during pregnancy, aspirin is not considered sufficient thromboprophylaxis. Since aspirin does not appear to confer benefit in terms of pregnancy outcome in women without evidence of prothrombotic disorders and may increase the risk of miscarriage and fetal abnormality, the use of empirical aspirin in the periconceptual period should be strongly resisted.

### Heparin and Antiphospholipid syndrome

Historically, heparin has been used as a thromboprophylactic agent in the treatment of pregnant women with APS and other thrombophilic defects. However, it is now recognized that heparin and the structurally related heparin sulphate (which is ubiquitously distributed on the surfaces of animal cells and in the extracellular matrix) have several other biological properties which are important at the feto–maternal interface. It appears that heparin is capable of binding

to aPL and also of antagonizing the action of the Th-1 cytokine interferon gamma, thereby protecting the trophoblast and maternal vascular endothelium from damage in early pregnancy. Later in pregnancy, when the inter-villous circulation has been established, the anticoagulant properties of heparin are beneficial in reducing the risk of placental fibrin deposition, thrombosis and infarction.

To date, there has been no large randomized controlled trial (RCT) comparing heparin treatment with placebo in pregnant women with APS. However there have been several small trials that have compared pregnancy outcome in women with APS treated with aspirin and heparin. A recent Cochrane review of 13 studies involving 849 participants showed that unfractionated heparin combined with LDA reduces the incidence of pregnancy loss by 54% (relative risk (RR) 0.46, 95% CI 0.29–0.71) when compared with LDA alone. This meta-analysis further suggested that low molecular weight heparin (LMWH) also has a beneficial effect, when compared with LDA alone (RR 0.78, 95% CI 0.39–1.57). However, uncertainty remains, since at present the published studies are too small for this finding to have reached clinical significance [64].

Two randomized trials have found that LDA and unfractionated heparin improves the live-birth rate in women with APS when compared with aspirin alone [59,60]. In the trial performed by Rai *et al.* in 1997, 90 women were randomized at the time of a positive urinary pregnancy test to receive either LDA or LDA and heparin daily until the time of miscarriage or 34 weeks' gestation [60]. The live-birth rate with LDA and heparin was 71% compared with 42% with LDA alone (OR 3.37, 95% CI 1.40–8.10). Most importantly, there was no difference in live-birth rates between the two treatment groups in those pregnancies which advanced beyond 13 weeks. This implies that the beneficial effect of adjuvant heparin therapy is conferred in the first trimester of pregnancy, at a time when the inter-villous circulation has not been fully established and hence cannot be due to the anticoagulant actions of heparin. It appears that the combination of aspirin and heparin promotes successful embryonic implantation in the early stages of pregnancy by protecting the trophoblast from attack by aPL. Later in pregnancy the combination therapy helps protect against subsequent thrombosis of the uteroplacental vasculature.

Combination therapy with aspirin and heparin significantly reduces the severity of the defective endovascular trophoblastic invasion in women with APS, allowing them to achieve a live birth. However it is important to remember that a proportion of pregnant women with aPL will remain at risk for late pregnancy complications due to the underlying uteroplacental vasculopathy. In a prospective series of 150 treated women with APS, a high risk for pre-term delivery, placental abruption, fetal growth retardation and the development of pregnancy-induced hypertension was found [19]. Once the pregnancy advances beyond the first trimester, specialist antenatal surveillance is required. Uterine artery Doppler ultrasonography at 22–24 weeks, followed by serial fetal growth and Doppler scans during the third trimester are useful tools with which to predict pre-eclampsia and intrauterine growth restriction in APS pregnancies. Women with a circulating lupus anticoagulant or high titres of IgG anticardiolipin antibodies are at particularly high risk of these complications [71].

Two recent studies have challenged the view that aspirin and heparin is the treatment of choice for pregnant women with APS, but both are methodologically flawed. Farquharson et al. [62] reported that LDA alone can be as effective as LMWH, but they included women with low positive titres for anticardiolipin antibodies, who were randomly assigned to treatment at a late stage in the first trimester, when pregnancy outcome was more likely to be successful. In addition, nearly 25% of the study participants switched treatment groups. The study by Laskin et al. [72] aimed to investigate whether treatment with LMWH plus aspirin results in an increased rate of live births compared with treatment with aspirin alone, but the study group was highly heterogeneous. The authors included women with two or more unexplained pregnancy losses prior to 32 weeks' gestation, accompanied by one or more of the following: positive aPL, positive antinuclear antibody (ANA) or an inherited thrombophilic defect. A total of 88 women were recruited to the study over a 4-year period, but the RCT was then stopped prematurely when an interim analysis showed no difference in live-birth rates in the two groups and a lower rate of pregnancy loss in the aspirin group than expected. Whether heparin should be denied to women with APS on the basis of the results of these two recent studies given the flawed designs mentioned above, is highly questionnable.

Heparin is well tolerated by pregnant women, despite the inevitable side effect of localized bruising at the injection sites. The optimal type and dose of heparin to maximize benefit and minimize potential side effects during pregnancy is uncertain. Higher doses of unfractionated heparin do not appear to reduce pregnancy morbidity when compared with lower doses. Heparin-induced thrombocytopenia was either not reported or did not occur [19,59,60] except for in one study where it was described as mild in two participants receiving LMWH [73]. Significant hemorrhage has not been reported to occur in mother or neonate.

There has been no trial comparing the efficacy of unfractionated heparin (UFH) and LMWH for treatment of APS in pregnant women. However, in the studies undertaken at St Mary's London, we have observed that UFH and LMWH preparations were equally beneficial in the treatment of APS [19,60]. Although more expensive, LMWH offers the significant practical advantage of a single daily subcutaneous injection.

It is now possible to reassure patients and their clinicians of the safety of prolonged low-dose heparin during pregnancy. The possibility of osteoporosis developing whilst receiving long-term therapy has been a source of concern. Maternal fractures have not been reported but they may have been missed. One longitudinal study of bone mineral density (BMD) measurements during pregnancy documented a median decrease of 3.7% in the lumbar spine in one study using UFH which is similar to that which occurs physiologically during pregnancy [74]. No change was noted in a further study which used LMWH [73] and in a multicenter multinational randomized trial designed to compare the effect of LMWH prophylaxis on pregnancy outcomes in thrombophilic pregnant women, the use of long-term prophylactic LMWH in pregnancy was not associated with a significant decrease in bone mineral density [75].

There may be clinical differences between unfractionated and low molecular weight heparin agents when used prophylactically for the management of thrombophilia associated with pregnancy, for example, in their ability to bind to thrombin and other proteins. However, clinical trials show them to be at least of equivalence as antithrombotic agents in non-pregnant women [76].

In summary, a combination of aspirin and heparin therapy for pregnant women with APS reduces pregnancy loss by 54%. This means that APS is currently the most important treatable cause of recurrent miscarriage.

### Intravenous immunoglobulin and Antiphospholipid syndrome

Intravenous immunoglobulin (IvIg) is a fractionated blood product made from pooled human plasma and is a non-specific immunosuppressant. It has been used to treat a number of medical disorders associated with an autoimmune etiology. It has been reported to suppress and neutralize auto antibodies, reduce natural killer cell activity, modify cytokine production, inhibit complement binding and both activate and inhibit super antigens [77]. The US Food and Drug Administration has approved the use of IvIg for auto-immune thrombocytopenia, but has declared that recurrent miscarriage, antiphospholipid antibody syndrome and repeated unexplained IVF failure to be invalid indications.

Given the widespread unlicensed use of IvIg in recent years, its high cost, short supply and extensive side-effect profile (which includes anaphylaxis, fever, muscle pains, nausea and headache [78]) the publication of a systematic review in 2007 [79] was particularly welcomed. Their review concluded that IvIg is not an effective therapy for women with primary recurrent miscarriage but that further randomized trials for women with secondary idiopathic miscarriage may be warranted [79]. A subsequent randomized double-blinded, placebo-controlled study reported that IvIg treatment offers no benefit over placebo in improving the ongoing pregnancy rates of women with secondary unexplained recurrent miscarriage [80].

One study that enrolled a total of 42 women with recurrent miscarriage associated with aPL showed that combination therapy with LDA and heparin is a superior treatment to IvIg [73]. Monitoring of pregnancy outcomes following treatment indicated that women receiving combination therapy with LDA and heparin achieved an improved rate of live births ($16/19 = 84\%$) relative to the IvIg group ($12/21 = 57\%$) (OR 0.25, 95% CI 0.05–1.13). The IvIg group suffered more fetal losses during the first trimester of pregnancy ($6/21 = 28.6\%$) than the comparison group ($2/19 = 10.5\%$) and the risk of premature delivery was also increased two-fold. Mean birth weights were found to be comparable between groups.

There was no reduction in pregnancy loss in any of the IvIg studies included in this analysis, however one of the studies had no pregnancy loss in either the treatment or the control group [81]. This was a small study ($n = 16$) and all participants received heparin and aspirin in addition to the study/control medication.

This study demonstrated a significant increase in premature delivery in the IvIg group (RR 3.00, 95% CI 1.19–7.56). In contrast, the outcome of pregnancy after IvIg did not significantly differ from outcome following prednisone and aspirin therapy [57]. In conclusion, IvIg treatment for aPL-associated pregnancy loss has no evidence base and should only be performed in the context of a randomized trial.

### Antiphospholipid syndrome and recurrent implantation failure

Whether thrombophilic disorders are causally linked to subfertility and recurrent implantation failure following IVF treatment is a topical and highly controversial issue. Since defective implantation during the early weeks of pregnancy is one of the underlying mechanisms accounting for the high pregnancy loss rate in women with aPL, it has been suggested that primary implantation may be adversely affected in women who are aPL positive.

The prevalence of aPL antibodies (both the lupus anticoagulant and anticardiolipin antibodies) is increased among women with infertility and implantation failure [82]. Both a prospective observational study [83] and a recently published meta-analysis [84] concluded that overall, the presence of aPL do not have an adverse effect on the outcome of IVF treatment cycles, as estimated by clinical pregnancy rate in seven studies (OR 0.99, 95% CI 0.64–1.53) or by live-birth rate in five studies (OR 1.07, 95% CI 0.66–1.75) [84]. Hence, universal screening of IVF patients for aPL cannot be justified on the basis of current evidence.

## Hyperhomocysteinemia

Hyperhomocysteinemia – which may be inherited or acquired – is a condition associated with deep venous thrombosis, placental vascular thrombosis (in particular pre-eclampsia and placental abruption), stillbirth, neural tube defects and recurrent pregnancy loss [85]. The inherited form results from the C to T substitution at nucleotide position 677 in the methylene tetrahydrofolate reductase (MTHFR) gene that converts an alanine to a valine residue [12]. Individuals that are homozygous for the mutation have significantly elevated plasma homocysteine levels and are prone to the early development of arteriosclerosis. Some 40% of Whites carry the mutation as a heterozygote and although they have an increased lifetime risk of venous and arterial thrombosis, a meta-analysis of multiple thrombophilic factors and their impact on fetal loss, has concluded there is little evidence that the mutation has significant adverse reproductive sequelae [16].

A variety of environmental conditions may lead to hyperhomocysteinemia including a reduced intake of folate, vitamin B12 or vitamin B6, excessive smoking and coffee consumption and certain medical conditions such as renal impairment and hypothyroidism. A meta-analysis of ten studies concluded that acquired hyperhomocystinemia is a risk factor for recurrent miscarriage [86]. The calculated risks attributable to elevated fasting and after load total plasma homocystinemia were 8.4% (95% CI 4.0–12.7) and 11.5% (95% CI 6.95–16.2) respectively.

A variety of pathophysiological mechanisms for hyperhomocysteinemia have been suggested. Inhibition of protein C activation or reduced antithrombin activity could be responsible for increasing the reported risk of venous thrombosis and theoretically the risk of placental pathology leading to pregnancy loss. Endothelial dysfunction or apoptosis mediated by impaired nitric oxide bioavailability, alteration of platelet reactivity, smooth muscle proliferation and disruption of prostacyclin pathway are the possible mechanisms described by the Homocysteine Lowering Trial Collaboration [87].

Plasma homocysteine levels are significantly lower in all trimesters of pregnancy compared with non-pregnant control values, with the lowest values found in the second trimester [88]. High-dose folic acid 5 mg daily and vitamin B12 at a dose of 0.5 mg per day reduce plasma homocysteine levels by 25% and 7% respectively [89].There has been no RCT in recurrent miscarriage women with hyperhomocysteinemia, looking at the effect of variable doses of folic acid on future pregnancy outcome.

## Acquired protein C resistance

Protein C is a key component in the anticoagulant pathway. When activated, protein C inhibits the actions of coagulation factors V and VIII. Resistance to the anticoagulant properties of activated protein C (APC resistance) was first reported in 1993 [90]. It was later demonstrated that APC resistance may either be inherited or acquired. Inherited APC resistance is mainly due to a single point mutation (G→A) at nucleotide position 1691 in the factor V gene. This results in a mutated form of factor V, which is resistant to inactivation by APC and known as factor V Leiden [91]. This mutation is common, being present in 5% (1 in 20) Whites and

leads to increased thrombin generation and a hyper-coagulable state.

Acquired APC resistance is a recognized risk factor for systemic venous thrombosis and is associated with lupus anticoagulant, high concentrations of coagulation factor VIII [92], pregnancy and the combined oral contraceptive pill. The prevalence of factor V Leiden and acquired APC resistance among women with recurrent miscarriage has been variably reported to be either similar to or increased compared with parous controls [93]. This uncertainty reflects the fact that most studies have included small numbers of women, have been prone to selection bias and have not differentiated between women with a history of recurrent miscarriage and those with late pregnancy complications.

A large observational study including more than 1000 consecutive non-pregnant women attending a specialist recurrent miscarriage clinic has demonstrated that acquired APC resistance is significantly more common among women with recurrent early miscarriage (80/904; 8.8%: $P = 0.02$) and those with a previous late miscarriage (18/207; 8.7%: $P = 0.04$) compared with parous controls (17/150; 3.3%) [93]. Furthermore, the women with acquired APC resistance were significantly less likely to have had a previous live birth ($P < 0.01$) compared with those with a normal APC ratio. In contrast, the frequency of inherited APC resistance due to the factor V Leiden allele, among women with a history of early and late miscarriage was similar to that amongst appropriately matched parous controls [90]. Of note is that in a previous much smaller study, in which APC resistance was assessed among women with recurrent miscarriage but no differentiation was made between congenital and acquired causes, the same researchers reported that the frequency of APC resistance was similar among women with early miscarriage compared with controls [39]. This omission emphasizes the importance of discriminating between the inherited and acquired forms of APC resistance.

These data suggest that acquired APC resistance contributes to the burden of recurrent pregnancy loss, the mechanism of which is likely to be thrombosis of the placental vasculature. Since a degree of APC resistance develops during normal pregnancy [94], it is possible that among women who are APC resistant prior to pregnancy that this effect is amplified when they become pregnant again. This theory has prompted the use of thromboprophylactic treatment regimens for women with recurrent miscarriage and APC resistance (both the inherited and acquired forms) during the next pregnancy, in order to improve the live-birth rate and protect the mother from the risk of venous thrombosis during the pregnancy and puerperium. Although it has not been possible to conduct a randomized controlled therapeutic trial to assess the potential benefits of low-dose heparin therapy during pregnancy in these women, current clinical practice favors the use of thromboprophylaxis from early in the first trimester until 6–12 weeks postpartum.

## Global markers of prothrombotic disorders

Several studies have suggested that some women with recurrent pregnancy loss exhibit prothrombotic features in the non-pregnant state. Vincent *et al.* [95] measured the levels of thrombin-antithrombin (TAT) complexes, a global marker of thrombin generation, in 86 non-pregnant women with recurrent miscarriage and a control group of 34 age-matched, parous women with no previous history of pregnancy loss. The TAT levels were significantly higher among the recurrent miscarriage women compared with the control group. This relationship was independent of the gestation of previous miscarriages – women with both first- and second-trimester fetal losses were found to have significantly higher levels of TAT complexes. Further, the TAT levels were unaffected by the women's aPL status. These observations suggest that a subgroup of women with RM, irrespective of aPL status, are in a prothrombotic state that is detectable even in the non-pregnant state. Potentially, this is an important group of women to identify since the further hypercoagulable state of pregnancy may be the "hit" that places them at risk of fetal loss due to thrombosis of the uteroplacental vasculature, and/or a maternal thrombotic event. It may also confer an increased risk of ischemic heart disease and stroke in later life [96].

Using different markers of thrombin generation, it has also been reported that women with recurrent miscarriage are in a chronic state of endothelial stimulation associated with activation of the coagulation system [97]. Furthermore, elevated levels of circulating procoagulant microparticles have been described in the peripheral circulation of women with both early and late unexplained miscarriages [98]. It has been proposed that, in addition to their direct effect on the coagulant cascade, these microparticles may also exert a proinflammatory and/or proapoptotic action which disturbs successful implantation and subsequent fetal growth.

Despite the improved understanding that a variety of thrombophilic and prothrombotic disorders make an important contribution to the problem of pregnancy loss, a consensus view has not been reached as to which investigations should be performed in these patients. We need to determine how best to screen women with a history of pregnancy loss for hemostatic abnormalities that (a) are predictive of poor future pregnancy outcome and (b) are amenable to treatment. Conventional tests for acquired and inherited coagulation defects are expensive, time consuming and take no account of the fact that hemostasis in vivo is a dynamic process which involves the interaction of coagulation and fibrinolytic pathways together with cellular elements such as endothelial cell surfaces. Hence, the measurement of individual coagulation factors is of limited use in establishing a woman's thrombophilic risk, particularly during pregnancy.

The potential of thromboelastography as a clinical tool to overcome many of the above limitations in hemostasis testing in our recurrent pregnancy-loss population is promising. The thromboelastogram (TEG) is a cheap, effective and reproducible method of assessing the kinetics, strength and stability of whole blood coagulation [99,100]. It is a highly sensitive global test for hemostatic defects and measures the visco-elastic properties of blood as it is induced to clot under a low shear environment resembling sluggish venous flow. The TEG print-out (a pictorial envelope; see Figure 13.1) provides measurements for the different stages of clot formation from the initial platelet–fibrin interaction, through platelet aggregation, clot strengthening and fibrin cross-linkage to clot lysis. Thromboelastogram parameters are abnormal in patients with established thrombophilic defects, such as antithrombin deficiency, as well as in a proportion of patients with unexplained recurrent systemic thrombosis [101].

Our recent studies have shown that TEG is a useful tool with which to identify a prothrombotic state in women with a history of previously unexplained recurrent miscarriage. The maximum clot amplitude (MA) was significantly greater among recurrent miscarriage women compared with normal parous controls. Furthermore, increases in the MA were more marked in women with a history of late miscarriage

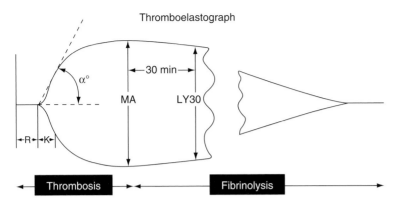

Thromboelastograph

**Figure 13.1** The thromboelastograph pictorial envelope. MA = maximum clot amplitude

compared with women with a history of only early pregnancy losses. None of the women in these studies smoked, was taking the oral contraceptive pill or had a history of thromboembolic disease [102].

The MA is a reflection of the absolute strength of the fibrin clot formed and hence is a dynamic test of fibrin and platelet function. Some 30% of non-pregnant RM women have an MA that is more than two standard deviations above the mean of a control parous population, adding further weight to our hypothesis that a significant proportion of RM women are in a prothrombotic state outside of pregnancy. Furthermore, the pre-pregnancy MA was predictive of future pregnancy outcome, being significantly higher amongst those RM women whose next pregnancy ended in a further miscarriage as opposed to a live birth [102]. Once pregnancy is confirmed, serial TEG testing during the first trimester can identify increases in the MA that precede the clinical evidence of impending miscarriage by several weeks. Our initial studies suggest that variable doses of aspirin can normalize the raised MA levels in early pregnancy and improve the live-birth rate (Regan & Rai unpublished data).

The great advantage of TEG testing compared with conventional coagulation assays is that it provides information about the interaction of platelets with the protein coagulation cascade. Hence, a complete evaluation of the process of clot initiation, formation, stability and lysis is obtained. Most importantly, it reliably identifies hypercoaguability that would only be detectable in conventional hemostasis assays when the platelet count or fibrinogen levels are markedly raised. In summary, a subgroup of recurrent miscarriage women are in a thrombophilic state outside pregnancy which predisposes them to future pregnancy loss.

Serial thromboelastography during pregnancy allows the detection of the developing hypercoaguability prior to pregnancy loss, which may prove to be amenable to correction with thromboprophylaxis.

## Future pregnancy management in recurrent miscarriage patients with thrombophilia

Couples with recurrent miscarriage are understandably anxious and need support and reassurance throughout the first trimester of pregnancy. Ultrasound is valuable in the management of early pregnancy to confirm viability, and after fetal heart activity has been detected, to provide ongoing maternal reassurance. Using transvaginal ultrasound, an intrauterine gestation sac will be visible at 5 weeks, a yolk sac at approximately 5.5 weeks and fetal heart activity at 6 weeks. Thereafter, a scan to check fetal heart activity may be obtained every week or every 2 weeks, until the end of the first trimester. The demonstration of normal sequential fetal growth and activity is very reassuring for many couples.

Women with APS should be offered a combination of aspirin and heparin treatment during the pregnancy. Low-dose aspirin (75 mg/day) should be commenced as soon as the patient has a positive urinary pregnancy test result. Daily subcutaneous injection of low molecular weight heparin (enoxaparin [Clexane] [Lovenox] 20 mg or dalteparin [Fragmin] 2500 unit) or twice-daily injections of unfractionated heparin ([Calciparine] 5000 IU) should be started as soon as an intrauterine gestational sac is confirmed by ultrasound scan. Some clinicians prefer to commence the heparin therapy as soon as the pregnancy test is positive. Although UFH is equally beneficial, LMWH offers the advantage of a once-daily injection due to its longer half-life and increased bioavailability. A platelet count should be done at the start of treatment and repeated 2 weeks later to exclude the rare complication of heparin-induced thrombocytopenia.

Despite significant improvement in live-birth rates, pregnant women who have APS and are treated with aspirin plus heparin until 34 completed weeks of gestation remain at risk for later pregnancy complications, including pre-eclampsia, intrauterine growth restriction, placental abruption and pre-term delivery [19]. Some clinicians prefer to continue treatment until the time of delivery in the belief that this reduces the risk of these late pregnancy complications, but there is no hard evidence to support this view. Indeed, the RCT by Rai *et al.* [60] emphasized that the main benefit of combination therapy with aspirin and heparin is to improve the quality and depth of embryonic implantation during the first trimester of pregnancy. After 13 weeks of gestation the number of pregnancies ending in live births did not differ significantly by treatment group [60].

Uterine artery Doppler ultrasonography at 22–24 weeks may be useful in predicting pre-eclampsia and intrauterine growth restriction in pregnancies complicated by APS and other thrombophilias. Women with circulating lupus anticoagulant or high titres of IgG anticardiolipin antibodies are at increased risk for these complications and sequential growth scans and Doppler studies during the third trimester should be undertaken [71]. Many women with a history of recurrent miscarriage will become anxious towards the end of the pregnancy and request early delivery either by induction of labor or elective cesarean section. For those women being treated with aspirin and or heparin it is important to plan regional anesthesia to minimize the risk of epidural hematoma. Current guidelines recommend that regional techniques should not be used until at least 12 hours after the previous prophylactic dose of LMWH and 6 hours after a dose of UFH. Heparin should not be given for at least 4 hours after the epidural catheter is removed. There are no prospective data on the risk of systemic thrombosis to determine the optimal management of asymptomatic women with inherited thrombophilia. Current Royal College of Obstetricians and Gynaecologists guidelines based on expert opinion recommend that postnatal thromboprophylaxis is indicated for women with known inherited thrombophilias (e.g. factor V Leiden and prothrombin gene mutations), but individual assessment will be guided by the type of

thrombophilia and the presence of other thrombotic risk factors. Similarly, in women with APS and no symptoms other than recurrent miscarriage, there is no evidence to justify routine postnatal thromboprophylaxis.

## Unexplained recurrent miscarriage and the role of supportive care

A significant proportion of cases of recurrent miscarriage remain unexplained, despite detailed investigation. These women can be reassured that the prognosis for a future successful pregnancy outcome with supportive care alone is in the region of 70% although the prognosis worsens with increasing maternal age and number of miscarriages (range 50–89%) [65,103–105]. The value of psychological support in improving pregnancy outcome has not been tested in an RCT. However, data from several non-randomized studies [103,104,106] have suggested that attendance at a dedicated early pregnancy clinic has a beneficial effect, although the underlying mechanism is unclear.

The success of thromboprophylactic treatment for women with recurrent miscarriage associated with APS has resulted in women with unexplained recurrent miscarriage frequently demanding similar treatment. Some clinicians have extrapolated the beneficial effect of aspirin and heparin therapy in women with APS to all women with recurrent miscarriage. A recently published Cochrane review [107] has explained the paucity of published intervention trials of anticoagulant agents in women with recurrent miscarriage without APS. The authors identified a total of 20 studies in their literature search, but only two randomized controlled studies could be included in their systematic review. Neither the study comparing LDA and placebo [63] nor the one comparing enoxaparin with aspirin [108] showed improvement in pregnancy outcome. However, this may be due to the fact that women with two losses were included in the study. Nonetheless, at the present time the use of LDA and heparin to prevent miscarriage in women with two or more unexplained miscarriages cannot be recommended. Prospective randomized placebo-controlled studies of sufficient magnitude are needed to establish the efficacy of this treatment intervention for women with unexplained recurrent miscarriage of unknown cause [109]. The results of the Scottish Pregnancy Intervention Study (SPIN) and thrombophilia in pregnancy prophylaxis study (TIPPS) are eagerly awaited.

# Conclusion

Recurrent miscarriage is a distressing condition that affects at least 1% of couples trying to achieve a successful pregnancy. The hypothesis that some cases of recurrent miscarriage are due to a defective or exaggerated hemostatic response to pregnancy is now supported by a substantial body of evidence. This has led to the introduction of new treatment options that have made a significant contribution to improving pregnancy outcomes.

Primary Antiphospholipid syndrome is an acquired thrombophilia and is found in 15% of women with recurrent miscarriage. In subsequent untreated pregnancies the miscarriage rate may be as high as 90%. Although recent studies have queried the need for heparin in addition to aspirin therapy, a Cochrane meta-analysis has shown that a combination of heparin and aspirin improves pregnancy outcome by 54%, to achieve a live-birth rate of over 70% in women with the syndrome. This means that APS is currently the most important treatable cause of recurrent pregnancy loss.

The prevalence of thrombophilic defects among the general population is high and the presence of a detectable defect does not necessarily preclude an uncomplicated pregnancy and term delivery. Nonetheless, recent reports have highlighted the fact that the presence of multiple prothrombotic risk factors are associated with poorer pregnancy outcome. In conclusion it appears that there is a complex interaction between the currently recognized acquired and inherited prothrombotic disorders that determine the reproductive risk. The challenge for the researchers in this field is the development of both global and specific assessments of hemostatic abnormality that may better predict those women who are at high risk of miscarriage and late pregnancy complications, in order that treatment can be more effectively targeted.

# Acknowledgments

We (LR and AH) are grateful for support from the NIHR Biomedical Research Centre Funding scheme.

# References

1. Regan L, Rai R. Epidemiology and the medical causes of miscarriage. *Baillieres Best Pract Res Clin Obstet Gynaecol* 2000; **14**(5): 839–54.

2. Drakeley AJ, Quenby S Farquharson RG. Mid trimester loss – appraisal of a screening protocol. *Hum Reprod* 1998; **13**(7): 1975–80.

3. Rai R, Regan L. Recurrent miscarriage. *Lancet* 2006; **368**: 601–11.

4. Stephenson MD, Awartani KA, Robinson WP. Cytogenetic analysis of miscarriages from couples with recurrent miscarriage: a case-control study. *Hum Reprod* 2002; **17**(2): 446–51.

5. Hogge WA, Byrnes AL, Lanasa MC, Surti U. The clinical use of karyotyping spontaneous abortions. *Am J Obstet Gynecol* 2003; **189**(2): 397–400.

6. Christiansen OB, Nybo Andersen AM, Bosch E *et al.* Evidence-based investigations and treatments of recurrent pregnancy loss. *Fertil Steril* 2005; **83**(4): 821–39.

7. Clifford K, Rai R, Watson H, Regan L. An informative protocol for the investigation of recurrent miscarriage: preliminary experience of 500 consecutive cases. *Hum Reprod* 1994; **9** (7): 1328–32.

8. Bick RL. Recurrent miscarriage syndrome and infertility caused by blood coagulation/platelet defects. In RL Brick, EP Frankel *et al* (eds.), *Hematological Complications of Obstetrics, Pregnancy and Gynaecology*. Cambridge: Cambridge University Press, 2006, pp. 55–74.

9. Egeberg O. Inherited antithrombin deficiency causing thrombophilia. *Thromb Diath Haemorrh* 1965; **13**: 516–30.

10. Bertina RM, Koeleman BP, Koster T *et al.* Mutation in blood coagulation factor V associated with resistance to activated protein C. *Nature* 1994; **369**: 64–7.

11. Poort SR, Rosendaal FR, Reitsma PH, Bertina RM. A common genetic variation in the 3'-untranslated region of the prothrombin gene is associated with elevated plasma prothrombin levels and an increase in venous thrombosis. *Blood* 1996; **88**: 3698–703.

12. Frosst P, Blom HJ, Milos R *et al.* A candidate genetic risk factor for vascular disease: a common mutation in methylenetetrahydrofolate reductase. *Nature Genetics* 1995; **10**: 111–13.

13. Preston FE, Rosendaal FR, Walker ID *et al.* Increased fetal loss in women with heritable thrombophilia. *Lancet* 1996; **348**(9032): 913–16.

14. Sanson BJ, Friederich PW, Simioni P *et al.* The risk of abortion and stillbirth in antithrombin-, protein C-, and protein S-deficient women. *Thromb Haemost* 1996; **75**(3): 387–8.

15. Sarig G, Younis JS, Hoffman R *et al.* Thrombophilia is common in women with idiopathic pregnancy loss and is associated with late pregnancy wastage. *Fertil Steril* 2002; **77**: 342–7.

16. Rey E, Kahn SR, David M, Shrier I. Thrombophilic disorders and fetal loss: a meta-analysis. *Lancet* 2003; **361**: 901–8.

17. Harris EN, Chan JK, Asherson RA *et al.* Thrombosis, recurrent fetal loss, and thrombocytopenia. Predictive

125

value of the anticardiolipin antibody test. *Arch Intern Med* 1986; **146**(11): 2153–6.

18. Wilson WA, Gharavi AE, Koike T *et al.* International consensus statement on preliminary classification criteria for definite antiphospholipid syndrome: report of an international workshop. *Arthritis Rheum* 1999; **42**: 1309–11.

19. Backos M, Rai R, Baxter N *et al.* Pregnancy complications in women with recurrent miscarriage associated with antiphospholipid antibodies treated with low-dose aspirin and heparin. *Br J Obstet Gynaecol* 1999; **106**: 102–7.

20. Oshiro BT, Silver RM, Scott JR, Yu H, Branch DW. Antiphospholipid antibodies and fetal death. *Obstet Gynecol* 1996; **87**(4): 489–93.

21. Rai RS, Clifford K, Cohen H, Regan L. High prospective fetal loss rate in untreated pregnancies of women with recurrent miscarriage and antiphospholipid antibodies. *Hum Reprod* 1995; **10**(12): 3301–4.

22. Dentali F, Crowther M. Acquired thrombophilia during pregnancy. *Obstet Gynecol Clin North Am* 2006; **33**(3): 375–88.

23. Robert JM, Macara LM, Chalmers EA, Smith GC. Inter-assay variation in antiphospholipid antibody testing. *BJOG* 2002; **109**(3): 348–9.

24. Lupus Anticoagulant Working Party on behalf of the BCSH Haemostasis and Thrombosis Task Force. Guidelines on testing for the lupus anticoagulant. *J Clin Pathol* 1991; **44**(11): 885–9.

25. Khamashta M, Hughes GR. Antiphospholipid syndrome. *Br Med J* 1993; **307**(6909): 883–4.

26. Miyakis S. International consensus statement on an update of the classification criteria for definite antiphospholipid syndrome. *J Thromb Haemost* 2006; **4**: 295–306.

27. Vinatier D, Dufour P, Cosson M *et al.* Antiphospholipid syndrome and recurrent miscarriages. *Eur J Obstet Gynecol Reprod Biol* 2001; **96**: 37–50.

28. Lockwood CJ, Romero R, Feinberg RF *et al.* The prevalence and biologic significance of lupus anticoagulant and anticardiolipin antibodies in a general obstetric population. *Am J Obstet Gynecol* 1989; **161**: 369–73.

29. Pattison NS, Chamley LW, Birdsall M *et al.* Does aspirin have a role in improving pregnancy outcome for women with the antiphospholipid syndrome? A randomized controlled trial. *Am J Obstet Gynecol* 2000; **183**(4): 1008–12.

30. Branch DW, Silver RM. Criteria for antiphospholipid syndrome: early pregnancy loss, fetal loss, or recurrent pregnancy loss? *Lupus* 1996; **5**(5): 409–13.

31. Tebo AE, Jaskowski TD, Hill HR, Branch DW. Clinical relevance of multiple antibody specificity testing in anti-phospholipid syndrome and recurrent pregnancy loss. *Clin Exp Immunol* 2008; **154**: 332–8.

32. Perez MC, Wilson WA, Brown HL, Scopelitis E. Anticardiolipin antibodies in unselected pregnant women. Relationship to fetal outcome. *J Perinatol* 1991; **11**(1): 33–6.

33. Rai RS, Clifford K, Cohen H, Regan L. High prospective fetal loss rate in untreated pregnancies of women with recurrent miscarriage and antiphospholipid antibodies. *Hum Reprod* 1995; **10**(12): 3301–4.

34. Kupferminc MJ, Eldor A, Steinman N *et al.* Increased frequency of genetic thrombophilia in women with complications of pregnancy. *New Engl J Med*, 1999; **340**: 9–13.

35. Middeldorp S. Thrombophilia and pregnancy complications: cause or association? *J Thromb Haemost* 2007; **5**(Suppl 1): 276–82.

36. Out HJ, Kooijman CD, Bruinse HW, Derksen RH. Histopathological findings in placentae from patients with intra-uterine fetal death and anti-phospholipid antibodies. *Eur J Obstet Gynecol Reprod Biol* 1991; **41**(3): 179–86.

37. Peaceman AM, Rehnberg KA. The effect of immunoglobulin G fractions from patients with lupus anticoagulant on placental prostacyclin and thromboxan production. *Am J Obstet Gynecol* 1993; **169**: 1403–6.

38. Carp HJ. Thrombophilia and recurrent pregnancy loss. *Obstet Gynecol Clin North Am* 2006; **33**(3): 429–42.

39. Rai RS, Regan L, Chitolie A, Donald JG, Cohen H. Placental thrombosis and second trimester miscarriage in association with activated protein C resistance. *Br J Obstet Gynaecol* 1996; **103**(8): 842–4.

40. Dizon-Townson DS, Meline L, Nelson LM, Varner M, Ward K. Fetal carriers of the factor V Leiden mutation are prone to miscarriage and placental infarction. *Am J Obstet Gynecol* 1997; **177**(2): 402–5.

41. Van Horn JT, Craven C, Ward K, Branch DW, Silver RM. Histologic features of placentas and abortion specimens from women with antiphospholipid and antiphospholipid-like syndromes. *Placenta* 2004; **25**(7): 642–8.

42. Sebire NJ, Backos M, El Gaddal S, Goldin RD, Regan L. Placental pathology, antiphospholipid antibodies, and pregnancy outcome in recurrent miscarriage patients. *Obstet Gynecol* 2003; **101**(2): 258–63.

43. Mousa HA, Alfirevic1 Z. Do placental lesions reflect thrombophilia state in women with adverse pregnancy outcome? *Hum Reprod* 2000; **15**(8): 1830–3.

44. Mak IY, Brosens JJ, Christian M *et al.* Regulated expression of signal transducer and activator of transcription, Stat5, and its enhancement of PRL expression in human endometrial stromal cells in vitro. *J Clin Endocrinol Metab* 2002; **87**(6): 2581–8.

45. Bose P, Black S, Kadyrov M et al. Heparin and aspirin attenuate placental apoptosis in vitro: implications for early pregnancy failure. *Am J Obstet Gynecol* 2005; **192**(1): 23–30.

46. Di Simone N, Caliandro D, Castellani R et al. Low-molecular weight heparin restores in-vitro trophoblast invasiveness and differentiation in presence of immunoglobulin G fractions obtained from patients with antiphospholipid syndrome. *Hum Reprod* 1999; **14**(2): 489–95.

47. Bose P, Black S, Kadyrov M et al. Adverse effects of lupus anticoagulant positive blood sera on placental viability can be prevented by heparin in vitro. *Am J Obstet Gynecol* 2004; **191**(6): 2125–31.

48. Quenby S, Mountfield S, Cartwright JE, Whitley GS, Vince G. Effects of low-molecular-weight and unfractionated heparin on trophoblast function. *Obstet Gynecol* 2004; **104**(2): 354–61.

49. Salmon JE, Girardi G, Holers V. Activation of complement mediates antiphospholipid antibody-induced pregnancy loss. *Lupus* 2003; **12**: 535–8.

50. Pierangeli SS, Vega-Ostertag V, Liu X, Girardi G. Complement activation – a novel pathogenic mechanism in the antiphospholipid syndrome. *Ann NY Acad Sci* 2005; **1051**: 413–20.

51. Girardi G, Redecha P, Salmon JE. Heparin prevents antiphospholipid antibody-induced fetal loss by inhibiting complement activation. *Nature Med* 2005; **10**(11): 1222–6.

52. Empson M, Lassere M, Craig JC, Scott JR. Recurrent pregnancy loss with antiphospholipid antibody: a systematic review of therapeutic trials. *Obstet Gynecol* 2002; **99**(1): 135–44.

53. Harris EN. Syndrome of the black swan. *Br J Rheumatol* 1987; **26**(5): 324–6.

54. Porter TF, LaCoursiere Y, Scott JR. Immunotherapy for recurrent miscarriage. *Cochrane Database Syst Rev* 2006; **2**: CD000112. DOI: 10.1002/14651858. CD000112.pub2.

55. Laskin CA, Bombardier C, Hannah ME et al. Prednisone and aspirin in women with autoantibodies and unexplained recurrent fetal loss. *New Engl J Med* 1997; **337**(3): 148–53.

56. Silver RK, MacGregor SN, Sholl JS et al. Comparative trial of prednisone plus aspirin versus aspirin alone in the treatment of anticardiolipin antibody-positive obstetric patients. *Am J Obstet Gynecol* 1993; **169**: 1411–17.

57. Vaquero E, Lazzarin N, Valensise H et al. Pregnancy outcome in recurrent spontaneous abortion associated with antiphospholipid antibodies: a comparative study of intravenous immunoglobulin versus prednisolone plus low dose aspirin. *Am J Reprod Immunol* 2001; **45**: 174–9.

58. Cowchock FS, Reece EA, Balaban D, Branch DW, Plouffe L. Repeated fetal losses associated with antiphospholipid antibodies: a collaborative randomized trial comparing prednisone with low-dose heparin treatment. *Am J Obstet Gynecol* 1992; **166**: 1318–23.

59. Kutteh WH. Antiphospholipid antibody-associated recurrent pregnancy loss: treatment with heparin and low-dose aspirin is superior to low-dose aspirin alone. *Am J Obstet Gynecol* 1996; **174**(5): 1584–9.

60. Rai R, Cohen H, Dave M, Regan L. Randomised controlled trial of aspirin and aspirin plus heparin in pregnant women with recurrent miscarriage associated with phospholipid antibodies (or antiphospholipid antibodies). *Br Med J* 1997; **314**(7076): 253–7.

61. James AH, Brancazio LR, Price T. Aspirin and reproductive outcomes. *Obstetric Gynecol Survey* 2007: **63**(1): 49–57.

62. Farquharson R, Quenby S, Greaves M. Antiphospholipid syndrome in pregnancy: a randomized controlled trial of treatment. *Obstet Gynecol* 2002; **100**(3): 408–13.

63. Tulppala M, Marttunen M, Soderstrom-Anttila V et al. Low-dose aspirin in prevention of miscarriage in women with unexplained or autoimmune related recurrent miscarriage: effect on prostacyclin and thromboxane A2 production. *Hum Reprod* 1997; **12**(7): 1567–72.

64. Empson M, Lassere M, Craig J, Scott J. Prevention of recurrent miscarriage for women with antiphospholipid antibody or lupus anticoagulant. *Cochrane Database Syst Rev* 2005; **2**: CD002859.

65. Rai R, Backos M, Baxter N, Chilcott I, Regan L. Recurrent miscarriage – an aspirin a day? *Hum Reprod* 2000; **15**(10): 2220–3.

66. Li DK, Liu L, Odouli R. Exposure to non-steroidal anti-inflammatory drugs during pregnancy and risk of miscarriage: population based cohort study. *Br Med J* 2003; **327**(7411): 368.

67. Patrono C, Garcia Rodriguez LA, Landolfi R, Baigent C. Low-dose aspirin for the prevention of atherosclerosis. *New Engl J Med* 2005; **353**: 2373–83.

68. Kozer E, Nifkar S, Costei A et al. Aspirin consumption during the first trimester of pregnancy and congenital abnormalities: a meta-analysis. *Am J Obstet Gynecol* 2002; **187**(6): 1623–30.

69. Werler MM, Sheehan JE, Mitchell AA. Maternal medication use and risks of gastroschisis and small intestinal atresia. *Am J Epidemiol* 2002; **155** (1): 26–31.

70. Alano MA, Ngougmna E, Ostrea EM Jr, Konduri GG. Analysis of nonsteroidal antiinflammatory drugs in meconium and its relation to persistent pulmonary hypertension of the newborn. *Pediatrics* 2001, **107**: 519–23.

71. Venkat-Raman N, Backos M, Teoh TG, Lo WT, Regan L. Uterine artery Doppler in predicting pregnancy outcome in women with antiphospholipid syndrome. *Obstet Gynecol* 2001; **98**(2): 235–42.

72. Laskin CA, Spitzer KA, Clark CA et al. Low molecular weight heparin and aspirin for recurrent pregnancy loss; results from the randomized controlled HepASA Trial. *J Rheumatol* 2009; **36** (2): 279–87.

73. Triolo G, Ferrante A, Ciccia F et al. Randomized study of subcutaneous low molecular weight heparin plus aspirin versus intravenous immunoglobulin in the treatment of recurrent fetal loss associated with antiphospholipid antibodies. *Arthritis Rheum* 2003; **48**(3): 728–31.

74. Backos M, Rai R, Thoms E et al. Bone density changes in pregnant women treated with heparin: a prospective longitudinal study. *Hum Reprod* 1999; **14**: 2876–80.

75. Le Templier G, Rodger MA. Osteoporosis and pregnancy. *Curr Opin Pulm Med* 2008; **14**(5): 403–7.

76. Hirsh J, Warkentin TE, Raschke R et al. Heparin and low-molecular-weight heparin: mechanisms of action, pharmacokinetics, dosing considerations, monitoring, efficacy, and safety. *Chest* 1998; **114**(5 Suppl): 489S–510S.

77. Omwandho CO, Gruessner SE, Roberts TK, Tinneberg HR. Intravenous immunoglobulin (IVIG): modes of action in the clinical management of recurrent pregnancy loss (RPL) and selected autoimmune disorders. *Clin Chem Lab Med* 2004; **42**(4): 359–70.

78. Sherer Y, Levy Y, Langevitz P et al. Adverse effects of intravenous immunoglobulin therapy in 56 patients with autoimmune diseases. *Pharmacology* 2001; **62**(3): 133–7.

79. Hutton B, Sharma R, Fergusson D et al. Use of intravenous immunoglobulin for treatment of recurrent miscarriage. *Br J Obstet Gynaecol* 2007; **114**: 134–42.

80. Stephenson MD, Kutteh W, Purkiss S et al. Intravenous immunoglobulin (IVIG) for treatment of idiopathic secondary recurrent miscarriage (ISRM). *Fertil Steril* 2009; **92**: S67–8.

81. Branch DW, Peaceman AM, Druzin M et al. A multicenter, placebo-controlled pilot study of intravenous immune globulin treatment of antiphospholipid syndrome during pregnancy. The Pregnancy Loss Study Group. *Am J Obstet Gynecol* 2000; **182** (1 Pt 1): 122–7.

82. http://www.rcog.org.uk/files/rcog-corp/uploaded-files/SACI5 mmunologicalTesting2008.pdf

83. Chilcott IT, Margara R, Cohen H et al. Pregnancy outcome is not affected by antiphospholipid antibody status in women referred for in vitro fertilization. *Fertil Steril* 2000; **73**(3): 526–30.

84. Practice Committee of American Society for Reproductive Medicine Anti-phospholipid antibodies do not affect IVF success. *Fertil Steril* 2008; **90**(5 Suppl): S172–3.

85. Dentali F, Crowther M. Acquired thrombophilia during pregnancy. *Obstet Gynecol Clin N Am* 2006; **33**(3): 375–88.

86. Nelen WL, Blom HJ, Steegers EA, den Heijer M, Eskes TK. Hyperhomocysteinemia and recurrent early pregnancy loss: a meta-analysis. *Fertil Steril* 2000; **74**(6): 1196–9.

87. Clarke R, Armitage J, Lewington S, Collins R. B-vitamin treatment trialists' collaboration homocysteine-lowering trials for prevention of vascular disease: protocol for a collaborative meta-analysis. *Clin Chem Lab Med* 2007; **45**(12): 1575–81.

88. Cikot RJ, Steegers-Theunissen RP, Thomas CM et al. Longitudinal vitamin and homocysteine levels in normal pregnancy. *Br J Nutr* 2001; **85**(1): 49–58.

89. MRC Vitamin Study Research Group. Prevalence of neural tube defects. *Lancet* 1991; **338**(8760): 131–7.

90. Dahlback B, Carlsson M, Svensson PJ. Familial thrombophilia due to a previously unrecognized mechanism characterized by poor anticoagulant response to activated protein C: prediction of a cofactor to activated protein C. *Proc Natl Acad Sci USA*, 1993; **90**: 1004–8.

91. Bertina RM, Koeleman BP, Koster T et al. Mutation in blood coagulation factor V associated with resistance to activated protein 1C. *Nature*, 1994; **369**: 64–7.

92. Laffan MA, Manning R. The influence of factor VIII on measurement of activated protein C resistance. *Blood Coagul Fibrinolysis* 1996; **7**(8): 761–5.

93. Rai R, Shlebak A, Cohen H et al. Factor V Leiden and acquired activated protein C resistance among 1000 women with recurrent miscarriage. *Hum Reprod* 2001; **16**(5): 961–5.

94. Cumming AM, Tait RC, Fildes S et al. Development of resistance to activated protein C during pregnancy. *Br J Haematol* 1995; **90**(3): 725–7.

95. Vincent T, Rai R, Regan L, Cohen H. Increased thrombin generation in women with recurrent miscarriage. *Lancet* 1998; **352**(9122): 116.

96. Smith GC, Pell JP, Walsh D. Spontaneous loss of early pregnancy and risk of ischaemic heart disease in later life: retrospective cohort study. *Br Med J* 2003; **326**(7386): 423–4.

97. Gris JC, Ripart-Neveu S, Maugard C et al. Respective evaluation of the prevalence of haemostasis abnormalities in unexplained primary early recurrent miscarriages. The Nimes Obstetricians and Haematologists (NOHA) Study. *Thromb Haemost* 1997; **77**(6): 1096–103.

98. Laude I, Rongieres-Bertrand C, Boyer-Neumann C et al. Circulating procoagulant microparticles in women with unexplained pregnancy loss: a new insight. *Thromb Haemost* 2001; **85**: 18–21.

99. Mallett SV, Cox DJ. Thrombelastography. *Br J Anaesth* 1992; **69**(3): 307–13.

100. Chandler WL. The thromboelastography and the thromboelastograph technique. *Semin Thromb Hemost* 1995; **21**(Suppl. 4): 1–6.

101. Handa ACDJ, Pasi KJ, Perry DJHG. Thromboelastography: An effective screening test for prothrombotic states. *Phlebology* 1997; **12**: 159–60.

102. Rai R, Tuddenham E, Backos M *et al.* Thromboelastography, whole-blood haemostasis and recurrent miscarriage. *Hum Reprod* 2003; **18**(12): 2540–3.

103. Clifford K, Rai R, Regan L. Future pregnancy outcome in unexplained recurrent first trimester miscarriage. *Hum Reprod* 1997; **12**(2): 387–9.

104. Brigham SA, Conlon C, Farquharson RG. A longitudinal study of pregnancy outcome folowing idiopathic recurrent miscarriage. *Hum Reprod* 1999; **14**(11): 2868–71.

105. Lindqvist PG, Merlo J. The natural course of women with recurrent fetal loss. *J Thromb Haemost* 2006; **4**(4): 896–7.

106. Liddell HS, Pattison NS, Zanderigo A. Recurrent miscarriage – outcome after supportive care in early pregnancy. *Aust N Z J Obstet Gynaecol* 1991; **31**: 320–2.

107. Kaandorp S, Di Nisio M, Goddijn M, Middeldorp S. Aspirin or anticoagulants for treating recurrent miscarriage in women without antiphospholipid syndrome. *Cochrane Database Syst Rev* 2009; **1** : CD004734.

108. Dolitzky M, Inbal A, Segal Y *et al.* A randomized study of thromboprophylaxis in women with unexplained consecutive recurrent miscarriages. *Fertil Steril* 2006; **86**(2): 362–6.

109. DiNisio M, Peters L, Middledorp S. Anticoagulants for the treatment of recurrent pregnancy loss in women without antiphospholipid syndrome. *Cochrane Database Syst Rev* 2005; **2**: CD004734.

# Inherited thrombophilia and early pregnancy

Saskia Middeldorp

## Thrombophilia

The term thrombophilia is most often used to describe a laboratory phenomenon that is associated with an increased tendency to venous thromboembolism, either acquired or inherited [1].

The most clearly established acquired thrombophilia is the antiphospholipid syndrome. This is a non-inflammatory auto-immune disease characterized by thrombosis or pregnancy complications in the presence of antiphospholipid antibodies [2]. In this chapter, primary antiphospholipid syndrome is considered, i.e. in the absence of systemic lupus erythematodes. Antiphospholipid antibodies are a wide and heterogeneous group of immunoglobulins that include, among others, lupus anticoagulants and anticardiolipin antibodies. Antiphospholipid antibodies recognize plasma proteins bound to suitable anionic surfaces. Preliminary criteria for the diagnosis of definite antiphospholipid syndrome were formulated at an international consensus meeting in 1999 and updated in 2005 [3,4]. Clinical criteria include having one or more clinical episodes of thrombosis, one or more unexplained fetal deaths (later than 10 weeks of gestation), or having three or more unexplained consecutive miscarriages (before 10 weeks of gestation). Laboratory criteria include lupus anticoagulant present in plasma, or medium or high titers of anticardiolipin antibody of IgG or IgM isotype in serum or plasma, or anti-$\beta$2 glycoprotein-I antibody of IgG or IgM in serum or plasma. Antiphospholipid syndrome is diagnosed if at least one of the clinical criteria and one of the laboratory criteria are met. To prevent the detection of transiently present antiphospholipid antibodies, laboratory tests should be performed twice, 12 weeks apart, and should be positive on both occasions. Since the clinical criteria as described above are prevalent in the general population, the diagnosis of antiphospholipid syndrome is largely based on laboratory tests. The prevalence of persistent lupus anticoagulant or antibodies against phospholipid in the general population is not well known. Although some population-based studies have estimated the prevalence of one or more positive tests, in most studies these were only assessed once [5–8].

Well-established hereditary thrombophilias can be categorized into abnormalities of the natural anticoagulant system and elevation of plasma levels of activated coagulation factors. In Figure 14.1, the current, highly simplified insight into the regulation of the coagulation system is depicted. Coagulation is initiated by a tissue factor (TF)-activated factor VII (FVIIa) complex that can activate factor IX or factor X. At high tissue factor concentrations, factor X is activated primarily by the TF–FVIIa complex, whereas at low tissue factor concentrations the contribution of the factor IXa–factor VIIIa complex to the activation of factor X becomes more pronounced. Coagulation is maintained through the activation of factor XI by thrombin. The coagulation system is regulated by the protein C pathway. Thrombin activates protein C. With protein S as a cofactor, activated protein C (APC) inactivates factors Va and VIIIa, which results in a downregulation of thrombin generation and consequently in an upregulation of the fibrinolytic system. Antithrombin is the other important natural anticoagulant that inhibits not only thrombin but also factor Xa and other coagulation factors by forming irreversible complexes.

Most laboratories include in their work-up of acquired thrombophilia tests that detect lupus anticoagulant and anticardiolipin antibodies of the IgG and IgM type; less routinely, levels of anti-$\beta$2 glycoprotein-I antibody of IgG and IgM type are measured. For inherited thrombophilia, the panel usually

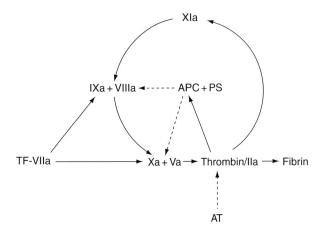

**Figure 14.1** Regulation of blood coagulation. Coagulation is initiated by a tissue factor (TF)–factor VIIa complex that can activate factor IX or factor X. At high tissue factor concentrations, factor X is activated primarily by the TF–VIIa complex, whereas at low tissue factor concentrations the contribution of the factor IXa–factor VIIIa complex to the activation of factor X becomes more pronounced. Coagulation is maintained through the activation by thrombin of factor XI. The coagulation system is regulated by the protein C pathway. Thrombin activates protein C. Together with protein S, activated protein C (APC) is capable of inactivating factors Va and VIIIa, which results in a down-regulation of thrombin generation and consequently in an up-regulation of the fibrinolytic system. The activity of thrombin is controlled by the inhibitor antithrombin. The solid arrows indicate activation and the broken arrows inhibition.

consists of plasma activity levels of antithrombin, protein C and protein S, factor V Leiden, and the prothrombin 20210A mutation; less common are factor VIII activity and homocysteine. Deficiencies of the natural anticoagulants antithrombin, protein C, or protein S are relatively strong risk factors for venous thromboembolism, but are rare, whereas the gain of function mutations factor V Leiden (that causes resistance of factor Va inactivation by activated protein C, APC resistance) and prothrombin 20210A are less strong but more prevalent. Mild hyperhomocysteinemia is associated with both venous thromboembolism and atherosclerosis and often occurs within families. However, there is no association between venous thromboembolism and specific mutations that cause hyperhomocysteinemia, and interventions to lower homocysteine levels do not have clinical benefit [9–11]. This suggests that hyperhomocysteinemia may be a marker rather than a risk factor for venous and arterial disease. Persistently elevated levels of coagulation factor VIII are also associated with an increased risk of venous thromboembolism and also occur within families. Although the cause of the elevation in factor VIII is unclear, it appears that factor VIII levels are, in part, determined genetically.

## The risk of venous thromboembolism in pregnancy

Normal pregnancy leads to extensive changes in hemostasis, increasing the procoagulant side of the coagulation balance. These changes in pregnancy are thought to be part of a complex physiological adaptation, which ensures control of bleeding from the placental site at the time of placental separation, while allowing the expansion of the maternal and fetal circulations at the uteroplacental interface during pregnancy [12]. These adaptations are the likely explanation for the increased risk of venous thromboembolism during pregnancy. Approximately two-thirds of all pregnancy-related venous thromboembolisms occur during pregnancy, and about one-third in the puerperium. Although the risk increases with gestational age, 22% of thrombotic episodes occur during the first trimester of pregnancy, followed by 34% and 44% during the second and third trimester [13].

Women with thrombophilia have an increased baseline risk of venous thromboembolism. For women who are diagnosed to have antiphospholipid syndrome based on complications in pregnancy, the risk of venous thromboembolism in a subsequent pregnancy is not well known. The few studies that have been published show a low risk, but these estimates are obtained in women who often have received various heparin regimens to prevent other pregnancy complications [14,15]. A cohort study amongst women with recurrent miscarriage did not show a significantly different risk for venous thrombotic events between women with antiphospholipid syndrome (4/1000 women–years) and women in whom the miscarriages were unexplained (1/1000 women–years) [14].

For women who were tested for inherited thrombophilia in the context of a family history of venous thromboembolism, risk estimates of venous thromboembolism overall, as well as during transient risk factors have been obtained in family studies. The overall risks, as well as the risk per pregnancy and per year of oral contraceptive use are listed in Table 14.1. It should be noted that the setting of testing matters, since it is assumed that in these families concomitant,

**Table 14.1** Incidences of first venous thromboembolism during pregnancy and oral contraceptive use in women with thrombophilia, as opposed to overall incidences in men and women.

| | Antiphospholipid syndrome diagnosed, based on pregnancy morbidity | Antithrombin, protein C or protein S deficiency | Factor V Leiden | Prothrombin 20210A | Elevated FVIII:c levels | Mild hyperhomo-cysteinemia |
|---|---|---|---|---|---|---|
| Pregnancy (%/pregnancy, 95%CI) | | 4.1 (1.7–8.3) [69] 1.2 (0.3–4.2) | 2.1 (0.7–4.9) [69,70] | 2.3 (0.8–5.3) [71] 0.5 (0.1–2.6) | 1.3 (0.4–3.4) [72] 0.3 (0.1–1.8) | 0.5 (0.0–2.6) [73] 0.0 (0.0–1.8) |
| • during pregnancy | 0.0 (0.0–3.4) [15] | 3.0 (1.3–6.7) | 0.4 (0.1–2.4) | 1.9 (0.7–4.7) | 1.0 (0.3–2.9) | 0.5 (0.0–2.6) |
| • during puerperium | 1.1 (0.6–5.5) [15] | | 1.7 (0.7–4.3) | | | |
| Oral contraceptive use (%/year of use) | unknown | 4.3 (1.4–9.7) [69] | 0.5 (0.1–1.4) [69,70] | 0.2 (0.0–0.9) [71] | 0.6 (0.2–1.5) [70] | 0.1 (0.0–0.7) [73] |
| Overall (%/year) | 0.4 (0.1–1.0) [14] | 1.5 (0.7–2.8) [74] | 0.5 (0.1–1.3) [69,75] | 0.4 (0.1–1.1) [76] | 1.3 (0.5–2.7) [72] | 0.2 (0.1–0.3) [73] |

Notes: The risk estimates for women with antiphospholipid syndrome are for women without history of venous thromboembolism, and are obtained with various antithrombotic approaches including heparin prophylaxis.

The risk estimates for inherited thrombophilia were obtained in women with a family history of venous thromboembolism, defined as at least one first degree symptomatic relative in studies of factor V Leiden, prothrombin 20210A, elevated levels of FVIIIa and hyperhomocysteinemia; at least one first- or second-degree relative in studies of antithrombin, protein C, or protein S deficiency.

but yet unknown, inherited thrombophilias are present. Thus, the risk is likely to be lower if women have been tested for other reasons, most notably for pregnancy failure.

## Association between thrombophilia and pregnancy failure

In antiphospholipid syndrome, lupus anticoagulant is more strongly related to venous thrombosis and pregnancy complications than antibodies against phospholipids [16,17]. For recurrent pregnancy loss, the importance of anti-β2 glycoprotein-I antibodies is not clearly established [17]. The association between inherited thrombophilic disorders and miscarriage was first observed in women from families with venous thrombosis [18–20]. In these cohort studies, probands were identified because of venous thromboembolism and a specific inherited thrombophilic disorder. A detailed history of previous pregnancies and miscarriages was taken in all women. Relatives were also investigated, and a standardized history was taken before the thrombophilia status was determined. It

was found that the risk of pregnancy loss was higher in carriers as compared to non-carriers. Since then, the association with both single and recurrent pregnancy loss has been confirmed in many studies, mostly with a case-control design [21,22].

The concept that recurrent miscarriage is a multi-causal disease is well established. Structural chromosomal abnormalities in the parents, antiphospholipid antibody syndrome of the woman, random numerical fetal chromosomal abnormalities, infectious, endocrine and immunological factors, as well as uterine anomalies are considered to play a role in the etiology of recurrent miscarriage [23]. In approximately half of the patients, recurrent miscarriage remains unexplained. It is difficult to estimate the prevalence of thrombophilia in women with recurrent miscarriage, since there is poor standardization of tests of antibodies against phospholipid, and the prevalence of inherited thrombophilia varies between populations. Furthermore, in published studies, patients have been selected based on different criteria.

A single late fetal loss and severe preeclampsia are also associated with inherited thrombophilia,

**Table 14.2** Assocation between various forms of thrombophilia and several forms of pregnancy failure

| Thrombophilia defect | Sporadic miscarriage OR (95% CI) | Recurrent miscarriage[*] OR (95% CI) | Intra-uterine fetal death[*] OR (95% CI) |
|---|---|---|---|
| **1a. Family studies** | | | |
| Antithrombin, protein C, or protein S deficiency | 2.0 (1.2–3.3) [18] 1.3 (0.9–1.7) [19] | 2.6 (0.8–8.0) [18] | 3.6 (0.5–7.7) [19] |
| Factor V Leiden mutation | 1.0 (0.6–1.7) [19] 2.0 (1.1–3.8) [20] | 2.6 (1.0–7.0) [20] | 1.4 (0.5–4.0) [20] |
| Prothrombin 20210A mutation | 1.3 (0.7–2.6) [71] | 0.9 (0.3–3.3) [71] | – |
| Homozygous defects or combinations of defects | 0.8 (0.2–3.6)[§] [19] 2.9 (1.5–5.8)[#] [20] | – | 14.3 (2.4–86)[§] [19] 6.4 (1.0–39)[#] [20] |
| Mild hyperhomocysteinemia | 0.8 (0.5–1.5) [77] | 1.1 (0.2–6.2) [77] | – |
| Elevated FVIII:c levels | 1.2 (0.7–1.9) [77] | 1.1 (0.4–3.1) [77] | – |
| **1b. Case-control studies** | | | |
| Antiphospholipid syndrome, lupus anticoagulant | – | 7.8 (2.3–26.5) [17] | 1.4 (0.72–0.80) [78][†] |
| Antiphospholipid syndrome, anticardiolipin antibodies | – | IgG 3.6 (2.3–5.7) [17] IgM 5.6 (1.3–25.0) [17] | |
| Antiphospholipid syndrome, anti-β2 glycoprotein-I antibodies | – | 2.1 (0.7–6.5) [17] | |
| Antithrombin deficiency | 1.5 (1.0–2.5) [21] | 0.9 (0.2–4.5) [21] | 7.6 (0.3–196)(22) |
| Protein C deficiency | 1.4 (1.0–2.1) [21] | 1.6 (0.2–10.5) [21] | 3.1 (0.2–38.5) [22] |
| Protein S deficiency | Heterogeneous data [21] | 14.7 (1.0–218.0) [21] | 7.4 (1.3–42.8) [21] 20.1 (3.7–109.2) [22] |
| Factor V Leiden mutation | 1.7 (1.2–2.5) [21] 1.7 (1.1–2.6) [22] | 2.0 (1.1–3.6) [21] 1.9 (1.0–3.6) [22] | 3.3 (1.8–5.8) [21] 2.1 (1.1–3.9) [22] |
| Prothrombin 20210A mutation | 2.1 (1.2–3.5) [21] 2.5 (1.2–5.0) [22] | 2.3 (1.1–4.8) [21] 2.7 (1.4–5.3) [22] | 2.3 (1.1–4.9) [21] 2.7 (1.3–5.5) [22] |
| Homozygous defects or combinations of defects | 2.7 (1.3–5.6) [22] | – | – |
| Mild hyperhomocysteinemia | 6.3 (1.4–28.4) [22] | 2.7 (1.4–5.2) [79] 4.2 (1.3–13.9) [22] | 1.0 (0.2–5.6) [22] |

[*] definition varies across studies.
[§] combined thrombophilia defects vs. no defect.
[#] homozygous Factor V Leiden vs. normal genotype.
[†] single intra-uterine fetal death.

[21,22,24], whereas an association is controversial in women with intra-uterine growth restriction and placental abruption [22,25].

Table 14.2 lists the strengths of the associations among various forms of pregnancy loss. The association between recurrent miscarriage and the presence of lupus anticoagulant and anticardiolipin antibodies was investigated in a meta-analysis and showed homogeneous results among the 25 included case-control studies, despite varying definitions of recurrent pregnancy loss, assays, and cut-off values used [17]. For inherited thrombophilia, the association tends to be stronger in the more "severe" forms of pregnancy loss, i.e. recurrent, or late losses. It should be noted that significant heterogeneity between studies was found in the two meta-analyses [21,22]. Also, it is important to bear in mind that most studies on the association between inherited thrombophilia and pregnancy loss have used definitions in which early pregnancy loss was defined quite variably, as loss before 10 weeks' gestational age until later than 20 weeks, without using ultrasound criteria. The association between factor V Leiden and recurrent miscarriage was robust when other potential underlying causes of fetal loss were excluded [21].

Although causality of the relationship is difficult to assess [26,27], this knowledge has further increased the number of investigations in couples with recurrent miscarriage, although the therapeutic consequences of a positive test result are yet uncertain [28]. The mechanisms of how thrombophilia leads to pregnancy complications remain obscure. It is attractive to hypothesize that hypercoagulability with thrombosis of placental vasculature is the pathophysiological substrate for the association between both acquired (antiphospholipid antibody syndrome) and inherited thrombophilia. However, it is likely that inflammatory mechanisms are implicated, in particular for early miscarriage in the context of antiphospholipid antibody syndrome [29]. In vitro experiments have shown that antiphospholipid antibodies inhibit extravillous trophoblast differentiation and subsequent placentation [30]. Although tissue factor activation seems to play a central role, this appears independent of its role in coagulation [31]. This "non-prothrombotic theory" is supported by the observation that both heparin and aspirin attenuate trophoblast apoptosis in vitro [32]. Based on these observations, it is not biologically plausible that a thrombotic component in women with inherited thrombophilia plays a key role. Furthermore, the placental vasculature has not been developed until 10 to 12 weeks' gestational age, and thus the thrombosis hypothesis leaves unexplained why the vast majority of women with recurrent miscarriage have early losses. For the common forms of inherited thrombophilia, experimental models for studying trophoblast differentiation and early placentation are not readily available. However, thrombomodulin-deficient mice, who are lacking the important natural anticoagulant protein C pathway, are unable to carry their fetuses beyond 8.5 weeks' gestational age, and dead fetuses are usually resorbed within 24 hours [33]. Fetal demise is caused by tissue factor-dependent activation of blood coagulation at the feto-maternal interface, and activated coagulation factors were found to induce cell death and inhibit growth of trophoblast cells. Administration of heparin or aspirin

to the mice delayed absorption of their embryos, but was unable to restore trophoblast differentiation and overcome the growth defect of these thrombomodulin deficient embryos.

Thus, mere hypercoagulability is unlikely to be the sole mechanism by which thrombophilia, either acquired or inherited, increases the risk for early pregnancy failure.

## Clinical implications of thrombophilia in early pregnancy

A general consideration is whether it is indicated to test women with a history of venous thromboembolism or with pregnancy failure for inherited thrombophilia. Although this is often performed, consequences of a positive or negative test are uncertain, whereas potential harms include complications of intensified anticoagulant treatment or prophylaxis, as well as the psychological impact of the knowledge of having a genetic defect, and costs [34].

In the next paragraphs, the evidence regarding potential clinical implications of acquired and inherited thrombophilia are reviewed for both venous thromboembolism and for pregnancy failure.

## Prevention of venous thromboembolism in women with thrombophilia without prior venous thromboembolism

In general, high-grade evidence regarding prophylaxis of venous thromboembolism in pregnancy and the postpartum period is lacking [35]. The optimal management for asymptomatic pregnant women with thrombophilia is uncertain and also depends on how the absolute risk of VTE (0.3%–1.2%, Table 14.1) is perceived by an individual woman and her treating physician, and weighed against the drawbacks of thrombosis prophylaxis. Women with antiphospholipid syndrome and recurrent pregnancy loss are generally treated with aspirin and low-molecular-weight heparin with the objective of improving pregnancy outcome in a subsequent pregnancy (see next section). This approach likely decreases the risk of venous thromboembolism as well. The common nuisances consist of the daily subcutaneous injections of low-molecular-weight heparin, which give rise to a high prevalence of aspecific itching skin reactions [36]. The risk of heparin-induced thrombocytopenia is considered to be too low to recommend regular platelet counts, but women using low-molecular-weight heparin are less likely to receive epidural catheters for pain relief during delivery due to the fear of epidural bleeding [37]. The weak level of recommendations in guidelines reflects the absence of evidence with its inherent uncertainty [38]. It seems generally justified to withhold anticoagulant prophylaxis in pregnancy in women with inherited thrombophilia. Although antithrombin deficiency is considered as giving a very high risk of pregnancy-related venous thromboembolism, which is also reflected by the recommendation to install prophylaxis with low-molecular-weight heparin, this common perception is not supported by studies within families that were not subject to selection bias [39–41]. In the puerperium the risk of thrombosis is higher (1.0%–3.0%, Table 14.1), so prophylaxis with anticoagulants (either vitamin K antagonists or low-molecular-weight heparin) should be considered, in particular for women with one of the deficiencies of the natural anticoagulants or combined thrombophilic defects [38]. Whether the low absolute risks in asymptomatic women with inherited thrombophilia justify testing all women or those with a family history of thrombosis or a known thrombophilia in the family, is widely debated [42,43]. The optimal dose of low-molecular-weight heparin is also uncertain, and in most centers asymptomatic women will be prescribed low-dose low-molecular-weight heparin for 4 to 6 weeks' postpartum.

## Prevention of venous thromboembolism in women with thrombophilia and a history of venous thromboembolism

There are no management studies for prophylaxis in pregnant women with thrombophilia and a history of deep-venous thrombosis. In two observational studies, the risk of antepartum recurrent VTE in women with a history of VTE ranged between 2.4% and 6.2% if no prophylaxis was installed [44,45]. In the first prospective study, an idiopathic first thromboembolic event as well as thrombophilia appeared to be risk factors for recurrence during the subsequent pregnancy [44], whereas this could not be confirmed in the second retrospective study [45]. In view of the high risk of recurrence, which was constant during all trimesters of pregnancy, anticoagulant prophylaxis with low-molecular-weight heparin from early pregnancy onwards should be strongly considered in women with an idiopathic first event or thrombophilia. It

should be noted that, in the prospective study [44], women with known thrombophilia were excluded. In particular, women with antiphospholipid syndrome are considered to be at high risk of recurrent venous thromboembolism and will generally either receive long-term anticoagulant therapy or prophylaxis during a subsequent pregnancy.

Some observational studies showed that recurrent venous thromboembolism tends to occur most often in women treated with lower doses of low-molecular-weight heparin [45–47]. This finding suggests that intermediate (75–150 anti-Xa units/kg/per day) or even therapeutic dosages may be preferred. Heparins should be discontinued at least 12 hours before delivery and restarted afterwards to avoid peripartum hemorrhage [38].

Women who are using vitamin K antagonists for secondary thrombosis prophylaxis outside pregnancy and who intend to become pregnant, should be bridged with therapeutic dose low-molecular-weight heparin throughout the entire pregnancy. Vitamin K antagonists used in the first trimester of pregnancy may lead to serious warfarin embryopathy. However, this does not occur if the induced maternal vitamin K deficiency is restored before 6 weeks after the first day of the last menstruation [48]. Therefore, a practical approach is to advise women to perform frequent urine pregnancy tests from the day of expected menstruation and to immediately discontinue vitamin K antagonists as soon as the test is positive. At the same time, they should start therapeutic dose low-molecular-weight heparin based on body weight, and take vitamin K (for instance 5 mg) by mouth for 3 consecutive days. If they are taking vitamin K antagonists with a long half-life, it can be considered to switch to shorter-acting coumadin derivates before they are pregnant.

## Women with thrombophilia and recurrent miscarriage

Given the observed association between thrombophilia and recurrent miscarriage, it is tempting to speculate about a potential benefit of anticoagulant therapy in these women. A Cochrane review on its efficacy in women with antiphospholipid syndrome performed in 2005 evaluated various (anticoagulant or aspirin) treatment regimens and concluded that only half of the trials had adequate concealment of allocation, a key component of study quality [49]. Two trials investigated aspirin alone and did not demonstrate a beneficial effect on a subsequent pregnancy outcome [50,51]. Two trials with a total of 140 patients showed a clear benefit of unfractionated heparin combined with aspirin as compared with aspirin alone, with a 54% relative risk reduction of pregnancy loss [52]. One trial in 98 women compared low-molecular-weight heparin combined with aspirin to aspirin alone and found no benefit (relative risk of pregnancy loss 0.78, 0.39–1.57) [53]. Recently, another trial was published that evaluated the same interventions in 88 women with recurrent miscarriage, half of whom had antiphospholipid syndrome [54]. Also, in this trial, no benefit was observed of one over the other treatment arm, with high live birth rates of 78% and 79%, respectively, regardless of presence of antiphospholipid syndrome or history of early vs. late recurrent pregnancy loss. Whether the differences in findings between unfractionated heparin and low-molecular-weight heparin are the result of different effects on, for instance, early placentation remains to be elucidated. It is interesting to note that women who were included in the trials where a treatment effect was observed had a markedly lower live birth rate in the comparator arm (42%–44% as compared with 68%–83% in the trials where no benefit was found from an intervention).

Treatment guidelines vary with regard to the administration of heparin for antiphospholipid syndrome and recurrent miscarriage. The American College of Chest Physicians (ACCP) guidelines recommend the combination of low-dose aspirin *and* a low dose of either unfractionated or low molecular weight heparin (LMWH) (level of evidence: 1B), whereas the European Society for Human Reproduction and Embryology (ESHRE) guidelines recommend the prescription of aspirin *with* or *without* LMWH (level of evidence: 2B) [38,55]. Noteworthy, based on the findings of the beforementioned Cochrane review, there is no evidence that aspirin has any benefit at all [49].

For women with inherited thrombophilia, evidence regarding the effectiveness of anticoagulant therapy or aspirin is still lacking [26,27]. The main problem is that arguments in favor of heparin are based either on case series or on randomized controlled trials without a placebo or no treatment arm. However, using a woman's history as the comparator in uncontrolled case series results in a bias toward positive outcome of any investigational treatment in the next pregnancy, as the prognosis of women with recurrent miscarriage appears good in many

reports [56]. This phenomenon of "regression to the mean" is nicely illustrated in a population study. Amongst 2480 pregnant women, 37 had a history of recurrent miscarriage; nevertheless their live birth rate was 89% without any intervention, whereas this rate before the index pregnancies was 28% [57]. This was not separately assessed for women with thrombophilia. In a report from a tertiary recurrent miscarriage clinic in the United Kingdom, the outcome of untreated pregnancies amongst 19 women heterozygous for the factor V Leiden mutation who had a history of recurrent early miscarriage was much lower compared with women with a similar pregnancy history without factor V Leiden (38% vs. 69%; OR 3.8, 95%CI 1.3–10.9) [58].

A randomized experimental approach is absolutely necessary for establishing whether anticoagulant therapy is beneficial in women with thrombophilia and pregnancy complications, in order to avoid the problem of confounding by indication. Only one randomized trial has been published in which two doses of enoxaparin (40 mg and 80 mg) were compared in women with inherited thrombophilia and recurrent pregnancy loss [59]. There was no difference between both treatment arms, with live birth rates of 84% and 78%. Unfortunately, this trial did not have a no treatment or placebo arm, which is the only appropriate comparator given the uncertainty about the natural history of recurrent miscarriage in thrombophilic women.

Recently, two trials in women with unexplained recurrent miscarriages failed to demonstrate a beneficial effect of aspirin, or aspirin combined with low-molecular-weight heparin as compared to placebo or no treatment [60, 66]. In one of those trials, an a priori subgroup analysis of women with thrombophilia did not show a significant effect of this intervention either, although the study was not powered for subgroup analyses [60].

## Women with inherited thrombophilia and a single pregnancy loss

In one trial women with one unexplained pregnancy loss after the tenth week of gestation and who were carriers of the factor V Leiden mutation, the factor II G20210A mutation, or had protein S deficiency, were randomized to low-molecular-weight heparin (enoxaparin, 40 mg/day) or low-dose aspirin (100 mg/day), given from the beginning of the eighth week of gestation [62]. In the enoxaparin group, 69 out of 80 women (86%) had a healthy live birth, which was remarkably different from 23 out of 80 women (29%) in the aspirin group (absolute risk difference 58%, 95%CI 43%–68% [60]. However, several methodological issues were raised, which included a quasi-randomized design and inadequate concealment of allocation [63,64]. Also, the prognosis of the women treated with aspirin was unexpectedly poor and in contrast to findings from another study. Here, patients with documented venous thromboembolism or premature atherosclerosis and carriership of the factor V Leiden or prothrombin 20210A mutation were included, as well as their first-degree relatives [65]. The live birth rates of the second pregnancy following a first loss were 77% (95%CI 62–87) in carriers and 76% (95%CI 57–89) in non-carriers after a first early miscarriage. After a late miscarriage in the first pregnancy, the live birth rate of the second pregnancy was 68% (95%CI 46–85) in carriers and 80% (95%CI 49–94) in non-carriers (OR 0.9, 95%CI 0.5–1.3).

Given the current evidence, women with a single pregnancy loss and inherited thrombophilia should be reassured that they have a high chance of a successful subsequent pregnancy without intervention with low-molecular-weight heparin.

## Other observations in women with inherited thrombophilia

Two prospective observational, non-randomized studies in women with familial thrombophilia assessed the effect of thrombosis prophylaxis on fetal loss, which was primarily given for the indication of thrombosis prophylaxis [66,67]. Such an assessment appears valid, assuming that there is no link between the decision to prescribe heparin and the perceived prognosis of fetal loss [68]. In the first study that included 83 women with thrombophilia who received thrombosis prophylaxis at some point during the first pregnancy in prospective follow-up, only 20 women (28%) received thrombosis prophylaxis to prevent fetal loss [66]. Among 21 women with thrombophilia who used heparin or oral anticoagulants before week 5 of the pregnancy until the end of the pregnancy, five (24%) experienced fetal loss, with an unadjusted relative risk of fetal loss associated with thrombosis prophylaxis of 1.1 (95% CI 0.4, 3.3), and a relative risk adjusted for center, total number of pregnancies, history of fetal loss and maternal age at gestation of 0.7 (95% CI 0.2, 3.2). In the second study, 26 of 37 women (70%) with a deficiency of antithrombin, protein C or protein S received thrombosis prophylaxis during pregnancy, mostly to prevent recurrent venous thromboembolism [67]. Prophylaxis was refused by 11 deficient women, most of whom had no history of venous thromboembolism. None of 26 deficient women with thrombosis prophylaxis experienced fetal loss, in contrast to five of 11 deficient women (45%) without thromboprophylaxis, with a relative risk adjusted for clustering of women in families of 0.07 (95% CI 0.01–0.7). The very different results from these studies cannot be easily explained by differences in study design or selection of patients.

## Conclusions

Women with thrombophilia are at increased risk for pregnancy-related venous thromboembolism. In general, antepartum anticoagulant prophylaxis can be withheld in women without a history of venous thromboembolism, whereas prophylaxis with at least intermediate doses of low-molecular-weight heparin throughout pregnancy are likely to be the best choice in women who have experienced venous thromboembolism in the past. Postpartum prophylaxis should be considered in asymptomatic women with inherited thrombophilia, and definitely in women with a thrombotic history.

Pregnancy failure and other vascular pregnancy complications are associated with the presence of both acquired and inherited thrombophilia. Mechanisms are likely to involve effects on trophoblast differentiation rather than mere hypercoagulability. For women with antiphospholipid syndrome, the evidence regarding the efficacy of aspirin with or without the addition of low-molecular-weight heparin is not solid, whereas two small trials have shown a clear benefit of unfractionated heparin. For women with inherited thrombophilia, low-molecular-weight heparin to prevent pregnancy loss is definitely experimental as solid evidence is not yet available. Aspirin alone or combined with low-molecular-weight heparin does not improve pregnancy outcome in women with unexplained recurrent pregnancy loss. Randomized controlled trials with an appropriate control group of either no treatment or placebo are currently being carried out and results should be awaited before anticoagulant prophylaxis of pregnancy failure in women with inherited thrombophilia can be implemented.

## References

1. Coppens M, Kaandorp SP, Middeldorp S. Inherited thrombophilias. *Obstet Gynecol Clin N Am* 2006; **33**(3): 357–74.

2. Urbanus RT, Derksen RH, de Groot PG. Current insight into diagnostics and pathophysiology of the antiphospolipid syndrome. *Blood Rev* 2008; **22**(2): 93–105.

3. Wilson WA, Gharavi AE, Koike T *et al.* International consensus statement on preliminary classification criteria for definite antiphospholipid syndrome: report of an international workshop. *Arthritis Rheum* 1999 Jul; **42**(7): 1309–11.

4. Miyakis S, Lockshin MD, Atsumi T, Branch DW, Brey RL, Cervera R *et al.* International consensus statement on an update of the classification criteria for definite antiphospholipid syndrome (APS). *Thromb Haemost* 2006; **4**(2): 295–306.

5. Ginsburg KS, Liang MH, Newcomer L, *et al.* Anticardiolipin antibodies and the risk for ischemic stroke and venous thrombosis. *Ann Int Med* 1992; **117**(12): 997–1002.

6. Runchey SS, Folsom AR, Tsai MY, Cushman M, McGovern PD. Anticardiolipin antibodies as a risk factor for venous thromboembolism in a population-based prospective study. *Br J Haematol* 2002; **119**(4): 1005–10.

7. de Groot PG, Lutters B, Derksen RH, Lisman T, Meijers JCM, Rosendaal FR. Lupus anticoagulants and the risk of a first episode of deep venous thrombosis. *J Thromb Haemost* 2005; **3**(9): 1993–7.

8. Naess IA, Christiansen SC, Cannegieter SC, Rosendaal FR, Hammerstroem J. A prospective study of anticardiolipin antibodies as a risk factor for venous thrombosis in a general population (the HUNT study). *J Thromb Haemost* 2006; **4**(1): 44–9.

9. Ray JG, Shmorgun D, Chan WS. Common C677T polymorphism of the methylenetetrahydrofolate reductase gene and the risk of venous thromboembolism: meta-analysis of 31 studies. *Pathophysiol Haemost Thromb* 2002; **32**(2): 51–8.

10. Rosenberg IH, Mulrow CD. Trials that matter: should we routinely measure homocysteine levels and "treat" mild hyperhomocysteinemia? *Ann Int Med* 2006; **145**(3): 226–7.

11. den Heijer M, Willems HP, Blom HJ *et al.* Homocysteine lowering by B vitamins and the secondary prevention of deep-vein thrombosis and pulmonary embolism. A randomized, placebo-controlled, double blind trial. *Blood* 2007; **109**: 139–44.

12. O'Riordan MN, Higgins JR. Haemostasis in normal and abnormal pregnancy. *Best Pract Res Clin Obstet Gynaecol* 2003; **17**(3): 385–96.

13. Ray JG, Chan WS. Deep vein thrombosis during pregnancy and the puerperium: a meta-analysis of the period of risk and the leg of presentation. *Obstet Gynecol Surv* 1999; **54**: 265–71.

14. Quenby S, Farquharson RG, Dawood F, Hughes AM, Topping J. Recurrent miscarriage and long-term thrombosis risk: a case-control study. *Hum Reprod* 2005; **20**(6): 1729–32.

15. Clark CA, Spitzer KA, Crowther MA *et al.* Incidence of postpartum thrombosis and preterm delivery in women with antiphospholipid antibodies and recurrent pregnancy loss. *J Rheumatol* 2007; **34**(5): 992–6.

16. Galli M, Luciani D, Bertolini G, Barbui T. Lupus anticoagulants are stronger risk factors for thrombosis than anticardiolipin antibodies in the antiphospholipid syndrome: a systematic review of the literature. *Blood* 2003; **101**(5): 1827–32.

17. Opatrny L, David M, Kahn SR, Shrier I, Rey E. Association between antiphospholipid antibodies and recurrent fetal loss in women without autoimmunie disease: a metaanalysis. *J Rheumatol* 2006; **33**(11): 2214–21.

18. Sanson BJ, Friederich PW, Simioni P *et al.* The risk of abortion and stillbirth in antithrombin-, protein C-, and protein S-deficient women. *Thromb Haemost* 1996; **75**(3): 387–8.

19. Preston FE, Rosendaal FR, Walker ID *et al.* Increased fetal loss in women with heritable thrombophilia. *Lancet* 1996; **348**: 913–6.

20. Meinardi JR, Middeldorp S, de Kam PJ *et al.* Increased risk for fetal loss in carriers of the factor V Leiden mutation. *Ann Int Med* 1999; **130**(9): 736–9.

21. Rey E, Kahn SR, David M, Shrier I. Thrombophilic disorders and fetal loss: a meta-analysis. *Lancet* 2003; **361**: 901–8.

22. Robertson L, Wu O, Langhorne P *et al.* Thrombophilia in pregnancy: a systematic review. *Br J Haematol* 2006; **132**(2): 171–96.

23. Rai R, Regan L. Recurrent miscarriage. *Lancet* 2006; **368**(9535): 601–11.

24. Morrison ER, Miedzybrodzka ZH, Campbell DM *et al.* Prothrombotic genotypes are not associated with pre-eclampsia and gestational hypertension: results from a large population-based study and systematic review. *Thromb Haemost* 2002; **87**: 779–85.

25. Pabinger I, Vormittag R. Thrombophilia and pregnancy outcomes. *J Thromb Haemost* 2005; **3**(8): 1603–10.

26. Middeldorp S. Thrombophilia and regnancy complications: cause or association? *J Thromb Haemost* 2007; **5**(Suppl. 1): 276–82.

27. Rodger MA, Paidas MJ, Mclintock C *et al.* Inherited thrombophilia and pregnancy complications revisited: association not proven causal and antithrombotic prophylaxis is experimental. *Obstet Gynecol* 2008; **112**(2): 320–4.

28. Norrie G, Farquharson RG, Greaves M. Screening and treatment for heritable thrombophilia in pregnancy failure: inconsistencies among UK early pregnancy units. *Br J Haematol* 2009; **144**(2): 241–4.

29. Sebire NJ, Regan L, Rai R. Biology and pathology of the placenta in relation to antiphospholipid antibody-associated pregnancy failure. *Lupus* 2002; **11**(10): 641–3.

30. Quenby S, Mountfield S, Cartwright JE, Whitley GS, Chamley L, Vince G. Antiphospholipid antibodies prevent extravillous trophoblast differentiation. *Fertil Steril* 2005; **83**(3): 691–8.

31. Redecha P, Franzke CW, Ruf W, Mackman N, Girardi G. Neutrophil activation by the tissue factor/Factor VIIa/PAR2 axis mediates fetal death in a mouse model of antiphospholipid syndrome. *J Clin Invest* 2008; **118**(10): 3453–61.

32. Bose P, Black S, Kadyrov M *et al*. Heparin and aspirin attenuate placental apoptosis in vitro: implications for early pregnancy failure. *Am J Obstet Gynecol* 2005; **192**(1): 23–30.

33. Isermann B, Sood R, Pawlinski R *et al*. The thrombomodulin-protein C system is essential for the maintenance of pregnancy. *Nat Med* 2003; **9**(3): 331–7.

34. Cohn DM, Vansenne F, Kaptein AA, de Borgie CA, Middeldorp S. The psychological impact of testing for thrombophilia: a systematic review. *J Thromb Haemost* 2008; **6**: 1099–104.

35. Gates S, Brocklehurst P, Davis LJ. Prophylaxis for venous thromboembolic disease in pregnancy and the early postnatal period. *Cochrane Database Syst Rev* 2002; (2): CD001689.

36. Bank I, Libourel EJ, Middeldorp S, van der Meer J, Buller HR. High rate of skin complications due to low-molecular-weight heparins in pregnant women. *J Thromb Haemost* 2003; **1**(4): 859–61.

37. Greer IA, Nelson-Piercy C. Low-molecular-weight heparins for thromboprophylaxis and treatment of venous thromboembolism in pregnancy: a systematic review of safety and efficacy. *Blood* 2005; **106**(2): 401–7.

38. Bates SM, Greer IA, Pabinger I, Sofaer S, Hirsh J. Venous thromboembolism, thrombophilia, antithrombotic therapy, and pregnancy: American College of Chest Physicians Evidence-Based Clinical Practice Guidelines (8th Edition). *Chest* 2008; **133**(6 Suppl): 844S-86S.

39. Friederich PW, Sanson BJ, Simioni P *et al*. Frequency of pregnancy-related venous thromboembolism in anticoagulant factor-deficient women: implications for prophylaxis. *Ann Int Med* 1996; **125**: 955–60.

40. Bucciarelli P, Rosendaal FR, Tripodi A, *et al*. Risk of venous thromboembolism and clinical manifestations in carriers of antithrombin, protein C, protein S deficiency, or activated protein C resistance: a multicenter collaborative family study. *Arterioscler Thromb Vasc Biol* 1999; **19**(4): 1026–33.

41. Vossen CY, Conard J, Fontcuberta J *et al*. Familial thrombophilia and lifetime risk of venous thrombosis. *J Thromb Haemost* 2004; **2**: 1526–32.

42. Vandenbroucke JP, van der Meer FJ, Helmerhorst FM, Rosendaal FR. Factor V Leiden – Should we screen oral contraceptive users and pregnant women? *BMJ* 1996; **313**(7065): 1127–30.

43. Cohn DM, Roshani S, Middeldorp S. Thrombophilia and venous thromboembolism: implications for testing? *Semin Thromb Hemost* 2007; **33**(6): 573–81.

44. Brill-Edwards P, Ginsberg JS, Gent M, Hirsh J *et al*. Safety of withholding heparin in pregnant women with a history of venous thromboembolism. *N Eng J Med* 2000; **343**(20): 1439–44.

45. Pabinger I, Grafenhofer H, Kaider A *et al*. Risk of pregnancy-associated recurrent venous thromboembolism in women with a history of venous thrombosis. *J Thromb Haemost* 2005; **3**(5): 949–54.

46. Sanson BJ, Lensing AW A, Prins MH *et al*. Safety of low-molecular-weight heparin in pregnancy: a systematic review. *Thromb Haemost* 1999; **81**: 668–72.

47. Lepercq J, Conard J, Borel-Derlon A *et al*. Venous thromboembolism during pregnancy: a retrospective study of enoxaparin safety in 624 pregnancies. *BJOG* 2001; **108**(11): 1134–40.

48. Wesseling J, van Driel D, Heymans HS *et al*. Coumarins during pregnancy: long-term effects on growth and development of school-age children. *Thromb Haemost* 2001; **85**(4): 609–13.

49. Empson M, Lassere M, Craig JC, Scott JR. Prevention of recurrent miscarriage for women with antiphospholipid antibody or lupus anticoagulant. *Cochrane Database Syst Rev* 2005; (2): CD002859.

50. Pattison NS, Chamley LW, Birdsall M, Zanderigo AM, Liddell HS, McDougall J. Does aspirin have a role in improving pregnancy outcome for women with the antiphospholipid syndrome? A randomized controlled trial. *Am J Obstet Gynecol* 2000; **183**(4): 1008–12.

51. Tulppala M, Marttunen M, Soderstrom-Anttila V *et al*. Low-dose aspirin in prevention of miscarriage in women with unexplained or autoimmune related recurrent miscarriage: effect on prostacyclin and thromboxane A2 production. *Hum Reprod* 1997; **12**(7): 1567–72.

52. Rai R, Cohen H, Dave M, Regan L. Randomised controlled trial of aspirin and aspirin plus heparin in pregnant women with recurrent miscarriage associated with phospholipid antibodies (or antiphospholipid antibodies) [see comments]. *BMJ* 1997; **314**(7076): 253–7.

53. Farquharson RG, Quenby S, Greaves M. Antiphospholipid syndrome in pregnancy: a randomized, controlled trial of treatment. *Obstet Gynecol* 2002; **100**(3): 408–13.

54. Laskin CA, Spitzer KA, Clark CA *et al*. Low molecular weight heparin and aspirin for recurrent pregnancy

loss: results from the randomized, controlled HepASA Trial. *J Rheumatol* 2009; **36**(2): 279–87.

55. Jauniaux E, Farquharson RG, Christiansen OB, Exalto N. Evidence-based guidelines for the investigation and medical treatment of recurrent miscarriage. *Hum Reprod* 2006; **21**(9): 2116–222.

56. Brigham SA, Conlon C, Farquharson RG. A longitudinal study of pregnancy outcome following idiopathic recurrent miscarriage. *Hum Reprod* 1999; **14** (11): 2868–71.

57. Lindqvist PG, Merlo J. The natural course of women with recurrent fetal loss. *J Thromb Haemost* 2006; **4**(4): 896–7.

58. Rai R, Backos M, Elgaddal S, Shlebak A, Regan L. Factor V Leiden and recurrent miscarriage-prospective outcome of untreated pregnancies. *Hum Reprod* 2002; **17**(2): 442–5.

59. Brenner B, Hoffman R, Carp H, Dulitzky M, Younis J, for the LIVE-ENOX Investigators. Efficacy and safety of two doses of enoxaparin in women with thrombophilia and recurrent pregnancy loss: the LIVE-ENOX study. *J Thromb Haemost* 2005; **3**(2): 227–9.

60. Kaandorp SP *et al.* Aspirin plus heparin or aspirin alone in women with recurrent miscarriage. *The New England Journal of Medicine* 2010; **362**(17): 1586–96.

61. Clark P *et al.* SPIN: the Scottish Pregnancy Intervention Study: a multicentre randomised controlled trial of low molecular weight heparin and low dose aspirin in women with recurrent miscarriage. *Blood* 2010; **115** (21): 4162–7.

62. Gris JC, Mercier E, Quere I *et al.* Low-molecular-weight heparin versus low-dose aspirin in women with one fetal loss and a constitutional thrombophilic disorder. *Blood* 2004; **103**: 3695–9.

63. Rodger M. Important publication missing key information. *Blood* 2004; **104** (10): 3413 ; author reply 3413 -4 2004; **104**: 3413–4.

64. Kaandorp SP, Di Nisio M, Goddijn M, Middeldorp S. Aspirin or anticoagulants for treating recurrent miscarriage in women without antiphospholipid syndrome. *The Cochrane Library* 2009; (1): CD004734.

65. Coppens M, Folkeringa N, Teune M *et al.* Natural course of the subsequent pregnancy after a single loss in women with and without the factor V Leiden or prothrombin 20210A mutations. *J Thromb Haemost* 2007; **5**: 1444–8.

66. Vossen CY, Preston FE, Conard J *et al.* Hereditary thrombophilia and fetal loss: a prospective follow-up study. *J Thromb Haemost* 2004; **2**(4): 592–6.

67. Folkeringa N, Brouwer JL, Korteweg FJ *et al.* Reduction of high fetal loss rate by anticoagulant treatment during pregnancy in antithrombin, protein C or protein S deficient women. *Br J Haematol* 2007; **136**(4): 656–61.

68. Vandenbroucke JP. When are observational studies as credible as randomised trials? *Lancet* 2004; **363**(9422): 1728–31.

69. Simioni P, Sanson BJ, Prandoni P *et al.* The incidence of venous thromboembolism in families with inherited thrombophilia. *Thromb Haemost* 1999; **81**(2): 198–202.

70. Middeldorp S, Henkens CM A, Koopman MM W *et al.* The incidence of venous thromboembolism in family members of patients with factor V Leiden mutation and venous thrombosis. *Ann Int Med* 1998; **128**(1): 15–20.

71. Bank I, Libourel EJ, Middeldorp S *et al.* Prothrombin 20210A mutation: a mild risk factor for venous thromboembolism but not for arterial thrombotic disease and pregnancy-related complications in a family study. *Arch Int Med* 2004; **164**(17): 1932–7.

72. Bank I, Libourel EJ, Middeldorp S *et al.* Elevated levels of FVIII:c within families are associated with an increased risk for venous and arterial thrombosis. *J Thromb Haemost* 2005; **3**(1): 79–84.

73. Van de Poel MH, Coppens M, Middeldorp S *et al.* Absolute risk of venous and arterial thromboembolism associated with mild hyperhomocysteinemia. Results from a retrospective family cohort study. *J.Thromb. Haemost.* **3** (Suppl.1), P0481. 2005.

74. Sanson BJ, Simioni P, Tormene D *et al.* The incidence of venous thromboembolism in asymptomatic carriers of a deficiency of antithrombin, protein C, or protein S: a prospective cohort study. *Blood* 1999; **94**: 3702–6.

75. Middeldorp S, Meinardi JR, Koopman MM W *et al.* A prospective study of asymptomatic carriers of the factor V Leiden mutation to determine the incidence of venous thromboembolism. *Ann Int Med* 2001; **135**(5): 322–7.

76. Coppens M, van der Poel MH, Bank I *et al.* A prospective cohort study on the absolute incidence of venous thromboembolism and arterial cardiovascular disease in asymptomatic carriers of the prothrombin 20210A mutation. *Blood* 2006; **108**: 2604–7.

77. Middeldorp S, van der Poel MH, Bank I *et al.* Unselected women with elevated levels of factor VIII:c or homocysteine are not at increased risk for obstetric complications. *Thromb Haemost* 2004; **92**(4): 787–90.

78. Infante-Rivard C, David M, Gauthier R, Rivard GE. Lupus anticoagulants, anticardiolipin antibodies, and fetal loss. A case-control study. *N Eng J Med* 1991; **325** (15): 1063–6.

79. Nelen WL, Blom HJ, Steegers EA, den Heijer M, Eskes TK. Hyperhomocysteinemia and recurrent early pregnancy loss: a meta-analysis. *Fertil Steril* 2000; **74**: 1196–9.

# Thrombosis, air travel and early pregnancy

## Gillian Norrie and Mike Greaves

In October 2000, media interest in the concept of air travel as a risk factor for venous thromboembolism was enhanced by the tragic case of a 28-year-old woman who died from pulmonary embolism shortly after arrival at Heathrow airport, following a 20-hour journey from Australia. The media frenzy was particularly apparent in the UK. Widely read national newspapers carried banner headlines including "Could These Seats be the Death of You?" (referring to the limited leg room in economy class sections of airliners), "'Cattle Class Syndrome' Could Kill 2000 a Year," "Millions at Risk in New Long Haul Flight Scare," and "The Air-Death Gene" (all referring to the high prevalence of heritable thrombophilia in the general population). As a result of this sensational reporting one could be forgiven for concluding that air travel carries a unique and very high risk of promoting deep vein thrombosis and death from pulmonary embolism. The clinical and epidemiological facts do not support this conclusion at all, however. Nevertheless, some travelers may be at more than the average risk of venous thromboembolism due to the presence of additional risk factors. Pregnancy may be one such risk factor and it is worthwhile, therefore, to attempt to quantify the level of risk in order to provide evidence-based advice on risk reduction. However, there are no robust data which address specifically the issue of pregnancy and travel in relation to the occurrence of venous thromboembolism. As such, the only informative approach to the issue is through extrapolation from the limited amount of robust pathophysiological and epidemiological data relevant to pregnancy which have accumulated on the general topic of venous thromboembolism. Those data are reviewed here.

## Thrombosis risk and early pregnancy

As has been described in the preceding chapters, venous thromboembolism (VTE) has a multifactorial

pathogenesis involving genetic predisposition, acquired diseases and conditions, and lifestyle and environmental factors. The annual incidence of VTE is of the order of 1 in 1000 individuals in Western populations. However there is a very marked effect of increasing age; therefore, the incidence in non-pregnant women of childbearing age is much lower, perhaps around 1 in 10,000 per annum (Figure 15.1). Pregnancy is an independent risk factor for VTE. Overall, VTE complicates approximately 1 in 1000 pregnancies [1]. Although clinicians have tended to regard late pregnancy and the puerperium as high-risk periods, increased risk is present at all stages. For example, in a meta-analysis of 12 published studies of deep vein thrombosis during pregnancy in which the trimester of occurrence was reported, Ray and Chan [2] calculated a weighted event rate of 21.9% (95% CI 17.4–27.3) in the first trimester, 33.7% (28.1–39.8) in the second trimester and 47.6% (39.2–56.2) in the third trimester. It is important to have insight into the level of risk relative to the non-pregnant state. This can be estimated from case–control studies. In the MEGA study [3], a study of risk factors for VTE in 285 patients and 857 controls, the analysis suggested an approximately five-fold increased risk of VTE during pregnancy (Odds Ratio 4.6; 95% CI 2.7–7.8) which contrasts with a 60-fold increased risk in the 3 months after delivery (OR 60.1; 26.5–135.9). Most of the increased risk during pregnancy was indeed in the third trimester (OR 8.8; 4.5–17.3) with only a modest increased risk in the first two trimesters (OR 1.6; 0.7–3.7). Notably, but not surprisingly, women who are carriers of factor V Leiden had a greater than 50-fold increased risk of pregnancy-related VTE compared with non-pregnant non-carriers (OR 52.2; 12.4–219.5).

It is reasonable to conclude from these observations that there is an increased risk of VTE in early pregnancy.

*Early Pregnancy*, ed. Roy G. Farquharson and Mary D. Stephenson. Published by Cambridge University Press.
© Cambridge University Press 2010.

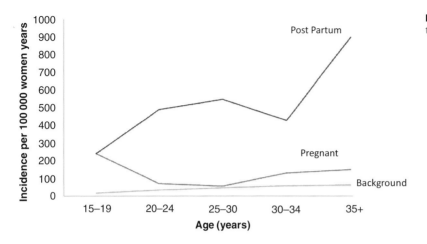

**Figure 15.1** Incidence of venous thromboembolism in women.

The relatively modest increase in risk, compared with later pregnancy and the puerperium, is consistent with the likely pathogenic mechanisms involved. Thus, the well-described increases in several coagulation factors in pregnancy, including factors V, VII, VIII, X and fibrinogen are most marked in the second and third trimesters. Nevertheless, some potentially prothrombotic changes begin to manifest in the first trimester. For example the pregnancy specific inhibitor of fibrinolysis, Plasminogen Activator Inhibitor 2 (PAI 2), is detectable in plasma during the first trimester [4]. Furthermore, markers of coagulation activation such as D-dimer and thrombin-antithrombin complex are significantly increased in plasma of women with healthy pregnancies by 12 weeks' gestation [5], and the fall in femoral venous blood flow velocity which is associated with pregnancy is said to be detectable by the end of the first trimester [1].

The data summarized above indicate an increased relative risk of VTE in pregnancy. However, the most important consideration for an individual is their subject-specific personal absolute risk, given their personal putative risk factors, rather than the population-averaged relative risk derived from epidemiological data. By extrapolation from the epidemiological evidence the absolute risk of VTE in a young woman during early pregnancy is low, certainly less than 1 in 1000. This risk is increased in the presence of additional risk factors, be they genetic or acquired. Nevertheless, even in a carrier of factor V Leiden who is pregnant the absolute risk of VTE remains low.

## Thrombosis risk and travel

Although the level of risk of VTE associated with air travel has been exaggerated through sensationalized

reporting in the mass media, it has nevertheless been established now that long-haul flights represent a risk factor for deep vein thrombosis and pulmonary embolism, including fatal events. However, despite the media focus specifically on air travel, there is ample evidence that the same applies to other modes of travel which enforce prolonged periods of immobility in relatively cramped conditions [6]. Indeed, these observations linking immobility to VTE are far from novel. For example, in 1940, Simpson [7] observed a six-fold increase in the rate of pulmonary embolism in Londoners seeking shelter in the confines of underground railway stations during bombing raids in World War II. It appears that the problem was resolved when mattresses were supplied to replace the deck chairs frequently used for sleeping, presumably allowing more leg movement and causing less compression of leg veins. After the early report by Homans [8], in 1954, of two cases of VTE apparently associated with air travel, there have been very many similar case reports, leading to the introduction of the terminology "economy class syndrome" as early as the 1970s.

Among the most compelling evidence which links symptomatic VTE with air travel, and emphasizes the duration of travel as a major factor, is the study by Lapostolle *et al.* [9]. They reviewed all recorded cases of pulmonary embolism, between 1993 and 2000, which occurred during or around the time of disembarkation from flights arriving at Charles de Gaulle airport, Paris, France. The total number of passengers on these flights amounted to 135 million. Among this population there were 53 episodes of hospitalization for pulmonary embolism, an incidence of <0.5 per million passengers. There was a very clear relationship to the duration of travel, fewer than 10% of cases occurring after flights of less than 8 hours duration. Other risk factors were frequently identifiable. Notably, in relation to the topic of this chapter, 18 were current users of an oral contraceptive or hormone replacement therapy, suggesting a link between female hormones and air travel-associated VTE which is supported by a study into pathogenesis referred to below. Other studies have supported these findings and, whilst the study design allows only a proportion of flight-related events to be captured (restricted to symptomatic pulmonary embolism within a few hours of long-haul air travel, whereas other data suggest that the risk persists for several weeks) they do confirm the association and the important contribution of combinations of risk factors.

Although there are no pregnancy-specific data, prospective cohort studies, in which evidence of the presence of lower limb deep vein thrombosis is sought by an objective test before and after air travel, have provided additional information. Such studies have employed ultrasound scanning of lower limb veins to detect thrombus; it is important to appreciate that small, localized thrombi may be detected and their clinical significance is not known. Some have used D-dimer assay, also. In five such studies [10–14], which all excluded subjects to be at high risk of VTE and were restricted to flights of at least 8 hours duration, the incidence of any deep vein thrombosis ranged from 1–12%. These results are difficult to reconcile but several features are worthy of comment. In the study by Scurr and colleagues [10] which demonstrated a 12% incidence, most thrombi were detected in isolated calf muscle veins and, as such, were not necessarily of any clinical significance. None was symptomatic. Furthermore, in half of the cases in this study the plasma D-dimer concentration was not raised. When the test is validated within the population to be studied, a low concentration of D-dimer has a high negative predictive value for exclusion of VTE in low-risk individuals. Hence, the likely clinical significance of some of the thrombi detected in this study is diminished further. If the results from this study are excluded from the analysis, of 2437 subjects included in the remaining studies, it appears that VTE was detected in 1.6% of low- or intermediate-risk travelers after flights of at least 8 hours. When the thrombi which were limited to isolated calf muscle veins (and which may not be clinically important) are excluded, just over 0.5% had any VTE, and symptomatic VTE

was present in just under 0.5%. Of course, this analysis makes no allowance for the background incidence of VTE detectable using the same methods in a cohort of non-travelers. When the data from the two studies which included a relevant control group are examined [11,12], the presence of isolated calf muscle vein thrombosis, the most prevalent finding, was only twice as common among flyers than in controls, and deep vein thrombosis only around four times more common. Overall, these types of studies have tended to confirm that subclinical leg vein thrombosis is somewhat increased after long-haul flights, with a modest increase in clinically apparent VTE also.

Additional insights into the level of risk of VTE associated with air travel come from case–control studies. Kuipers et al [15] have performed a methodologically robust systematic review of such studies. This included ten published studies in which the frequency of a history of any form of travel among subjects with VTE was compared with that in a control population without VTE. When data were analyzed from six studies in which results for air travel could be separated, the pooled odds ratio for air travel of any duration was 1.4 (95% CI 0.9–2.0); when three of these studies were excluded on the grounds of likely bias due to the methods employed, the pooled odds ratio of the remaining studies was 1.9 (95% CI 1.2–2.8). There was evidence for an effect of flight duration. When all ten studies were included in the analysis the pooled odds ratio for any travel was 1.7 (95% CI 1.4–2.1), consistent with the concept that the modest increase in risk of VTE is not restricted to travel by air [16]. In summary, from these data it is reasonable to conclude that travel is associated with an increased risk of VTE of around only two-fold.

What is the absolute risk of VTE after air travel? Kuipers et al. [15] estimated this using data from their own study of VTE among around 9000 employees of international companies and organizations – that is, frequent flyers. Based on 22 episodes of VTE in this cohort they calculated an absolute risk of a symptomatic VTE occurring within 4 weeks of flights longer than 4 hours of 1 in 4600 flights. Of course, it is inappropriate to generalize this to the overall travelling population due to the highly selected nature of the cohort studied (generally healthy). Nevertheless, it seems likely that this level of risk, which is clearly modest, would apply also in the case of a healthy woman of child-bearing age.

In relation to the pathogenesis of VTE associated with air travel, the physiology of the venous circulation, the historical observations referred to above, and the indication that other forms of travel are implicated, together suggest that immobility is a major factor. However, it has been hypothesized that other features of the aircraft cabin environment may play a role. The cabin pressure in passenger aircraft is around 76 kPa, which approximates to an altitude of 2500 m above sea level. At this pressure the oxygen saturation in arterial blood can fall to around 90% and hypobaric hypoxia has been considered to have the potential to activate blood coagulation. Although some limited evidence has been published in support of this, in a comprehensive study of 73 healthy volunteers exposed for 8 hours to hypobaric hypoxia comparable to that encountered by air travelers Toff et al. [17] found no evidence for any prothrombotic change in an extensive range of sensitive assays of blood coagulation and hemostasis. Due to the complexities of conducting such a study, coagulation activation during actual air travel has been studied infrequently. However Schreijer et al. [18] conducted a well-designed and executed cross-over study on 71 healthy volunteers in whom coagulation activation was assessed during an 8-hour flight, an 8-hour session watching movies and also whilst engaged in normal daily activities. Although no coagulation activation was detected in the majority, some evidence for increased thrombin generation was found in 17% during the flight, compared with 3% whilst watching movies and 1% whilst ambulatory. Of note, the evidence of coagulation activation was principally among women with factor V Leiden who were using oral contraception, a population which was not strongly represented in the study by Toff et al [17]. This observation lends biological plausibility to the findings. Taken together, these data suggest that hypobaric hypoxia of a degree associated with passenger air travel does not activate coagulation in most healthy individuals. However, when other procoagulant factors are present, increased blood coagulability may be triggered. The observation that one such factor is the use of contraceptive hormones has clear implications in relation to pregnancy and air travel. For example, acquired resistance to the anticoagulant activity of protein C is a major contributor to the prothrombotic effect of the combined oral contraceptive [19] and is also a feature of normal pregnancy [20]. Although there are no data available on the effect of hypobaric hypoxia on blood coagulation during pregnancy, it is reasonable to hypothesize that there may be an additive or even a synergistic effect. Finally, in relation to pathogenesis, whilst it has been hypothesized that dehydration resulting from the low atmospheric humidity on board passenger aircraft may predispose to VTE there is no evidence to support this [21].

## Estimating the thrombosis risk from travel during early pregnancy

Based on the data reviewed in the preceding sections, the absolute risk of symptomatic VTE in a healthy pregnant woman is low – much less than 1 in 1000 in early pregnancy. In a healthy non-pregnant woman of child-bearing age the risk of symptomatic VTE following a flight of 4 hours or longer is low also, again probably much less than 1 in 1000, and some other types of travel may carry a similar risk. Although there are no data available on the absolute risk of VTE a woman who undertakes a long-haul flight during early pregnancy, even if the two risk factors are synergistic, it seems unlikely that the risk of VTE is as great as 1 in 100 for example, although it may possibly approach this level during the puerperium. However, as always in this multifactorial condition, the potential impact of additional risk factors should not be overlooked. These heritable and acquired risk factors have been described elsewhere in this book. As an example, an obese woman who has a personal history of unprovoked VTE, is no longer treated with anticoagulant and who is 12 weeks pregnant almost certainly has a relatively high absolute risk of travel-related VTE even if this cannot be adequately quantified. The crucial question is whether there are interventions of proven efficacy in reducing the risk of VTE associated with travel and, if so, which pregnant women should be offered those interventions.

## Prevention of travel-related VTE

Potentially effective measures to reduce the risk of travel-related VTE include enhanced mobility, use of graduated compression hosiery and pharmacological interventions.

Improved mobility may be facilitated by increased leg room whilst seated. This generally requires placement in the higher grade and more expensive areas of the aircraft. Whether this strategy is effective in reducing the risk of VTE is not known of course, although there are well-recorded case reports of VTE occurring in business class passengers. Interestingly, in one epidemiological study, an excess of air-travel related VTE occurred in the tallest and shortest passengers, compatible with an effect of seating arrangements on risk

[6]. The efficacy of the seated leg exercises promoted by some airlines to reduce risk of VTE has been questioned [22] but, based on the physiology of venous return, and some evidence that foot exercises against resistance increase blood flow in the popliteal vein [23], their adoption seems reasonable, as do recommendations to avoid remaining seated throughout the journey.

A Cochrane review has addressed the question of efficacy of graduated compression stockings in the prevention of deep vein thrombosis in airline passengers [24]. However, of the ten publications, the majority have been criticized in relation to quality and other issues [15] and we do not feel that they should be considered further here. The remaining two randomized controlled trials were small. In one, participants were randomized to dried vine leaves or diuretics also. In the second, the study by Scurr et al. described above [10], 12 of the 100 low-risk passengers allocated to the no-stockings arm suffered asymptomatic deep vein thrombosis compared with none of the 100 allocated to the class I compression stocking arm. The limitations of this study have been referred to already. In summary there are insufficient well-conducted studies to determine whether graduated compression stockings are effective in the prevention of travel-related deep vein thrombosis. The use of full-length compression hosiery is believed to reduce the risk of subclinical deep vein thrombosis after surgical procedures [25,26], and there is evidence that below-knee stockings are no less effective in this population [27]. However these observations may not be generalizable to the distinctive situation of reduced mobility due to seating arrangements within an airplane passenger compartment.

There are no robust data available on the safety and efficacy of pharmacological interventions for the prevention of travel-related thrombosis. The principal pharmaceuticals which could be considered are heparins and aspirin, also some "complementary" preparations have been promoted [28]. Low molecular weight heparin (LMWH) is effective in reducing the incidence of VTE post-operatively (by 50–60%) as well as in hospitalized subjects more generally, with little increased risk of bleeding. Low molecular weight heparin does not cross the placenta and may be safely employed during pregnancy. Although it seems likely that prophylactic LMWH would reduce the risk of travel-related VTE, and is occasionally prescribed for this purpose, this is by extrapolation from its proven efficacy in these other situations and is not fully evidence-based. In our opinion, based on the low absolute risk of travel-related VTE in the overwhelming majority of women during early pregnancy, pharmacological thromboprophylaxis with LMWH can be justified only extremely rarely. Aspirin has, at best, limited efficacy in the prevention of VTE. Perioperative prophylaxis with aspirin appears to reduce the risk of VTE by around 25% in high-risk surgical patients [29]. There are no robust data on its efficacy in prevention of travel-related thrombosis. Although low dose aspirin use appears to be safe in pregnancy, in any patient taking aspirin there is an increased risk of clinically important gastric bleeding. As such, the risk–benefit ratio of aspirin as an antithrombotic in the context of travel-related VTE, a rare complication in healthy travelers, is likely to be narrow. It is somewhat perplexing, therefore, that in a questionnaire-based postal survey of members of the Royal College of Obstetricians and Gynaecologists [30], 53% of respondents indicated that they would recommend thromboprophylaxis with aspirin 75 mg (and 6% with aspirin 300 mg) to pregnant women intending to travel by air.

## Advice to women who undertake long-haul travel during early pregnancy

Based on the evidence where available, coupled with pragmatism, we recommend:

Women should be advised that there may be no additional risk associated with short journeys, for example flights of less than 3 hours duration.

For longer flights the absolute risk is low for most individuals, and the increased risk is not restricted to travel by air. On the grounds that restricted mobility is probably an important pathogenic factor, women should be advised to maintain mobility, when appropriate and possible, before, during and after the journey, and to perform leg exercises intermittently while seated.

Whilst below-knee compression stockings are not of proven efficacy in the context of travel, their use is unlikely to be harmful.

In women considered to be at the highest risk, due to the co-existence of multiple risk factors, pharmacological thromboprophylaxis could be considered, but this should be exceptional.

Although not based on evidence from relevant clinical trials, LMWH could be given in a prophylactic dose prior to embarkation for each leg of the journey.

In our opinion, use of aspirin for the prevention of travel-related thrombosis is not justified.

# References

1. Clark P. Maternal venous thrombosis. *Eur J Obstet Gynecol Reprod Biol* 2008; **139**(1): 3–10.

2. Ray JG, Chan WS. Deep vein thrombosis during pregnancy and the puerperium: a meta-analysis of the period of risk and the leg of presentation. *Obstet Gynecol Surv* 1999; **54**(4): 265–71.

3. Pomp ER, Lenselink AM, Rosendaal FR, Doggen CJ. Pregnancy, the postpartum period and prothrombotic defects: risk of venous thrombosis in the MEGA study. *J Thromb Haemost* 2008; **6**(4): 632–7.

4. Wright JG, Cooper P, Astedt B et al. Fibrinolysis during normal human pregnancy: complex inter-relationships between plasma levels of tissue plasminogen activator and inhibitors and the euglobulin clot lysis time. *Br J Haematol* 1988; **69**(2): 253–8.

5. Eichinger S, Weltermann A, Philipp K et al. Prospective evaluation of hemostatic system activation and thrombin potential in healthy pregnant women with and without factor V Leiden. *Thromb Haemost* 1999; **82**(4): 1232–6.

6. Cannegieter SC, Doggen CJ, van Houwelingen HC, Rosendaal FR. Travel-related venous thrombosis: results from a large population-based case control study (MEGA study). *PLoS Med* 2006; **3**(8): e307.

7. Simpson K. Shelter deaths from pulmonary embolism. *Lancet* 1940; **11**: 744.

8. Homans J. Thrombosis of the deep leg veins due to prolonged sitting. *New Engl J Med* 1954; **250**(4): 148–9.

9. Lapostolle F, Surget V, Borron SW et al. Severe pulmonary embolism associated with air travel. *New Engl J Med* 2001; **345**(11): 779–83.

10. Scurr JH, Machin SJ, Bailey-King S et al. Frequency and prevention of symptomless deep-vein thrombosis in long-haul flights: a randomised trial. *Lancet* 2001; **357**(9267): 1485–9.

11. Schwarz T, Langenberg K, Oettler W et al. Deep vein and isolated calf muscle vein thrombosis following long-haul flights: pilot study. *Blood Coagul Fibrinolysis* 2002; **13**(8): 755–7.

12. Schwarz T, Siegert G, Oettler W et al. Venous thrombosis after long-haul flights. *Arch. Intern.Med.* 2003; **163**(22): 2759–64.

13. Hughes RJ, Hopkins RJ, Hill S et al. Frequency of venous thromboembolism in low to moderate risk long distance air travellers: the New Zealand Air Traveller's Thrombosis (NZATT) study. *Lancet* 2003; **362**(9401): 2039–44.

14. Jacobson BF, Munster M, Smith A et al. The BEST study – a prospective study to compare business class versus economy class air travel as a cause of thrombosis. *S Afr Med J* 2003; **93**(7): 522–8.

15. Kuipers S, Schreijer AJ, Cannegieter SC et al. Travel and venous thrombosis: a systematic review. *J Intern Med* 2007; **262**(6): 615–34.

16. Trujillo-Santos AJ, Jimenez-Puente A, Perea-Milla E. Association between long travel and venous thromboembolic disease: a systematic review and meta-analysis of case-control studies. *Ann Hematol* 2008; **87**(2): 79–86.

17. Toff WD, Jones CI, Ford I et al. Effect of hypobaric hypoxia, simulating conditions during long-haul air travel, on coagulation, fibrinolysis, platelet function, and endothelial activation. *J Am Med Assoc* 2006; **295**(19): 2251–61.

18. Schreijer AJ, Cannegieter SC, Meijers JC et al. Activation of coagulation system during air travel: a crossover study. *Lancet* 2006; **367**(9513): 832–8.

19. Rosing J, Tans G, Nicolaes GA et al. Oral contraceptives and venous thrombosis: different sensitivities to activated protein C in women using second- and third-generation oral contraceptives. *Br J Haematol* 1997; **97**(1): 233–8.

20. Mahieu B, Jacobs N, Mahieu S et al. Haemostatic changes and acquired activated protein C resistance in normal pregnancy. *Blood Coagul Fibrinolysis* 2007; **18**(7): 685–8.

21. Schreijer AJ, Cannegieter SC, Caramella M et al. Fluid loss does not explain coagulation activation during air travel. *Thromb Haemost* 2008; **99**(6): 1053–9.

22. Schreijer AJ, Cannegieter SC, Doggen CJ, Rosendaal FR. The effect of flight-related behaviour on the risk of venous thrombosis after air travel. *Br J Haematol* 2008; **144**: 425–9.

23. Hitos K, Cannon M, Cannon S, Garth S, Fletcher JP. Effect of leg exercises on popliteal venous blood flow during prolonged immobility of seated subjects: implications for prevention of travel-related deep vein thrombosis. *J Thromb Haemost* 2007; **5**(9): 1890–5.

24. Clarke M, Hopewell S, Juszczak E, Eisinga A, Kjeldstrom M. Compression stockings for preventing deep vein thrombosis in airline passengers. *Cochrane Database Syst Rev* 2006; **2**(2): CD004002.

25. Allan A, Williams JT, Bolton JP, Le Quesne LP. The use of graduated compression stockings in the prevention

of postoperative deep vein thrombosis. *Br J Surg* 1983; **70**(3): 172–4.

26. Wille-Jorgensen P, Rasmussen MS, Andersen BR, Borly L. Heparins and mechanical methods for thromboprophylaxis in colorectal surgery. *Cochrane Database Syst Rev* 2001; **3**(3): CD001217.

27. Sajid MS, Tai NR, Goli G, Morris RW, Baker DM, Hamilton G. Knee versus thigh length graduated compression stockings for prevention of deep venous thrombosis: a systematic review. *Eur J Vasc Endovasc Surg* 2006; **32**(6): 730–6.

28. Scurr JH, Gulati OP. Zinopin – the rationale for its use as a food supplement in Traveller's thrombosis and motion sickness. *Phytother Res* 2004; **18**(9): 687–95.

29. Watson HG, Chee YL. Aspirin and other antiplatelet drugs in the prevention of venous thromboembolism. *Blood Rev* 2008; **22**(2): 107–16.

30. Voss M, Cole R, Moriarty T *et al.* Thromboembolic disease and air travel in pregnancy: a survey of advice given by obstetricians. *J Obstet Gynaecol* 2004; **24**(8): 859–62.

# Chapter 6

# Immunotherapy and early pregnancy

Ole B. Christiansen

## Introduction

Recurrent miscarriage (RM), defined as three or more consecutive miscarriages, affects 0.5–1% of all women. In a minority of couples causes such as parental chromosome abnormalities, significant uterine malformations, endocrine or thrombophilic disturbances can be found and some cases are probably the result of repeated *de novo* fetal chromosome aberrations in pregnancies of karyotypically normal parents [1]. In many cases immunological abnormalities can be identified in peripheral blood. A series of autoantibodies, a T-helper type I cytokine bias or increased natural killer (NK) cell activity have been reported to be found with increased prevalence in these patients [2–5] although none of these biomarkers has been documented per se to be sufficient to cause miscarriage/RM. Furthermore, most of them do not reflect immunological conditions inside the uterus. Immunological disease is often caused by cell-mediated autoimmune reactions exclusively localized in the target organ (e.g. insulin dependent diabetes mellitus, multiple sclerosis), and the diagnosis is not dependent on the demonstration of particular immunological reactions/biomarkers in peripheral blood. The knowledge that multiple sclerosis is an autoimmune disease is mainly based on genetic epidemiological studies e.g. the finding of associations to particular HLA class II alleles. The demonstration of specific immunological disturbances in peripheral blood is thus not mandatory to propose an immunological etiology for a disease and the strongest evidence for the involvement of the immune system in RM indeed comes from genetic epidemiological studies. Genetic polymorphisms associated to deficiency of mannose-binding lectin, particular HLA class I and class II alleles and genetic polymorphisms of importance of NK cell interactions or cytokine production can be found with increased prevalence in RM patients or subsets of these [6–10]. Patients with secondary RM (the loss of three or more pregnancies to miscarriage following one successful pregnancy) seem to be more prone to have an immunological background than other RM patients. Recent results point towards a role for immunization against male-specific minor histocompatibility (HY) antigens in the etiology of secondary RM [11] and maternal carriage of the immunological high-responder allele HLA-DR3 is increased in women with secondary RM [9]. There is also support for the hypothesis that the chance of an immunological etiology for RM is increased in patients with a high number of previous miscarriages (≥4): the prevalence of particular HLA-DR alleles or HLA-G alleles and the frequency of mannose-binding lectin deficiency increase with the number of previous miscarriages [6,8,9]. Furthermore, the chance for fetal aneuploidy as an etiology to miscarriage decreases with the number of previous miscarriages [12].

If significant anatomical, chromosomal, endocrinological or coagulation disorders are excluded it may be assumed that the etiology of RM is mainly immunological primarily based on results from large genetic-epidemiological studies. This justifies that trials of immunotherapy in RM have often not included patients according to the presence of selected immunological biomarkers but rather according to the absence of non-immunological risk factors.

Three immunotherapeutic approaches have been tested in RM: prednisone, active immunization with allogeneic lymphocytes from the partner or third-party donors, and intravenous immunoglobulin (IvIg). Prednisone therapy has so far been tested in only one, although large placebo-controlled trial (PCT) in RM patients positive for autoantibodies [13].

In this trial prednisone was administered in large doses during all of pregnancy; a small but non-significant effect was found but the obstetric side effects were significant. More trials of prednisone using smaller doses in a shorter time period should be undertaken but until such studies are published, prednisone treatment cannot be recommended in RM. Since many more PCTs have been conducted regarding the other forms of immunotherapy these will be discussed in more detail.

## Allogeneic leukocyte immunization therapy

The thought that allogeneic leukocyte immunization therapy (ALT) could be beneficial in RM arose from the observation that injections of paternal lymphocytes into pregnant female mice in crosses of strains with a high fetal resorption rate could decrease the resorption rate [14]. Furthermore, pre-transplantation blood transfusions were reported to decrease the rejection rate in organ transplantation [15] – a condition with similarities to implantation of the semi-allogeneic fetal allograft in the uterus. The first PCT of ALT reported that injections of paternal lymphocytes (partner lymphocyte therapy, PLT) increased the pregnancy success rate significantly but subsequent PCTs provided conflicting results [16]. Partner lymphocyte therapy or infusion/injection of third-party donors (donor lymphocyte transfusions, DLT) became widely used within and outside controlled trials since 1985. In 1994, a meta-analysis of all PCTs (mainly PLT and a few DLT trials) showed that ALT significantly increased the chance of a live birth with 16.3% (95% CI 4.8–27.8%) among patients with primary RM and no auto- or alloantibodies, whereas no effect could be detected in patients with secondary RM [17,18]. In 1999, the results of a large PCT showed that PLT did not increase the chance of a live birth compared with placebo but rather tended to decrease it [19]. Subsequently, a Cochrane meta-analysis found that the odds ratio (OR) for live birth after PLT was 1.23 (95% CI 0.89–1.70) and for DLT 1.39 (95% CI 0.68–2.82) and it concluded that neither treatment provides significant beneficial effect over placebo in preventing further miscarriages [20].

Since the publication of the Cochrane review, ALT has been abandoned in most clinics and studies of this treatment option have had a very difficult course for being selected for presentation at meetings and for publication in medical journals.

## Heterogeneity of ALT trials

In the PCTs included in the Cochrane analysis, the live-birth rates ranged from 45.6% [19] to 84.0% [21] in the treatment groups and from 30.0% [21] and 46.7% [16] to 72.7% [22] and 78.6% [23] in the placebo groups. There was significant statistical heterogeneity ($P = 0.01$) between the outcomes in the trials of PLT in the Cochrane meta-analysis, throwing doubt on the rationale of calculating a pooled OR at all. This heterogeneity can be due to (a) heterogeneity of immunization protocols and (b) heterogeneity of patient populations.

### Heterogeneity of immunization protocols

Knowledge from general immunology tells us that the immunizing procedures used in the trials included in the Cochrane analysis of ALT differ so much in their mode of action that this alone can explain the heterogeneity of the results in the trials. In most ALT trials immunization had been done according to the protocol applied by Mowbray et al., administering a total of 5 ml partner lymphocyte suspension (c. $2 \times 10^8$ cells) in equal amounts intradermally, subcutaneously and intravenously before conception and in early pregnancy [16]. The DLT treatment, as used in the PCT carried out in my clinic, is completely different in terms of the amount, the origin and the route of administration of the immunizing agent than ALT used in almost all other trials [24]. In my trial intravenous infusions with 150 ml of buffycoat (leukocyte-enriched blood concentrate) from two red-cell-compatible blood donors were undertaken twice before conception with intervals of 1 month before conception. Transfusions were repeated every 5th month until conception but no transfusions were given during pregnancy. At each DLT a total of 1.5 to $4.6 \times 10^9$ white cells were exclusively infused intravenously. This is more than 10 times the number of cells given in most other protocols. The dose of the immunizing agent (number of cells administered) is known to be a very important factor in immunotherapy [25,26]: very low and very high doses will normally induce tolerance whereas intermediate doses induce immunization, which (in pregnancy) may harm the fetus. There is evidence that intravenous administration of high doses of an antigen, in the absence of additional co-stimulatory signal (as done in my protocol), is a much better way to induce tolerance than the subcutaneous/intradermal administration of smaller doses of antigen used in most ALT protocols [25].

In conclusion, ALT as performed in most trials, is prone to induce (potentially harmful) immunization whereas ALT, as done in my trial, in theory induces tolerance.

Storage of the immunizing agent may also be important. In one trial, cells for injection were stored overnight whereas in almost all other trials cells were injected within a few hours after being drawn from the partner/donor [19]. Storage of lymphocytes for 24 hours may alter their immunogenetic properties radically, which may impair the anti-abortive effect [27]. The much lower live-birth rate after PLT in one trial [19] compared with all other trials (46% vs 50–79%) may, in theory, be caused by this.

Whereas there is thus evidence that the way of administration, the amount of immunizing agent and storage of the immunizing cells are important for the effect after ALT there is no evidence that administration of cells from the partner results in different effects compared with administration of third-party donor cells (Table 16.1). If all trials of PLT or DLT were included in a common meta-analysis (which was not done in the Cochrane analysis), the OR for live birth after ALT would become 1.30 (95% CI 0.96–1.76), which is almost statistically significant (Figure 16.1).

### Heterogeneity of patient populations

The PCTs included in the Cochrane meta-analysis of ALT were very heterogeneous with respect to the frequency of secondary RM patients, ranging from 0% [23, 28] to 25.7% [19] and 31.8% [24], and also with regard to the mean number of previous miscarriages, ranging from 3.4 miscarriages [21] to 4.8 miscarriages [19]. However, ALT may display different effects in different subpopulations of RM patients (Table 16.1). As previously mentioned, ALT was found efficient in a previous meta-analysis of outcome in primary RM patients from eight PCTs but had no effect in secondary RM [17]. Furthermore, the effect of ALT significantly increased with the number of previous miscarriages in primary RM [18]. Such an effect gradient across several trials indicates that the number of

**Table 16.1** Importance of subsets of recurrent miscarriage (RM) or immunotherapy protocols and their consideration in the Cochrane meta-analysis of immunotherapy [20].

| Patient- or treatment-related parameter | Importance of parameter | Separate analysis in the Cochrane review |
|---|---|---|
| Primary vs secondary RM | Yes, in previous meta-analyses [17,39] | No |
| Few vs multiple miscarriages | Yes, in a previous meta-analysis [18] | No |
| Immunizing dose | Yes, well known in vaccination | No |
| Route of administration | Yes, well known in vaccination | No |
| Partner vs donor cells | No evidence that RM is partner-specific | Yes |

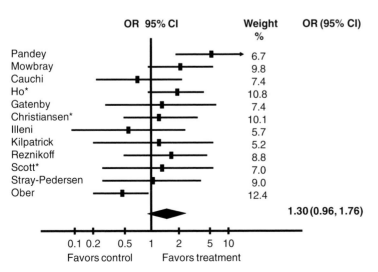

Figure 16.1 Pooled odds ratio for live birth after allogeneic lymphocyte immunization versus placebo calculated after combining trials using partner and/or third-party donor lymphocytes. *marks trials including patients receiving partner and/or third party donor lymphocytes.

miscarriages is an effect modifier, which should be taken into account when performing and interpreting meta-analyses of immunotherapy in RM [29]. This modifying effect may be explained by the fact that the probability of an immunological etiology for RM increases with the number of previous miscarriages, as previously discussed.

## Criticism of the Cochrane analysis on ALT

The Cochrane analysis only distinguishes between trials using paternal and donor cells but not between different immunizing doses and the route of administration, which, as discussed above, are the most important determinants for development of tolerance vs immunization (Table 16.1). Furthermore, no separate analysis in patients with primary RM was carried out, which is surprising since the previous meta-analysis of most relevant PCTs had given evidence for an effect only in primary RM [17]. There was neither any analysis according to the number of previous miscarriages, which is relevant since this parameter seems to be an important effect modifier [18].

Instead of completely rejecting the efficacy of immunotherapy, the authors of the Cochrane analysis on ALT should conclude that some types of immunotherapy in RM look promising but more PCTs should be carried out. New protocols of PCTs of ALT should take into account the lessons learned from the previous trials. If a new meta-analysis of PCTs of ALT is carried out, it should, as a minimum, look into effects according to doses of the immunization agent and the route of administration and it should evaluate the effect according to the number of miscarriages and in subsets of primary and secondary RM patients (Table 16.1).

## Intravenous immunoglobulin

Intravenous immunoglobulin (IvIg) is prepared by extracting the IgG fraction from plasma from normal blood donors. It exhibits a documented effect in many immunological disorders. The mode of action is probably multiple (Table 16.2) but some documented effects are modulation of cytokine production, blockage of lymphocyte receptors, inhibition of autoantibody formation, neutralization of activated complement components and induction of apoptosis of activated lymphocytes [30,31].

Knowing the association between many genes with immunological function and RM it is an obvious

**Table 16.2** Theories attempting to explain the effect of active (allogeneic lymphocyte therapy) and passive immunotherapy (intravenous immunoglobulin) in the prevention of recurrent miscarriage.

| Therapy | Theory |
|---------|--------|
| Allogeneic lymphocyte immunization | Production of anti-paternal antibodies or blocking antibodies<br>Dampening of natural killer (NK) cell activity<br>Modification of cytokine production<br>Establishment of microchimerism |
| Intravenous immunoglobulin | Suppression/neutralization of autoantibodies<br>Dampening of NK cell activity<br>Modification of cytokine production<br>Inhibition of complement binding and activation<br>Fc receptor modulation and blockade<br>Inhibition of superantigens<br>Modulation of adhesion molecules on T lymphocytes<br>Induction of apoptosis of activated cytotoxic lymphocytes |

thought that IvIg may be beneficial in the prevention of the disorder. In RM patients, a number of uncontrolled trials of IvIg treatment have been carried out with apparently favorable results. However, without an untreated control group the effect is impossible to evaluate. Seven PCTs of IvIg treatment including 345 RM patients have been published so far [32–38]. The results have been very different with one trial showing a significant treatment effect [34], another showing a strong trend towards a treatment effect [33] whereas the others did not demonstrate any beneficial effect at all. In the Cochrane meta-analysis, the pooled OR for live birth was 0.98 (95% CI 0.61–1.58) and it was concluded that there was no benefit of IvIg in the treatment of RM [20]. After the publication of this Cochrane analysis, IvIg treatment was abandoned in most clinics and further testing in PCTs virtually stopped since the pharmaceutical companies producing IvIg seem to be very reluctant to support further relevant trials because they accept the negative conclusion from the Cochrane review. In 2006 another meta-analysis of the published PCTs found that the overall live-birth rates for IvIg and placebo were 61.0% and 54.9%, respectively (OR = 1.28, 95% CI 0.78–2.10) [39]. However, in the secondary RM group (Figure 16.2), the respective live-birth rates were 63.8% and 38.6% (OR = 2.71, 95% CI = 1.09–6.73, $P = 0.03$) pointing towards a much better effect in secondary than in primary RM where no positive effect could be found at all.

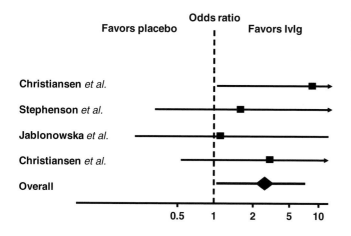

**Figure 16.2** Pooled odds ratio for live birth after intravenous immunoglobulin (IvIg) versus placebo calculated for patients with secondary recurrent miscarriage from four trials [33,36–39].

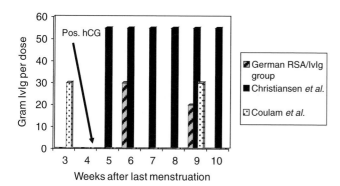

**Figure 16.3** Details of the infusion protocols from three placebo-controlled trials of intravenous immunoglobulin (IvIg) in patients with recurrent miscarriage [32,34,38].

## Heterogeneity of IvIg trials

In the seven PCTs, the live-birth rate after IvIg ranged from 45% [38] to 77% [37] but after placebo ranged even more from 29% [33] to 79–83% [35,37]. This stresses the fact that the trials are extremely heterogeneous. The heterogeneity can be due to (a) heterogeneity of treatment protocols and (b) heterogeneity of patient populations.

### Heterogeneity of treatment protocols

Since the mode of action of IvIg in most immunological disorders is not fully clarified, the doses used in these disorders are empirical and often lack consensus. Frequently used regimens are: 0.4 g/kg body weight daily for 5 consecutive days for idiopathic thrombocytopenic purpura or 1 g/kg body weight/day for 2 days at 4-week intervals for severe asthma [40,41]. The doses used in most RM trials have generally been much smaller than those used in autoimmune disorders (Figure 16.3) and only in my two trials have doses approaching the former mentioned doses been used [33,38].

There was also an extreme diversity between the trials with regard to the starting time of the first infusion, the number of infusions given and the amount of IvIg/placebo given at each infusion (Figure 16.3). The starting time of IvIg infusions may be crucial since obviously any therapy for RM should start before the embryo is dying or already dead. The majority of miscarriages occur before week 8 and in these cases the embryo very often exhibits signs of impaired growth from week 6 as measured by ultrasound or hormones. It takes weeks to obtain some of the immunomodulating effect of IvIg and it is probably therefore important to start IvIg infusions from gestational week 5 or before if a beneficial effect is to be obtained. In spite of this, in three trials infusions were only started in most of the patients in week 6–8 after the detection of fetal heart action [32,35,37]. Pregnancies being viable at this relatively late time of gestation display a fair spontaneous prognosis for being successful because a considerable part of the "at risk" time has passed at the time of the first infusion of IvIg or placebo [42]. The success rate in the placebo group is thus expected to be high, which is also evident in the relevant trials where live-birth rates in the placebo group of 68–83% were detected [32,35,37]. Start of IvIg in gestational week 5 may even be too late for many pregnancies and it is reasonable to believe that starting infusions some time before embryonic implantation might improve the effect. In two trials [34,36] this approach was indeed used (Figure 16.3) and a meta-analysis of these two trials showed a significant treatment effect [39].

### Heterogeneity of patient populations

The patient populations were very different in the various trials; in my two PCTs 74–100% of the patients had more than four previous miscarriages compared with only 19% [32], 21% [35] and 22% [37] of the patients in other PCTs. In two trials [32,35] patients with secondary RM were excluded whereas in the other trials patients with secondary RM comprised more than half of the patients. This heterogeneity of the trials may have great importance for the possibility of finding an effect of IvIg since, as previously discussed, there are many indications that women with ≥4 miscarriages and women with secondary RM are especially prone to have an immunological background for their problem.

## Criticism of the Cochrane analysis on IvIg

The treatment protocols used and the patient populations of the PCTs included in the Cochrane analysis of IvIg in RM were thus extremely heterogeneous and it is questionable how much information can be obtained by the combination of all patients from these trials in a meta-analysis [20]. The Cochrane meta-analysis of IvIg did not look into relevant subgroups of patients (Table 16.1) although there is plenty of evidence to suggest that the dose of IvIg and the timing of the first infusion are very important for the effect and evidence from a non-Cochrane meta-analysis suggests that the effect may be greatest in secondary RM [39].

To conclude that IvIg is inefficient in the treatment of RM based on a non-selective summary of data from the available PCTs would be comparable to concluding that treatment of women with infertility, regardless of the cause, with ovarian stimulation using a fixed low follicle-stimulating hormone (FSH) dose is inefficient because a trial of such a treatment modality would not be able to show any significant effect of FSH therapy over placebo. However, if the patients in such a trial were subdivided according to the causes of infertility and only those with anovulation and no other infertility causes were treated with adequate FSH doses adjusted by monitoring of the follicle growth, a significant treatment effect would be found.

## Negative aspects of immunotherapy in RM

### Allogeneic leukocyte immunization therapy

The use of ALT poses – in theory – serious side effects: transmission of viruses and prions, suppression of the immune defence against infections and maybe a long-term increased risk of some hematologic malignancies [43]. Infectious agents such as HIV and hepatitis B and C can be transmitted. The cell donors should be screened for these infections but such screening can never provide 100% certainty since the donors can be recently infected and the cellular suspensions cannot be virus-inactivated. In my trial many treated patients had significant influenza-like symptoms after intravenous DLT and major and minor postnatal complications were found in 8/29 (28%) of the children born after DLT compared with 1/10 (10%) children born after placebo [24]. However, looking at only major complications, the frequencies were equal in the two groups: 2/29 (7%) versus 1/10 (10%).

A study by Kling et al. evaluated maternal side effects in a large group of women with RM and recurrent implantation failure treated with intradermal PLT [44]. The occurrence of side effects was low and comparable to the frequency of side effects after vaccination for infectious diseases.

### Intravenous immunoglobulin

There are two negative aspects of IvIg therapy that must be considered when deciding whether to use IvIg therapy to RM patients or not: (a) the potential harm effects and (b) the economic costs of the drug.

#### Harm effects of IvIg

The harm effects can be divided into allergy, direct effects on organs and the risk of transmission of infectious agents. A severe immunological reaction against the (small) IgA content in IvIg can develop in IgA-deficient patients: however, by screening for IgA deficiency (found in approximately 1/800) before IvIg infusion this complication can be avoided. Allergic reactions against other components in IvIg are normally slight (skin rash, arthralgias).

A series of pathogens pose a confirmed or theoretical risk of transmission by plasma products. Hepatitis A, B and C, HIV 1 and 2, HTLV I/II and parvovirus 19 can be transmitted by blood products and the prions causing the variant form of Creutzfeldt – Jakob disease might be transferred by plasma products although it has never been documented. Considerable achievements have been reached in the reduction of the possible risk of transmission of infectious agents. The main steps in obtaining the current high safety of plasma products are: (1) rigid donor selection procedure, (2) screening of donations in order to exclude infectious donations and quarantining of batches of plasma for 60 days, and (3) validated steps for elimination and/or inactivation of potentially infectious agents. Using the procedures mentioned has resulted in a high pathogen safety of currently available plasma products. Indeed there has not been reported any transmission of pathogens after IvIg infusion since the early 1990s [45].

### The costs of IvIg

The economical costs of IvIg are unfortunately high due to the production process, which including screening for and inactivation of pathogens, is complex and expensive. In Denmark, the price for IvIg paid by the hospitals to the manufacturers is approximately 48 euros/g. A patient with secondary RM and at least four first-trimester miscarriages will in my clinic receive seven infusions of 25 g IvIg, which cost 8400 euros. According to my PCTs [33,38], the treatment will increase the live-birth rate from 23% to 58%. The number of patients needed to treat (NNT) to achieve one additional live birth can be calculated to 2.8 and each live birth will thus cost $2.8 \times 8400 = 23\,520$ euros. This amount is only slightly higher than the cost for each live birth after IVF/ICSI treatment provided that 60% of those starting treatment will end up having a live birth and that they on average will need two treatment cycles to achieve the live birth. IVF/ICSI treatment is today a generally accepted treatment and in Denmark and several other countries it is publicly funded. If full documentation for the efficacy of IvIg in subsets of RM can be provided there is thus no reason that this treatment should not be publicly funded too.

## Possible mechanisms of action of immunotherapy in RM

Initial theories proposed until 1990 claimed that "unexplained" RM was caused by inability of the patients to produce so-called antipaternal blocking antibodies – this inability was thought to be due to excessive sharing of HLA antigens between partners. Neither the theories of excessive HLA sharing nor the lack of blocking antibodies have been substantiated and this has been used as an argument from the opponents of immunotherapy for abandoning these therapies [46,47]. However, recent research indicates that the putative immunological background for many cases of RM is much more complex than suggested by the initial simple theories of an adverse alloimmune response. The potential mode of action of immunotherapy in RM is thus much more multifaceted than initially suggested.

In Table 16.2 are listed a number of plausible theories trying to explain how active immunotherapy with ALT and passive immunotherapy with IvIg may work in the prevention of pregnancy loss. Several of these theories have not been substantiated, for example in my PCT of IvIg [33] it was not possible to detect any short-term decrease in the levels of a series of autoantibodies. Other mechanisms, for example induction of apoptosis of activated lymphocytes or establishment of donor cell microchimerism have so far not been investigated in RM patients receiving ALT or IvIg [31,48].

## Conclusions

Overall, there is evidence that ALT increases the live-birth rate by 30% in unselected RM patients and even more in those with primary RM without auto- and alloantibodies. Since it may pose potential short- and long-term risks, patients must be thoroughly informed of the potential risk and the limited benefit of the treatment. More PCTs in the potential main target group with primary RM should be undertaken to get better documentation for the benefit and more information about the optimal doses and methods of administration and about harm effects. In my clinic we have not offered ALT for the last 4 years since many aspects of this treatment still need to be elucidated.

The current knowledge about IvIg treatment in RM is based on seven very heterogeneous PCTs. As discussed above, there are indeed many strong indications that IvIg display effects in subsets of RM patients using the right protocols (Figure 16.2) [39]. The first PCTs have provided enough information to enable us to prepare a protocol for a new large PCT, which would have a very good chance to document an effect. A new PCT focusing on patients with secondary RM and using an IvIg infusion protocol associated with a 23.5% therapeutic effect in this subgroup should be conducted and it may still be possible to recruit patients to such a trial [33]. A new US/Canadian PCT of IvIg in secondary RM is soon being concluded and in my clinic we have now initiated a PCT of IvIg focusing on the same patient subset. I am thus confident that within 3–4 years the possible benefit of IvIg in secondary RM will be unambiguously clarified.

Patients undergoing immunotherapy inside or outside PCTs should be monitored for changes of some of the immunological biomarkers that have drawn attention during recent years (Table 16.2). Finding a significant association between immunotherapy-induced changes in these biomarkers and successful pregnancy outcome will be of importance for our understanding of the mechanisms of action of immunotherapy in RM. More knowledge is required about the pathophysiological background of RM in order that both new and traditional immunological interventions can be tested in the right patients in the right way. In the future, immunotherapy for RM may comprise interventions that target the immune system more specifically than the treatments discussed in this chapter: injections with cytokines or cytokine inhibitors and treatments acting locally in the uterus. Such treatments, in addition, have the advantage that they do not pose any risk of infections. A long journey, however, remains before these interventions have undergone adequate testing in PCTs and before this is done, they should not be used in clinical practice.

# References

1. Christiansen OB. A fresh look at the causes and treatments of recurrent miscarriage, especially its immunological aspects. *Hum Reprod Update* 1996; **2**: 271–93.

2. Petri M, Golbus M, Anderson R *et al.* Antinuclear antibody, lupus anticoagulant and cardiolipin antibody in women with idiopathic habitual abortion. *Arthritis Rheum* 1987; **30**: 601–6.

3. Xu L, Chang V, Murphy A, *et al.* Antinuclear antibodies in sera of patients with recurrent pregnancy wastage. *Am J Obstet Gynecol* 1990; **163**: 1493–7.

4. Hill JA, Polgar K, Anderson DJ. T-helper 1-type immunity to trophoblast in women with recurrent spontaneous abortion. *J Am Med Assoc* 1995; **273**: 1933–6.

5. Quack KC, Vassiliadou N, Pudney J *et al.* Leukocyte activation in the decidua of chromosomally normal and abnormal fetuses from women with recurrent abortion. *Hum Reprod* 2001; **16**: 949–55.

6. Kruse C, Rosgaard A, Steffensen R, *et al.* Low serum level of mannan-binding lectin is a determinant for pregnancy outcome in women with recurrent spontaneous abortion. *Am J Obstet Gynecol* 2002, **187**: 1313–20.

7. Christiansen OB, Nielsen HS, Lund M *et al.* Mannose-binding lectin-2 genotypes and recurrent late pregnancy losses. *Hum Reprod* 2009; **24**(2): 291–9.

8. Pfeiffer KA, Fimmers R, Engels G *et al.* The HLA-G genotype is potentially associated with idiopathic recurrent spontaneous abortion. *Mol Hum Reprod* 2001; **7**: 373–8.

9. Kruse C, Steffensen R, Varming K, Christiansen OB. A study of HLA-DR and – DQ alleles in 588 patients and 562 controls confirms that HLA-DRB1*03 is associated with recurrent miscarriage. *Hum Reprod* 2004; **19**: 1215–21.

10. Christiansen OB, Steffensen R, Nielsen HS, Varming K. Multifactorial etiology of recurrent miscarriage and its scientific and clinical implications. *Gyn Obstet Invest* 2008; **66**: 257–67.

11. Nielsen HS, Nybo Andersen A-M, Kolte AM, Christiansen OB. A firstborn boy is suggestive of a strong prognostic factor in secondary recurrent miscarriage: a confirmatory study. *Fertil Steril* 2008; **89**: 907–11.

12. Ogasawara M, Aoki K, Okada S, Suzumori K. Embryonic karyotype of abortuses in relation to the number of previous miscarriages. *Fertil Steril* 2000; **73**: 300–4.

13. Laskin CA, Bombardier C, Hannah ME, *et al.* Prednisone and aspirin in women with autoantibodies and unexplained recurrent fetal loss. *New Engl J Med* 1997; **337**: 148–53.

14. Chaouat G, Kiger N, Wegmann TG. Vaccination against spontaneous abortion in mice. *J Reprod Immunol* 1983; **5**: 389–92.

15. Opelz G, Sengar DPS, Mickey MR, Terasaki PI. Effect of blood transfusions in subsequent kidney transplantations. *Transplant Proc* 1973; **5**: 253–9.

16. Mowbray JF, Gibbings CR, Lidell H *et al.* Controlled trial of treatment of recurrent spontaneous abortions by immunisation with paternal cells. *Lancet* 1085; **I**: 941–3.

17. Recurrent Miscarriage Immunotherapy Trialists Group. Worldwide collaborative observational study and meta-analysis on allogeneic leukocyte immunotherapy for recurrent spontaneous abortion. *Am J Reprod Immunol* 1994; **32**: 55–72.

18. Daya S, Gunby J and Recurrent Miscarriage Immunotherapy Trialists Group. The effectiveness of allogeneic leukocyte immunization in unexplained primary recurrent spontaneous abortion. *Am J Reprod Immunol* 1994; **32**: 294–302.

19. Ober C, Karrison T, Odem RR *et al.* Mononuclear-cell immunization in prevention of recurrent miscarriages: a randomized trial. *Lancet* 1999; **354**: 365–9.

20. Porter TF, LaCoursiere Y, Scott JR. Immunotherapy for recurrent miscarriage [Cochrane Review]. *Cochrane Database Syst Rev* 2006: **2**: CD000112.

21. Pandey MK, Agrawal S. Induction of MLR-Bf and protection of fetal loss: a current double blind randomized trial of paternal lymphocyte immunization for women with recurrent spontaneous abortion. *Int Immunopharmacol* 2004; **4**: 289–98.

22. Cauchi MN, Lim D, Young DE *et al.* Treatment of recurrent aborters by immunization with paternal cells – controlled trial. *Am J Reprod Immunol* 1991; **25**: 16–17.

23. Illeni MT, Marelli G, Parazzini F *et al.* Immunotherapy and recurrent abortion: a randomized clinical trial. *Hum Reprod* 1994; **9**: 1247–9.

24. Christiansen OB, Mathiesen O, Husth M *et al.* Placebo-controlled trial of active immunization with third party leukocytes in recurrent miscarriage. *Acta Obstet Gynecol Scand* 1994; **73**: 261–8.

25. Wood KJ, Jones ND, Bushell AR, Morris PJ. Alloantigen-induced specific immunological unresponsiveness. *Phil Trans R Soc Lond* 2001; **356**: 665–80.

26. Christiansen OB, Andersen A-MN, Bosch E *et al.* Evidence-based investigations and treatments of recurrent pregnancy loss. *Fertil Steril* 2005; **83**: 821–39.

27. Clark DA, Chaouat G. Loss of surface CD200 on stored allogeneic leukocytes may impair anti-abortive effect in vivo. *Am J Reprod Immunol* 2002; **53**: 13–20.

28. Reznikoff-Etievant MF. Abstracts of contributors' individual data submitted to the Worldwide Prospective Observation Study on Immunotherapy for Treatment of Recurrent Spontaneous Abortion. *Am J Reprod Immunol* 1994; **32**: 266–7.

29. Carp HJA, Toder V, Torchinsky A *et al.* Allogeneic leukocyte immunization after five or more miscarriages. *Hum Reprod* 1997; **12**: 250–5.

30. Bayry J, Misra N, Latry V *et al.* Mechanisms of action of intravenous immunoglobulin in autoimmune and inflammatory diseases. *Transfus Clin Biol* 2003; **10**: 165–9.

31. Prasad NK, Papoff G, Zeuner A *et al.* Therapeutic preparations of normal polyspecific IgG (IVIG) induce apoptosis in human lymphocytes and monocytes: a novel mechanism of action of IVIG involving the Fas apoptotic pathway. *J Immunol* 1998; **161**: 3781–90.

32. The German RSA/IVIG Group Intravenous immunoglobulin in the prevention of recurrent miscarriage. *Br J Obstet Gynaecol* 1994; **101**: 1072–7.

33. Christiansen OB, Mathiesen O, Husth M *et al.* Placebo-controlled trial of treatment of unexplained secondary recurrent spontaneous abortions and recurrent late spontaneous abortions with i.v. immunoglobulin. *Hum Reprod* 1995; **10**: 2690–5.

34. Coulam C, Krysa L, Stern J, Bustillo M. Intravenous immunoglobulin for treatment of recurrent pregnancy loss. *Am J Reprod Immunol* 1995; **34**: 333–7.

35. Perino A, Vassiliadis A, Vucetich A *et al.* Short-term therapy for recurrent abortion using intravenous immunoglobulins: results of a double-blind placebo-controlled Italian study. *Hum Reprod* 1997; **12**: 2388–92.

36. Stephenson MD, Dreher K, Houlihan E, Wu V. Prevention of unexplained recurrent spontaneous abortion using intravenous immunoglobulin: a prospective, randomized, double-blinded, placebo-controlled trial. *Am J Reprod Immunol* 1998; **39**: 82–8.

37. Jablonowska B, Selbing A, Palfi M *et al.* Prevention of recurrent spontaneous abortion by intravenous immunoglobulin: a double-blind placebo-controlled study. *Hum Reprod* 1999; **14**: 838–41.

38. Christiansen OB, Pedersen B, Rosgaard A, Husth M. A randomized, double-blind, placebo-controlled trial of intravenous immunoglobulin in the prevention of recurrent miscarriage: evidence for a therapeutic effect in women with secondary recurrent miscarriage. *Hum Reprod* 2002; **17**: 809–16.

39. Hutton B, Sharma R, Fergusson D *et al.* Use of intravenous immunoglobulin for treatment of recurrent miscarriage: a systematic review. *BJOG* 2006; **114**: 134–42.

40. Imbach P, Baradun S, d'Apuzzo V *et al.* High-dose intravenous gammaglobulin for idiopathic thrombocytopenic purpura in childhood. *Lancet* 1981; **1**: 1228–31.

41. Mazer BD, Gelfand EW. An open-label study of high dose intravenous immunoglobulin in severe childhood asthma. *J Allergy Clin Immunol* 1991; **87**: 976–83.

42. Brigham SA, Conlon C, Farquharson RG. A longitudinal study of pregnancy outcome following idiopathic recurrent miscarriage. *Hum Reprod* 1999; **14**: 2868–71.

43. Blajchman MA. Allogeneic blood transfusions, immunomodulation and postoperative bacterial infection: Do we have the answers yet? (Editorial). *Transfusion* 1997; **37**: 121–5.

44. Kling C, Steinmann J, Westphal E *et al.* Adverse efects of intradermal allogeneic lymphocyte immunotherapy: acute reactions and role of autoimmunity. *Hum Reprod* 2006; **21**: 429–35.

45. Späth PJ, Kempf C. Challenges and achievements in pathogen safety of intravenous immunoglobulin. In MC Dalakas, PJ Späth (eds.), *Intravenous Immunoglobulins in the Third Millennium*. Washington DC: Parthenon Publishing, 2004, pp. 9–20.

46. Coulam CB. Immunological tests in the evaluation of reproductive disorders: a critical review. *Am J Obstet Gynecol* 1992; **167**: 1844–51.

47. Porter TF, Scott JR. Alloimmune causes of recurrent pregnancy loss. *Semin Reprod Med* 2000; **18**: 393–400.

48. Starzl TE, Demetris AJ, Murase N *et al.* Donor cell chimerism permitted by immunosuppressive drugs: a new view of organ transplantation. *Immunol Today* 1993; **14**: 326–32.

# Endometrial receptivity

José A. Horcajadas

## Summary

The development of endometrial receptivity is a pre-requisite for successful embryonic implantation. Receptive status is only acquired during a short period of time in the mid-luteal phase, called the window of implantation (WOI). During this time, centered 7 days after the endogenous peak of LH (LH + 7), the endometrial epithelium acquires a functional ability to support blastocyst adhesion. To understand the basic mechanisms implicated in endometrial receptivity, researchers have investigated, during the last decade, the molecular events in the endometrium using the preferred molecular approach in animal and/or human models. The development of microarray technology has made it possible to analyze the expression of thousands of genes at the same time in a specific sample. In the last 7 years, an uncountable number of genes have been demonstrated to be regulated during the WOI in humans. However, the search for a potential informative marker of uterine receptivity to embryo implantation is still ongoing. This chapter summarizes the hormonal regulation and molecular bases of endometrial receptivity, its clinical implication and the possible models to study this complex process and to develop functional assays in vitro.

## Introduction

The human endometrium is a complex tissue and its cyclic regulation requires the successful interaction of a myriad of factors. This organ is hormonally regulated, being non-adhesive to embryos throughout most of the menstrual cycle in humans and other mammals. The endometrium undergoes dynamic reorganization during the menstrual cycle in preparation for implantation. If implantation does not occur, the superficial layer is partially or completely shed and remodeled for the next cycle [1]. In this environment,

endometrial receptivity refers to a hormone-limited period in which the endometrial tissue acquires a functional and transient ovarian steroid-dependent status allowing blastocyst adhesion [2].

Endometrial receptivity has been studied from the histological, biochemical and molecular point of view. Morphological changes include modifications in the plasma membrane [3] and cytoskeleton [4,5]. These changes occur as part of the complex decidualization process that takes place in the stromal compartment [6] and endometrial vasculature. Moreover, several biochemical markers for endometrial receptivity have been proposed over the years [7] although so far none of them has proved to be clinically useful.

The common classical approach to analyze this process has been the "fishing" strategy: attempts to determine a gene responsible for the receptive status by a one-by-one approach, meaning that researchers were focusing on a specific gene or a small group of genes and studying it from different perspectives. The recent advent of high-throughput microarray screening of the expression of human genes has permitted a new approach for identifying changes in global gene expression in a specific physiological or pathological situation [8]. As a result, an enormous amount of data is generated and the task of a researcher is to identify the desired markers by eliminating the unrelated genes and revealing the interesting ones by this elimination process.

This chapter focuses on the endometrial receptivity process taking into account other important aspects of the endometrial regulation, function and model of study.

## The endometrium as a tissue

The lining of the human uterus is a complex mucosa composed of two major compartments: a germinal or basal layer (basalis), which persists from cycle to cycle, and a transient superficial layer (functionalis). The function of the latter is to accommodate the implanting blastocyst and provide the maternal component of the placenta. The tissue components of the endometrium are a lining surface of epithelium and associated glands with a connective tissue stroma in which is embedded an elaborate vascular tree. Endometrial components' features change along the menstrual cycle [9].

Cyclic changes of the endometrium have been well described at the light microscopy level [1]. Although some authors prefer to simplify the menstrual cycle and divide it into two main phases, proliferative and secretory, it is much more exact to consider three different phases: the proliferative phase (days 5–14), the secretory phase (14–28) and menses (days 1–4) if no implantation occurs.

For more than 50 years, histological evaluation of the endometrium has been the gold standard for clinical diagnosis set on the basis of the morphological observations of Noyes and colleagues [10,11]. The authors described the "specific" morphological appearance of the different compartments of the endometrium throughout the menstrual cycle. They distinguished different phases of the cycle on the basis of histological features and even endometrial dating during the luteal phase. Here we present basic histological features of the endometrium along the menstrual cycle.

The early proliferative phase (days 5–7) is characterized by straight, fairly undifferentiated glands with circular cross-section lined by a columnar epithelium with basally located nuclei. Their luminal diameter (below 50 μm) changes little in the proliferative phase and the height of the cells remains fairly constant (around 21 μm). Few mitotic figures can be seen. By the mid-proliferative phase (days 8–10) the endometrial glands are longer with slight tortuosity. Mitotic figures are prominent and cells appear pseudostratified. In the late proliferative phase (11–14) the glands appear with a marked tortuosity and wider lumena. Pseudostratification increases and stromal edema starts to be evident. During secretory phase (LH + 2/3) there is still a moderate degree of glandular and stromal mitosis. The cells appear taller and less pseudostratified than before. At LH + 4 only occasional mitoses can be seen. Sub- and supra-nuclear vacuoles within the gland cells are maximal on this day. Gland cell size is also maximal on this day. At LH + 5 mitosis activity has ceased absolutely in glands although can be

visualized in stroma. Around 25% of the endometrium is occupied by glands in this phase. At LH + 7 the gland cells contain little secretory material and have acquired a low columnar to cuboidal appearance. This is the point of maximal receptivity for clinical and research purposes. The amounts of secretory product within the glands and stromal edema are both maximal by day LH + 8. In the last week of the secretory phase there are few changes and they mainly occur in stroma and blood vessels. The late secretory phase is characterized by regression and glandular involution. At day LH + 10 stromal edema has decreased and at LH+11 the stromal predecidual reaction is mainly confined to the perivascular regions, but may also extend to adjacent glands and there is lymphocytic infiltration. By day LH + 12 the predecidual reaction extends to beneath the luminal epithelium. There is an increase in the lymphocyte number. The predecidual reaction is extensive on days LH + 13/14, with a sheet-like formation in the stroma. Stroma disintegration and extravasation of erythrocytes are evident. If no implantation occurs, shedding of the functionalis layer of the endometrium ensues [9].

## Regulation of the endometrial gene expression profile

The human endometrium undergoes cyclical variation with every menstrual cycle during the reproductive years. The endometrial changes driven by the ovarian steroid hormones. Estradiol has a peak of expression at the end of the proliferative phase and progesterone starts to increase its concentration at the beginning of the secretory phase, peaking on day 21 (Figure 17.1). These elicit their actions by binding to specific high-affinity receptors, which, acting as transcriptional factors, modulate the transcription of a large number and variety of genes. Global gene expression analyses performed along the menstrual cycle have revealed a strong relationship between molecular profile and hormonal regulation. The major changes of gene expression levels occur in the mid-secretory phase.

Both estrogen receptor α (ERα) and β (ERβ) are expressed in the endometrium, being ERα dominant. This receptor is present in both the epithelial glands and stroma of the functionalis layer, with its expression maximal during the proliferative phase and declining during the secretory phase. Epithelial ERβ also decreases during the secretory phase but it is not

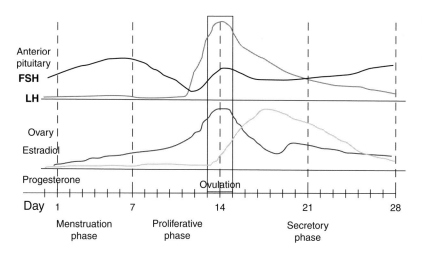

**Figure 17.1** Profile of expression of the hormones during the menstrual cycle. A color reproduction of this figure can be found in the color plate section.

detected in stroma. Progesterone receptor A and B are co-expressed in endometrium. Their expression is stimulated by estrogen during the proliferative phase and downregulated by progesterone in the secretory phase.

The coordinated action of steroids, acting through their nuclear receptors, in the endometrial cells, promotes the gene regulation of hundreds of genes, inducing the formation of a receptive phenotype. Endometrial cells undergo specific structural and functional changes that allow the embryo to implant. Detailed analyses, phase by phase, using microarray technology are published by Ponnampalam *et al.* [12] and Talbi *et al.*[13].

## Markers of endometrial receptivity

For decades, a large amount of research worldwide has been focused on the problem of finding a specific marker(s) of uterine (endometrial) receptivity – biomarkers that will predict functionality and that can be useful for the diagnosis and treatment of couples with infertility of endometrial origin. What are our requirements for these markers? They have to be present in fertile women with proven fertility during the window of implantation, have to be (relatively) easily measurable (preferably by non-invasive methods), correlate to successful implantation and be absent or significantly reduced in infertile women with unexplained (possible endometrial factor) infertility.

### Histological dating

The first approach to assess uterine receptivity was the histological dating by Noyes in 1950 [10], further revised by the same authors [11]. These classic papers

have been the most quoted in our field, cited thousands of times and followed as "the" diagnostic tool for endometrial dating and endometrial research worldwide. However, its accuracy and the functional relevance of this system based exclusively on histological observations as a predictor of receptivity have been questioned in recent randomized studies [14,15]. Murray and colleagues have demonstrated that histological features solely have high interobserver, intraobserver and intercycle variations [15]. The differences between pathologists depend on the day of the menstrual cycle when the endometrial biopsy is collected. Also, this methodology does not have the capability to discriminate between fertile and infertile couples [14]. These studies suggest that new technologies should be added for objective identification of endometrial samples and the study of endometrial development in health and disease.

## Pinopodes and immunohistochemical markers

With the advent of electron microscopy and immunological and molecular techniques, the number of potential biomarkers has increased dramatically over the last 20 years. The best recognized structure associated with the receptive endometrium is the pinopode. These structural adaptations of the luminal surface epithelium were first described in 1971 [16]. Nikas and colleagues reported that pinopodes are expressed for only 1–2 days and the appearance of these structures varies within the window of implantation [17]. It has been reported that variability between cycles and between patients and variations in the temporal and spatial distribution argue against

**Table 17.1** Different studies performed at the time of implantation in human using wide genomic analysis.

| Study | Samples | RNA pooled | First sample (day of cycle) | Second sample (day of cycle) | Fold change | UP | DOWN |
|---|---|---|---|---|---|---|---|
| Kao et al. [23] | 11 | No | Prolif. phase (8–10) | LH+(8–10) (21–23) | >2 | 156 | 377 |
| Carson et al. [22] | 6 | Yes | LH+(2–4) (15–17) | LH+(7–9) (20–22) | >2 | 323 | 370 |
| Borthwick et al. [24] | 10 | Yes | Prolif. phase (9–11) | LH+(6–8) (19–21) | >2 | 90 | 46 |
| Riesewijk et al. [25] | 10 | No | LH+2 (15) | LH+7 (20) | >3 | 153 | 58 |
| Mirkin et al. [26] | 8 | No | Early-luteal (16) | Mid-luteal (21) | >2 | 49 | 58 |

its usefulness as a specific biomarker of receptive endometrium.

Immunohistochemical assessment of the endometrium has identified a large number of endometrial proteins that present cycle-dependent expression around the time of implantation. These proteins show a controlled expression around day 20–24 of the menstrual cycle in fertile women. Among them are the 24 kDa heat shock protein [18], integrins (αvβ3, α1β1), MUC-1, glycodelin, CD44, Leukemia Inhibitory Factor (LIF), Heparin Binding EGF (HB-EGF), HOXA-10, prolactin, IGF-II, Cadherin-11 and calcitonin [19]. Other putative biomarkers of endometrial receptivity have been studied because of the results obtained with mouse knock-out (KO) models such as Leptin, Basigin or p53 [20].

## Gene expression markers

The strongest acceleration in the discovery of new markers has occurred with the advent of DNA microarray analyses. DNA microarray technology is so far one of the most widely used and potentially revolutionary research tools derived from the human genome project. This technique has been developed within the last decade and allows the assessment of the complete genomic expression profile in a given biological sample in a single experiment [8].

The technique is based on the complementarity of the DNA duplex and the capability of single-stranded DNA to bind to solid supports such as nylon membranes or glass. Usually, immobilized probes are hybridized with labeled cDNAs. This labeling can be carried out with fluorescence or radioactivity depending on the support chosen. There is a very wide range of microarrays commercially available, separated into two categories: cDNA arrays and high-density synthetic oligonucleotide microarrays [21].

In reproductive medicine, researchers started a race in this field and four studies on human endometrial gene expression were published in the period of 2002 and 2003 [22–25]. Two years later, another paper on this topic was published [26]. Although all of these studies used the same technology, many differences in experimental design and data analysis require attention. These include the day of the menstrual cycle for endometrial biopsy, the phases of the menstrual cycle compared, patient-to-patient genomic variation, number of endometrial biopsies and pooling or not pooling the isolated RNA (see Table 17.1). Furthermore, different data analysis and statistical methods were employed for considering a gene regulated. Four of them established a minimal two-fold increase to consider gene regulation evident. However, our group considered a more stringent criterion of a three-fold increase, and samples were obtained from the same patient on 2 different days of the menstrual cycle. This approach minimizes biological variability between samples [25].

All the studies focused on endometrial receptivity have generated long lists of genes with known and unknown potential roles in this critical process. The differences indicated in study designs and methodologies are reflected in the lack of a large list of consensus genes. Strikingly, only one gene, i.e. osteopontin, was consistently upregulated in all five studies at the time of implantation. There are several important molecules highlighted by their presence in four of five papers. Some of them are proteins previously identified in the endometrium with or without a described

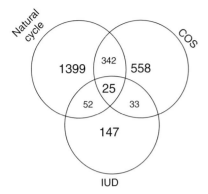

**Figure 17.2** Venn diagram comparing the three studies performed in our laboratory at the time of implantation in natural cycle [27], in COS [27] and in the presence of an inert IUD [28] to find the consensus genes in endometrial receptivity (with permission).

function. Genes were involved in lipid metabolism (apolipoprotein D), immune response (decay accelerating factor for complement, serine or cysteine proteinase, interleukin (IL)-15), regulation of cell cycle (growth arrest and DNA-damage-inducible, alpha), ion binding (annexin IV) or enzymes with different functions in different tissues (monoamine oxidase A).

In an attempt to create a user-friendly list of key genes, we decided to compare the results obtained in three different situations that included fertile conditions (natural cycle) [27], subfertile (COS) [27] and refractory conditions (IUD) [28]. After comparison of the three studies, we found that they only shared 25 WOI genes (Figure 17.2). Interestingly, all of them were regulated in one sense in the natural cycle, and on the contrary in COS and IUD (dys-regulated). However, it is not possible to assign the role of magic molecule in implantation to any of those molecules [29]. Endometrial receptivity has to be understood as a complex process produced by many genes in a coordinated way.

# Endometrial receptivity as a global process

The significant histological, biological and physiological features that occur in the endometrium throughout the menstrual cycle are ultimately the result of changes that occur at the gene transcription level, together with post-transcriptional modifications and epigenetic changes. Endometrial receptivity at the time of embryonic implantation is a crucial moment of the menstrual cycle with a fundamental relevance

and its understanding has been one of the main goals for researchers working in human reproduction.

Most of the laboratories have their favorite protein or molecule and have tried to elaborate its function in endometrial receptivity. But, at the moment, functional studies have not demonstrated the existence of a magic bullet for human endometrial receptivity as we have mentioned previously. Probably, we will never be able to understand this complex process with the narrow focus of one gene, because it is the result of an equilibrated expression of many genes that conform to pathways. For this reason, our laboratory, has analyzed the development of the luteal phase day by day (Figure 17.3) and we have compared the results with the ovarian-stimulated cycles performed in IVF clinics [30].

In order to understand how cellular functionalities are activated and deactivated along the WOI in natural and stimulated cycles, we analyzed their corresponding temporal functional profiles. To that end, we used the first day as reference and we compared each subsequent day to this reference time by a gene set enrichment analysis, as implemented in the FatiScan tool of Babelomics [31]. Many over-represented biological terms were shared in both natural and COS categories, particularly on days +3 and +5, suggesting a similar development on the first days of the WOI. On day +7 however, the natural cycle showed a higher number of over-represented biological terms, such as *localization, response to external stimulus, locomotion, response to biotic stimulus* and others [30]. Interestingly, most of these GO terms are not present in the transition from day hCG+5 to hCG+7 in COS cycles. Only two GO terms are conserved in the transition from the pre-receptive to receptive state in natural and COS cycles; these terms are the response to the stress and cellular physiological process.

We also found similarities in the biological terms under-represented in the pre-receptive endometrium, except on day +7 when more differences were observed. On day +7, no common biological term was identified in natural and COS cycles. Furthermore, some terms appeared to be under-represented in hCG+7 of COS cycles, such as response to external stimulus or organismal physiological process, which are over-represented in LH+7 of natural cycles [30]. These results show that we can consider a function or a dysfunction taking into account a gene, a couple of genes or a small number of genes. Endometrial

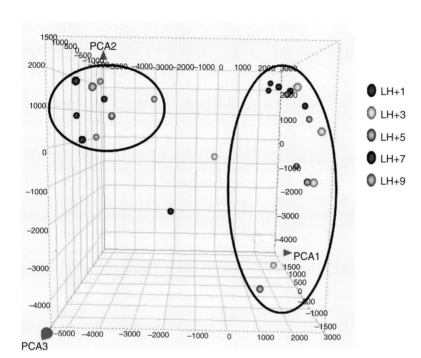

**Figure 17.3** Principal component analysis of human endometrium throughout the development of the secretory phase (after the endogenous pick of LH) in natural cycle (adapted from Horcajadas *et al.* [30]). A color reproduction of this figure can be found in the color plate section.

LH+1
LH+3
LH+5
LH+7
LH+9

receptivity is a complex process in which every regulated gene contributes to the global process in a particular manner.

## New methods for endometrial receptivity studies

The main techniques used to study the features of the receptive endometrium include microscopy for endometrial morphology [32], quantitative PCR, in situ hybridization and gene expression microarrays for gene expression in endometrial biopsy [29]. Other approaches have analyzed the proteomics and metabolomics of endometrial biopsies or endometrial flushings or secretions [33].

It is evident that evaluation of endometrial function must include new technologies. The histological studies previously discussed [14,15] suggest that new technologies should be added for objective identification of biological samples (biopsies or flushing) and the study of endometrial development in health and disease.

During the last 10 years many researchers have tried to create an objective and modern tool for endometrial evaluation. However, those kits currently commercially available have not demonstrated to be sufficiently useful for clinic use. Last year, our laboratory presented the ERA (Endometrial Receptivity

Array) [34]. During the last 5 years and using a whole genome microarray we analyzed the differential gene expression profile of endometria at LH + 1, LH + 3, LH + 5 (pre-receptive phase) versus LH + 7 (receptive phase) by a t-test. A list of 738 probes representing 293 genes was selected to create our ERA according to very strict criteria. The functional sense of these genes was assessed by FATIGO-GEPAS [31]. A significant number of these genes are implicated in the response to stress, defense response and cell adhesion. This molecular method that lists a gene selection for endometrial receptivity offers a new objective tool for endometrial diagnosis. We are now in the functional validation of this array using endometrial samples with specific pathologies such as implantation failure, endometriosis and others. While this model could be a useful tool for clinic use, the future of endometrial evaluation has to be directed to non-invasive methods such as endometrial fluids or serum markers. Researchers are now working on these two lines of investigation to provide non-invasive diagnostic tools.

An alternative approach to studying endometrial receptivity and also embryonic implantation has been culture models. We can divide these models into explants, monolayer cultures, co-cultures and three-dimensional cultures. Organ explants would appear to provide perfect models for mimicking the in vivo environment, as the three-dimensional structure and integrity of the endometrium is preserved and all layers of the endometrium are included. Landgren *et al.* [35] developed a model using endometrial biopsies taken 4, 5 and 6 days after the LH peak from healthy women with normal regular menstrual cycles. It was used for placing embryos on the lining epithelium of the explant within 3 hours of the biopsy being taken. Monolayer culture consists of single cultures of endometrial epithelial cells in flasks and wells. These cultures can be performed using primary cell culture coming from endometrial biopsies or established endometrial epithelial cell lines. These cultures have been used mainly for studying the response to drugs and for embryo adhesion assays [5]. A co-culture consists of a separated but communicated culture of epithelial and stromal endometrial cells. This has been used to get high rates of blastocyst formation in a clinical setting, especially as a salvage treatment option in couples with repeated implantation failures [36,37]).

The ultimate in vitro model to study endometrial receptivity and embryonic implantation therefore would contain all the cell types of the endometrium (epithelium, stroma, endothelial and immune cells) so that the complex interactions between the maternal tissue and the blastocyst could be characterized. However, mimicking the physiological three-dimensional architecture of the endometrium is clearly a challenge. Several approaches have been reported, consisting of layers of epithelial and stromal cells grown in and below tissue culture well inserts (reviewed in Mardon *et al.* [38]. One arrangement consists of endometrial stromal cells seeded into a collagen type I gel in culture well inserts, on top of which there is a thin layer of Matrigel, and upon which endometrial epithelial cells are seeded. In a second model stromal cells are seeded into a culture well below the insert, and epithelial cells are plated on the surface of Matrigel in the insert described. A third configuration consists of stromal cells seeded into a mixture of collagen type I and Matrigel, and epithelial cell clumps placed on the surface. However, human studies using the three-dimensional models in conjunction with blastocysts are still very limited but constitute part of the future in endometrial receptivity investigation. Clinically, co-culture systems may provide means of developing novel culture media, overcoming recurrent implantation failure and deepen the knowledge of the molecular basis of endometrial receptivity while on the other hand providing a tool for developing new contraceptive agents.

## Conclusions

The molecular basis of endometrial receptivity and of the reciprocal interactions that occur between the blastocyst and the endometrium are still poorly understood [39,40]. Temporally, the window of implantation in the human appears to be restricted between cycle days 20 and 24 [41]. Spatially, although the whole endometrium shows changes at gene expression level, the receptive endometrium is restricted to a specific area [42]. Researchers have found many molecules whose expression is directly related with receptive status. Gene by gene analyses and microarray technology have produced huge amounts of data. However, it has been demonstrated that endometrial receptivity does not depend on a single molecule. All the functional genomic studies have shown that endometrial receptivity is a very complex process, in which an uncountable number of genes are involved. These works have also demonstrated that a limited number of candidates are always present and endometrial receptivity could be explained with their modifications. Now is the time to learn about what the genomic era can add to our understanding of human endometrial receptivity. Future directions in endometrial receptivity studies will also require complementarity with proteomics and functionomics. Although non-primate animal models have distinct advantages in economic and temporal cost, with vast amounts of genetic information and the ability to be genetically modified, they remain inherently limited in their ability to elucidate the physiological mechanisms of endometrial receptivity. However, studies on non-human primates have shown high fidelity to human implantation, suggesting their potential as models for investigation in endometrial receptivity, embryo implantation and early pregnancy.

## References

1. Wynn RM. The human endometrium: cyclic and gestational changes. In RM Wynn, WP Jollie (eds.), *Biology of the Uterus*. 2nd edition. New York: Plenum, 1989, pp. 289–332.

2. Psychoyos A. Uterine receptivity for nidation. *Ann N Y Acad Sci* 1986; **476**: 36–42.

3. Murphy CR. Human implantation: recent advances and clinical aspects. *J Reprod Fertil Suppl* 2000; **55**: 23–8.

4.  Thie MB, Harrach-Ruprecht B, Sauer H *et al.* Cell adhesion to the apical pole of epithelium: a function of cell polarity. *Eur J Cell Biol* 1995; **66**: 180–91.

5.  Martin JC, Jasper D, Valbuena D *et al.* Increased adhesiveness in cultured endometrial-derived cells is related to the absence of moesin expression. *Biol Reprod* 2000; **63**: 1370–6.

6.  Irwin J, Kirk D, King R *et al.* Hormonal regulation of human endometrial stromal cells in culture: an in vitro model for decidualization. *Fertil Steril* 1989; **52**: 761–8.

7.  Giudice LC. Emerging concepts on human implantation. *Hum Reprod* 1999; **14**(Suppl.): 3–16.

8.  Schena M, Shalon D, Davis RW, Brown PO. Quantitative monitoring of gene expression patterns with a complementary DNA microarray. *Science* 1995; **270**: 467–70.

9.  Dockery B, Burke MJ. The fine structure of mature human endometrium: In JD Aplin, AT Fazleabas, SR Glasser, LC Giudice (eds.), *The Endometrium: Molecular, Cellular and Clinical Perspectives*. 2nd edition. London: Informa Healthcare, 2008, pp. 46–65.

10. Noyes RW, Hertig AT, Rock J. Dating the endometrial biopsy. *Fertil Steril* 1950; **1**: 3–17.

11. Noyes RW, Hertig AT, Rock J. Dating the endometrial biopsy. *Am J Obstet Gynecol* 1975; **122**: 262–3.

12. Ponnampalam AP, Weston GC, Trajstman AC, Susil B, Rogers PA. Molecular classification of human endometrial cycle stages by transcriptional profiling. *Mol Hum Reprod* 2004; **10**: 879–93.

13. Talbi S, Hamilton AE, Vo KC *et al.* Molecular phenotyping of human endometrium distinguishes menstrual cycle phases and underlying biological processes in normo-ovulatory women. *Endocrinology* 2006; **147**: 1097–121.

14. Coutifaris C, Myers ER, Guzick DS *et al.* Histological dating of timed endometrial biopsy tissue is not related to fertility status. *Fertil Steril* 2004; **82**: 1264–72.

15. Murray MJ, Meyer WR, Zaino RJ *et al.* A critical analysis of the accuracy, reproducibility, and clinical utility of histologic endometrial dating in fertile women. *Fertil Steril* 2004; **81**: 1333–43.

16. Psychoyos A, Mandon P. Study of the surface of uterine epithelium by scanning electron microscopy. *CR Hebd Seances Acad Sci D* 1971; **272**: 2723–5 (in French).

17. Nikas G, Drakakis P, Loutradis D *et al.* Uterine pinopodes as markers of the "nidation window" in cycling women receiving exogenous oestradiol and progesterone. *Hum Reprod* 1995; **10**: 1208–13.

18. Ciocca DR, Asch RH, Adams DJ, McGuire WL. Evidence for modulation of a 24 K protein in human endometrium during the menstrual cycle. *J Clin Endocrinol Metab* 1983; **57**: 496–9.

19. Lessey B, Glasser S. Endometrial receptivity: In JD Aplin, AT Fazleabas, SR Glasser, LC Giudice (eds.), *The Endometrium: Molecular, Cellular and Clinical Perspectives*. 2nd edition. London: Informa Healthcare, 2008, pp. 46–65.

20. Aghajanova L, Simon C, Horcajadas JA. Are favorite molecules of endometrial receptivity still in favor? *Expert Rev Obstet Gynecol* 2008; **3**: 487–501.

21. Barret JC, Kawasaki ES. Microarrays: the use of oligonucleotides and cDNA for the analysis of gene expression. *Drug Discov Today* 2003; **8**: 134–41.

22. Carson DD, Lagow E, Thathiah A *et al.* Changes in gene expression during the early to mid-luteal (receptive phase) transition in human endometrium detected by high-density microarray screening. *Mol Hum Reprod* 2002; **8**: 871–9.

23. Kao LC, Tulac S, Lobo S *et al.* Global gene profiling in human endometrium during the window of implantation. *Endocrinology* 2002; **143**: 2119–38.

24. Borthwick JM, Charnock-Jones DS, Tom BD *et al.* Determination of the transcript profile of human endometrium. *Mol Hum Reprod* 2003; **9**: 19–33.

25. Riesewijk A, Martin J, van Os R *et al.* Gene expression profiling of human endometrial receptivity on days LH+2 versus LH+7 by microarray technology. *Mol Hum Reprod* 2003; **9**: 253–64.

26. Mirkin S, Arslan M, Churikov D *et al.* In search of candidate genes critically expressed in the human endometrium during the window of implantation. *Hum Reprod* 2005; **20**: 2104–17.

27. Horcajadas JA, Riesewijk A, Polman J *et al.* Effect of controlled ovarian hyperstimulation in IVF on endometrial gene expression profiles. *Mol Hum Reprod* 2005; **11**: 195–205.

28. Horcajadas JA, Sharkey AM, Catalano RD *et al.* Effect of an intrauterine device on the gene expression profile of the endometrium. *J Clin Endocrinol Metab* 2006; **91**: 3199–207.

29. Horcajadas JA, Pellicer A, Simon C. Wide genomic analysis of human endometrial receptivity: new times, new opportunities. *Hum Reprod Update* 2007; **13**: 77–86.

30. Horcajadas JA, Mínguez P, Dopazo J *et al.* Controlled ovarian stimulation induces a functional genomic delay of the endometrium with potential clinical implications. *J Clin Endocrinol Metab* 2008; **93**: 4500–10.

31. Al-Shahrour F, Diaz-Uriarte R, Dopazo J. FatiGO: a web tool for finding significant associations of Gene Ontology terms with groups of genes. *Bioinformatics* 2004; **20**: 578–80.

32. Bourgain C, Devroey P. Histologic and functional aspects of the endometrium in the implantatory phase. *Gynecol Obstet Invest* 2007; **64**: 131–3.

33. Boomsma CM, Kavelaars A, Eijkemans MJ *et al.* Cytokine profiling in endometrial secretions: a non-invasive window on endometrial receptivity. *Reprod Biomed Online* 2009; **18**: 85–94.

34. Díaz-Gimeno P, Horcajadas JA, Martínez-Conejero JA *et al.* Development of a customized array for the molecular diagnosis of human endometrial receptivity. *Fertil Steril* 2008; **90** (Suppl. 1).

35. Landgren BM, Johannisson E, Stavreus-Evers A, Hamberger L, Eriksson H. A new method to study the process of implantation of a human blastocyst in vitro. *Fertil Steril* 1996; **65**: 1067–70.

36. Simón C, Mercader A, Garcia-Velasco J *et al.* Coculture of human embryos with autologous human endometrial epithelial cells in patients with implantation failure. *J Clin Endocrinol Metab* 1999; **84**: 2638–46.

37. Barmat LI, Liu HC, Spandorfer SD *et al.* Autologous endometrial co-culture in patients with repeated failures of implantation after in vitro fertilization-embryo transfer. *J Assist Reprod Genet* 1999; **16**: 121–7.

38. Mardon H, Grewal S, Mills K. Experimental models for investigating implantation of the human embryo. *Semin Reprod Med* 2007; **25**: 410–17.

39. Dey SK, Lim H, Das SK, Reese J *et al.* Molecular cues to implantation. *Endocr Rev* 2004; **25**: 341–73.

40. Yoshinaga K. Review of factors essential for blastocyst implantation for their modulating effects on the maternal immune system. *Semin Cell Dev Biol* 2008; **19**: 161–9.

41. Anderson TI. Window of uterine receptivity. In T Yoshinaga (ed.), *Blastocyst Implantation*. Boston: Serono Symposia USA, Adams Publishing Group, 1990, pp. 219–24.

42. Guzeloglu-Kayisli O, Basar M, Arici A. Basic aspects of implantation. *Reprod Biomed Online* 2007; **15**: 728–39.

# Chapter 8

# Clinical assessment of the endometrium

Kristin Holoch and Bruce A. Lessey

## Introduction

### Historical perspective

Endometrium lining the uterine cavity develops from Müllerian anlagen, and consists of epithelial, stromal and vascular elements that undergo complex patterns of growth and differentiation each month of reproductive life, in anticipation of pregnancy [1]. As an interface, the endometrium maintains a role in immune surveillance and is also a conduit for spermatozoa from the vagina to the fallopian tubes. The endometrium represents an endocrine organ, a site of active leukocyte trafficking and one of two sites in adults where angiogenesis normally can be found. The endometrium undergoes monthly and predictable developmental cycles in response to ovarian steroids. By virtue of these many attributes, the endometrium presents many opportunities for clinical assessment related to its function. Assessment of the endometrium has become a focus of the diagnostic workup for infertility, pregnancy loss and abnormal uterine bleeding, which together account for over half of all medical visits by reproductive aged women.

The study of the uterus dates back at least 2400 years. Hippocrates (460–377 BC) first mentioned the uterus as a cavernous structure. As recently reviewed by Okulicz [2], Aristotle described the human uterus as bicornuate. It was not until the early second century AD that Soranus of Ephesus correctly described the anatomy of the uterus. In the fifteenth century Vesalius produced detailed drawings of the uterine anatomy and during this time, Leonardo da Vinci produced a classic drawing of the pregnant uterus in 1489, opened to show the fetus and placenta *in situ* (Figure 18.1).While the primary function of the uterus relates to childbearing, a detailed understanding of its diverse physiology has been revealed only during the last century of study.

Endometrium lines the inner surface of the myometrium and is a steroid hormone target tissue, like the breast and prostate. The endometrium undergoes almost continuous developmental changes starting at menstruation, thickening in response to follicular estrogen, and becoming receptive toward embryo implantation in response to progesterone following ovulation and formation of a corpus luteum [3]. Easy access to the endometrium has fostered early interest and facilitated research related to its function. Markee's classic experiment in which cycling endometrium was transplanted to an intraocular location in primates provided direct observations related to menstruation [4]. In the early 1950s, Noyes and colleagues established the initial histological dating criteria for assessment of endometrial development. Those criteria led to the concept of luteal phase defect (LPD), a hypothetical disorder first suggested by Georgina Seegar Jones in 1949. The diagnosis of LPD evolved from other early studies [5,6], although not without significant controversy and debate [7]. It remains one of the most studied areas of endometrial assessment and yet is still an enigma of uncertain clinical importance [8].

Infertility and recurrent pregnancy loss are often attributable to implantation failure [9–12]. The success of an early pregnancy requires synchronous interactions between the endometrium, corpus luteum and embryo; delayed implantation for any reason might contribute to implantation failure [13,14]. Up to one half of all pregnancy failures during in-vitro fertilization (IVF) cycles are thought to be due to defects in uterine receptivity [12], although embryo quality takes on greater importance as women age [15]. To interpret endometrial changes associated with implantation failure, the timing of implantation first had to be established.

*Early Pregnancy*, ed. Roy G. Farquharson and Mary D. Stephenson. Published by Cambridge University Press.
© Cambridge University Press 2010.

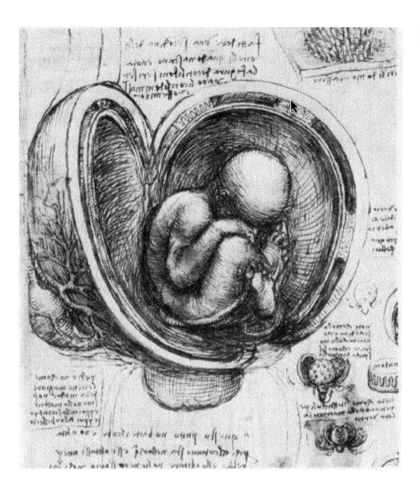

**Figure 18.1** Study of a womb, c. 1489 by Leonardo da Vinci.

During the 1950s, Hertig and colleagues examined hysterectomy samples from newly pregnant women; they identified and classified 34 embryos (eight free-floating before day 19 of the menstrual cycle and 26 attached, all after day 21) [16]. Not only did this landmark study suggest that a window of implantation existed, but it allowed these investigators access to early nidation sites, greatly advancing the field of implantation in humans. Other studies followed that further defined and refined the timing of endometrial receptivity [14,17–19].

With the availability of specific mono- and polyclonal antibodies, immuno-histochemistry supplanted histologic dating alone and this remains an active avenue for endometrial receptivity research [20–23]. In the last 10 years, DNA microarray techniques and other advanced molecular techniques have dramatically increased the number of candidate biomarkers of endometrial receptivity [11,24–26]. The use of non-invasive techniques including ultrasound, serum markers or the use of proteomics also promises to keep endometrial assessment in the foreground and an active area of research well into the future. The purpose of this chapter is to review available literature on the clinical assessment of the endometrium and to focus on those tools available to diagnose and treat both infertility and pregnancy loss.

## Implantation window and defects in uterine receptivity

The mechanism of implantation varies widely between species, reflecting the evolving conflicts between maternal and embryonic interests [27,28]. Hemochorial placentation as found in human and the higher primates begins with an initial interaction (apposition) between the embryo and the maternal endometrial lining [29,30]. Surface (luminal) epithelium of the endometrium is a barrier to embryo implantation throughout much of the menstrual cycle. Endometrial receptivity is acquired during the mid-secretory phase in normal fertile women and occurs about one week after ovulation, reflecting the acquisition of appropriate recognition factors and secretory proteins that permit and facilitate embryo–uterine adhesion, embryonic survival and subsequent invasion [31,32]. A concept of receptor-mediated implantation in humans is now well established [33–36] although epithelial–epithelial interaction at the apical surfaces between embryo and endometrium has long been described as a paradoxical event [37]. Attachment is an ephemeral process followed quickly by intrusive probing by the embryonic trophoblast [38], giving way to trophoblast invasion, along the loosened lateral luminal cell surfaces, digesting its way through the basement membrane into the underlying stroma (decidua) [39,40]. Based on classic studies, estimation of the window of endometrial receptivity extends from post-ovulatory days 6–10 (corresponding to cycle day 20–24).Wilcox and colleagues confirmed the timing of this window in normal fertile women and demonstrated that delayed implantation resulted in a higher risk of miscarriage [14].

If synchrony between the endometrium, ovary and embryo is essential, then histology delay in the endometrium could extend the time of non-receptivity and provide an explanation of how infertility and pregnancy loss occur. Jones was the first to suggest that endometrial inadequacy might be a cause of infertility or early pregnancy wastage [41]. While progesterone insufficiency and retarded histology was the primary and initial focus of investigations into endometrial receptivity defects, biochemical changes within the endometrium that are independent of histology also appear to contribute to poor reproductive outcome. In the 1990s it was widely reported that women with tubal disease and hydrosalpinges exhibited reduced implantation rates in the IVF setting [42–44]. This defect was treatable; salpingectomy reversed this deficit and improved subsequent implantation rates [45,46].

Endometriosis is a second condition associated with implantation defects that can also result in lower IVF success rates [47]. Aberrant expression of endometrial biomarkers in the endometrium of hydrosalpinx and endometriosis patients has been reported, suggesting that the endometrium is somehow affected by hydrosalpinx fluid or the inflammatory changes that accompany endometriosis [48–57]. Understanding how tubal fluid or peritoneal disease interferes with the establishment of endometrial receptivity is a separate question and beyond the scope of this review.

# Endometrial assessment

## Endometrial histology

Nearly 60 years ago Noyes and colleagues first described the criteria for endometrial dating [58]. Published as the first article in the first issue of *Fertility and Sterility*, this seminal article remains one of the most cited papers in the gynecological literature [59]. The initial study was carried out on endometrial biopsies obtained from infertile women. By definition, therefore, these tissues probably did not represent normal endometrium. The histological features used for endometrial dating are shown in Figure 18.2; in fairness these were presented as an idealized representation and can not be expected to have meaningful accuracy when applied to an individual case. Variability in these criteria between subjects and between observers produces unacceptable results that precludes accurate prospective chronological assignment of progression through the menstrual cycle [60,61]. Nevertheless, these criteria have been learned and applied as the primary tool for endometrial assessment over the past 60 years, despite their shortcomings.

The true incidence of LPD in fertile and infertile women remains uncertain, but is likely a common finding in both groups of women. In one study 4% of 1630 women evaluated for infertility had documented LPD, while no cases were identified in fertile women seeking tubal anastomosis [62]. Li and colleagues reported that 14% of infertility patients had LPD compared with only 4% of fertile controls [63]. Interestingly, this group found that women with endometriosis and unexplained infertility had significantly higher rates of LPD than women with other infertility diagnoses. Others have noted a wide range of LPD detection rates (1.9% to 60%) among infertile women [64]. Much of this variability derives from the subjective nature of reading biopsy material and the variability that changes depending on the cycle stage when the biopsy was obtained [65].

Technological advances during these past 60 years also changed the way histological dating criteria are applied. Before the availability of urinary LH surge predictors, endometrial biopsies were obtained late in the secretory phase and chronology determined by counting backwards from the next menstrual flow. Controversy also exists regarding how many days the endometrial biopsy need be delayed in order to be out of phase. Davis and colleagues reported an incidence

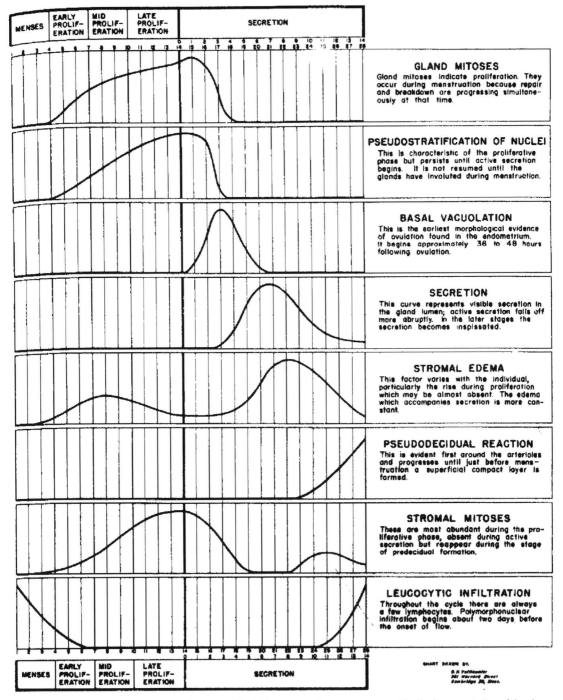

# DATING THE ENDOMETRIUM
## APPROXIMATE RELATIONSHIP OF USEFUL MORPHOLOGICAL FACTORS

**Figure 18.2** Endometrial dating criteria of Noyes *et al.* [58]. The patterns shown represent an idealized representation of the changes in endometrial cell characteristics throughout the secretory phase of the menstrual cycle.

of LPD in 26.7% of patients using a 2-day lag versus 6.6% if a 3-day lag was used [66]. Two consecutive out-of-phase biopsies are required to confirm the diagnosis of LPD. Studies of repeat biopsies found a second out-of-phase biopsy was highly variable, ranging from 20–80% out of phase [7]. As endometrial biopsies are uncomfortable for patients and could potentially disrupt a pregnancy, this uncertainty and need for repeat biopsies becomes less practical for routine assessment of the endometrium. Finally, evidence now suggests that endometrial receptivity can be abnormal even in the presence of normal histology [52,67,68]. Biochemical derangements in the endometrium that exist without histological delay greatly expand the possibilities of using the endometrium as an indicator of reproductive health [69].

## Hormonal assessment

Surrogate measures of endometrial receptivity have long been sought. Serum progesterone measurements are a mainstay of hormonal assessment to document ovulation and appear to correlate well with endometrial biopsy results [70–72]. The corpus luteum (CL) arising from a vacated follicle survives up to 14 days in a non-conception cycle. Deficiencies in progesterone leading to pregnancy loss or infertility could arise as a result of suboptimal follicular development [73]. Strott and colleagues showed that women with a short luteal phase exhibited reduced gonadotropin levels and LH surges of reduced magnitude [74]. The CL normally depends on a tonic level of LH secretion from the pituitary. In non-human primates, inactivation of LH using antiserum caused a prompt decline in circulating progesterone levels [75]. Similar decreases in progesterone levels were seen in women following administration of GnRH antagonists [76]. Progesterone is secreted in pulses, corresponding to the LH pulse frequency [77]. Changes in the pulse generator could theoretically alter progesterone secretion, leading to LPD. Soules et al. observed reduced LH concentrations at mid-cycle in women with documented LPD [78]. The major shortcoming of hormonal measurements arises if endometrial receptivity defects are independent of circulating progesterone levels [52,67].

Since the hormonal milieu can indirectly alter endometrial function, evaluation of women with infertility or recurrent pregnancy loss should also include assessment of the pituitary (prolactin and TSH), adrenal (testosterone and DHEA-S), and assessment of estradiol and FSH to evaluate ovary reserve. In addition, in patients with obesity or polycystic ovary syndrome (PCOS), assessment of insulin or androgen levels may also be indicated. Endocrinopathies like PCOS can disrupt hypothalamic–pituitary–ovarian function leading to alterations in the endometrium that contribute to implantation failure [79,80]. Direct effects of androgens or insulin may render the endometrium non-receptive [81–85]. Hyperprolactinemia, in particular, is associated with the disruption in GnRH pulsatility and reduction in ovarian steroid production [73]. Higher elevations in prolactin lead to anovulation, while subtle elevations in this hormone can indirectly disrupt endometrial function; a shortened luteal phase is associated with mildly elevated prolactin. Daly et al. reported 16% of women with LPD also had hyperprolactinemia [86]. Increased levels of androgens are also associated with LPD and alterations in endometrial function. Women with polycystic ovary syndrome (PCOS) and hyperandrogenism have poor reproductive outcome, including miscarriage and infertility, due to their underlying hyperandrogenism or hyperinsulinemia [87], though not all studies agree [88–90]. Identification and correction of endocrinopathies remain an important part of the work-up for any woman with suspected implantation failure.

Progesterone is critical to the success of an early pregnancy [91], reflected in its direct stimulatory action on key endometrial proteins [17,20,24,55,92–100]. Progesterone also downregulates endometrial steroid receptors (ER and PR) during the mid-secretory phase, resulting in three distinct patterns of endometrial gene expression in response to the combined effects of steroid hormones and changing receptor patterns [26]. Either inadequate progesterone or secondary progesterone resistance [67] can account for alterations in steroid receptor downregulation noted in the endometrium of some women with infertility. Persistent estrogen or progesterone receptors during the mid-luteal phase would alter that balance of estrogen and progesterone-mediated effects, and change the paracrine dynamics that underlie the acquisition of endometrial receptivity [55,96]. Thus, steroid receptors or the enzymes that metabolize steroids have been suggested as useful tools for the assessment of endometrial function [96,101–103]. Abnormalities in endometrial maturation [73] or differentiated function [67,104] would also be a consequence of reduced progesterone action. While these concepts appear sound, recent data suggest that the endometrium of women with infertility may be fundamentally different from that of normal fertile women; progesterone resistance may be an acquired defect in certain types of infertility (e.g. endometriosis). It appears that in normal endometrium, artificially lowered progesterone levels during a mock luteal phase failed to demonstrate observable effects on endometrial function and did not result in any delay in histology based on endometrial biopsy [8]. Such tantalizing data hint at the complexities that exist in different subsets of women and may explain the paradoxical reports that exist in the literature regarding assessment of the endometrium.

# Endometrial ultrastructure

## Glycocalyx

Initial interaction of the embryo with the endometrium occurs at the apical surface of the luminal epithelium [32,105,106]. Like the growing embryo that must hatch from its zona pellucida to expose surface receptors and/or adhesion molecules, the surface of the differentiating endometrium also undergoes changes that render it receptive to embryonic interaction. In rabbits, the surface epithelium undergoes differentiation with a loss of surface negativity and changes in the luminal glycocalyx [107]. Similar changes were noted in rat endometrium [108], although the precise basis for these changes in morphology were not initially understood. The glycocalyx was the first stage-specific alteration that coincides with establishment of endometrial receptivity. Initial characterizations included lectin-binding affinity studies [109], and similar changes were described on the embryonic epithelium, coincident with the acquisition of adhesiveness [110,111].

Glycocalyx is predominantly made up of the endometrial mucin, Muc-1 [112]. Mucins are high molecular weight glycoproteins with a protein core that contains tandem repeat domains enriched in serine, threonine and proline residues, attached to O-linked carbohydrate moieties. They may play a role in protecting the upper reproductive tract from bacterial colonization. In most species, Muc-1 appears to be a barrier to implantation. In the rabbit, Muc-1 is up-regulated by progesterone but removed at sites of implantation by actions of the blastocyst [113]. In the mouse and rat, Muc-1 is downregulated at the time of implantation [114,115]. In human endometrium, Muc-1 is present throughout the menstrual cycle, making its role during implantation somewhat enigmatic. One study suggested that Muc-1 is differentially expressed on ciliated cells [55]. Muc-1 also provides scaffolding for cell adhesion proteins that may be required for embryo attachment [116]. For more information on Muc-1's role in endometrial biology, see Carson *et al.* [33].

## Pinopods and ultrastructural organelles

Pinopods (translated from "drinking foot," also known as pinopodes, uterodomes) are bleb-like projections from the lumen surface of the endometrium (Figure 18.3A,B). These ultrastructural features were first described as markers of a receptive endometrium in the rat uterus [117]. The name derives from the fact that pinopods had pinocytotic activity in the rat uterus, taking up ferritin injected into the uterine cavity. Similar structures were subsequently described in human endometrium [118–125] and proposed as markers of receptivity. Although pinopods do not apparently possess pinocytotic activity in the human endometrium [126], these structures are similar in appearance to those described in the rat. While best viewed by electron microscopy, pinopods can be seen by light microscopy alone, using a 40× objective in formalin-fixed, paraffin-embedded sections [119,127]. Investigators have described pinopod expression in both fertile and infertile women [124,125,128–135] and in vitro in endometrial culture where they appear to be a preferred site for embryo attachment (Figure 18.3C) [136,137]. The putative value of pinopods is their temporal association with the window of implantation. The assessment of pinopod expression is arguably subjective; given the evanescent pattern of expression lasting only 1 or 2 days, absence of pinopods could occur if a biopsy was obtained even 1 day too early or late. In contrast to earlier reports, two prospective randomized studies did not confirm the expected pattern of pinopod expression [138,139]; a third study found no association at all between pinopods and the window of implantation [140]. Pinopod shape changes during the secretory phase [141], becoming "uterodomes," a name proposed by Murphy [142] which may contribute to these divergent views of pinopod timing. The location of pinopods on the apical surface of mid-secretory endometrium suggests a role in embryo/endometrial interaction. These expanded blebs of plasma membrane are the site of integrin

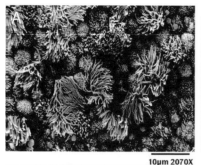
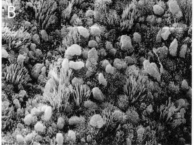
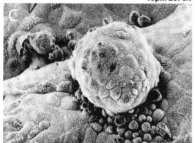
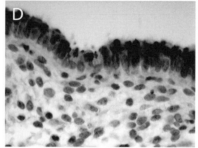

**Figure 18.3** Pinopods are present throughout the secretory phase but appear to undergo changes that reflect developmental progression. In the proliferative phase, few pinopods are seen (A). In the mid-secretory phase, pinopods become apparent, extending from the luminal epithelium (B). In vitro studies show that human embryos are capable of interacting with the pinopods, in support of their function during implantation (C). Pinopods can be visualized under light microscopy (D). Here the tips of pinopods are decorated with osteopontin, a ligand for the αvβ3 integrin, containing the arg-gly-asp (RGD) sequence thought to play a role during implantation. Panel C used with permission (Bentin-Ley *et al.,* 1999 [137]).

expression [130] coinciding temporally and spatially with expression of other key endometrial biomarkers including LIF, glycodelin, osteopontin and galectin-9 and galectin-3, L-selectin ligands and decay accelerating factor (DAF) (Figure 18.3D) [143–149]. Endowed with these key endometrial proteins, pinopods might serve as an important site of endometrial–embryo interaction, elevating a receptive luminal surface toward the implanting blastocyst. In addition, specialized surfaces on pinopods provide a potential explanation to the epithelial–epithelial paradox, previously raised by Denker [37].

Another feature of receptive endometrium are the nucleolar channel systems (NCSs). These are intranuclear organelles first described in transmission electron microscopy [150]. These channels are composed of more than 30 nucleoproteins that represent extensions of the endoplasmic reticulum through the nuclear pores, with proposed enzymatic roles within the nucleolus. The relevance of NCSs to this chapter relates to their association to the mid-secretory phase. Guffanti and colleagues recently described NCSs in both fertile and infertile women as being present only during a six-day period corresponding to the window of implantation between cycle day 19–24 [151]. The expression of these structures appears to be hormonally dependent and they were not observed in patients treated with high estrogen and low progesterone stimulation. It will be interesting to see data on

NCSs in infertile patients and to determine if they are indeed useful markers of receptivity. Based on other findings, NCSs could be lacking in women with endometriosis due to poor endometrial response to progesterone and an exaggerated response to estrogen reported in the endometrium of these women [67,102].

# Endometrial imaging

Imaging techniques are important for the clinical evaluation of the uterus and endometrium [152–155]. Women with a history of infertility, recurrent pregnancy loss or those with abnormal uterine bleeding or suspected intrauterine pathology seeking medical help should be offered ultrasound imaging. Although diagnostic and operative hysteroscopy are considered the gold standard for endometrial evaluation, cost and relative invasiveness of operative procedures makes transvaginal ultrasound, with or without color Doppler and three-dimensional imaging a favorable alternative screening modality. More advanced (and costly) imaging methods, including magnetic resonance imaging (MRI) have also been advocated. In this section we will review the clinical usefulness of imaging techniques for the clinical assessment of the endometrium.

## Ultrasound, Doppler flow and MRI

Transvaginal ultrasound is readily available in most practitioners' offices and offers a convenient method

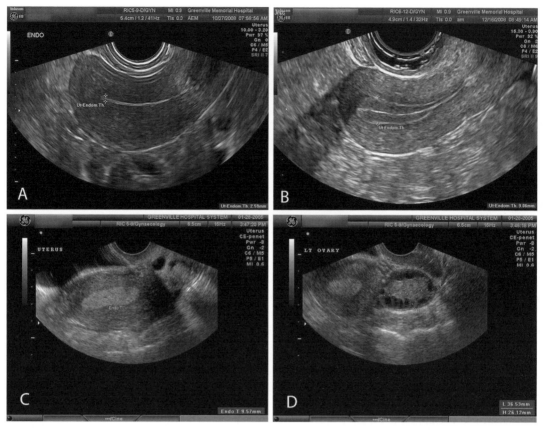

**Figure 18.4** Ultrasound is a useful tool for the evaluation of endometrium and uterine pathology. Endometrial thickness begins as a thin line in the proliferative phase (A) but rapidly grows to a thick, trilaminar appearance in most women (B). In some women, the echogenicity of the endometrium is abnormal. Although the secretory phase reflects this hyperechoic pattern some women with hyperandrogenism and polycystic ovary syndrome can also have inappropriately echogenic endometrium during the proliferative phase (C). In this case, polycystic appearing ovaries were also present (D).

to assess endometrial thickness, contour and pelvic anatomy. Ultrasound is a sensitive method to identify abnormalities that could interfere with embryo implantation or cause abnormal uterine bleeding in pre- or post-menopausal women. Compared to laparoscopy, ultrasound has been reported to have a sensitivity of 86%, a specificity of 98%, a positive predictive value of 99%, and a negative predictive value of 79% for detection of pathology [155]. Ultrasound has been primarily used to measure endometrial thickness, echogenicity and uterine blood flow. Advanced techniques also include three-dimensional ultrasound with or without sonohysterography.

The endometrium thickens during each cycle in response to follicular estrogen production by the ovary (Figure 18.4). During the proliferative phase the endometrium typically starts as a thin line (Figure 18.4A) but grows to a thickened strip with a

trilaminar appearance (Figure 18.4B). Endometrial thickness is measured at the endometrial–myometrial interface through the sagittal plane of the uterine body, 1 cm from the fundus [156]. Errors in endometrial thickness measurements can occur if an oblique section of the uterus is captured or if the uterus is not imaged along its entire length to achieve maximal fundal endometrial thickness. Limitations to transvaginal ultrasonography exist, since polyps or other intracavity lesions can be difficult to visualize and falsely increase the perceived endometrial thickness. Anovulatory women, especially women with longstanding amenorrhea and hyperandrogenism, may have hyperechoic linings that reflect the abnormal hormonal milieu and polycystic ovaries (Figure 18.4C, D). Thickness may vary depending on the type of stimulation; IVF cycles sometimes have greater endometrial thickness than untreated or IUI cycles [157]. Despite the dependence on steroid hormones, studies suggested that endometrial growth does not always correlate well with hormone levels [158], and that neither thickness nor echogenic pattern correlated well with endometrial histology [159].

A relationship between endometrial thickness and pregnancy has been well studied, but reports vary widely about the significance of this correlation [156]. Some investigators found that thin endometrium is associated with a poor outcome or reduced pregnancy rates [158,160–163], while others found no predictive value of endometrial thickness [157,164,165]. A thicker endometrium was associated with positive pregnancy outcome in early IVF studies [166–168], and in cycles where conception occurred, endometrial thickness was reported to increase, while it did not in non-conception cycles [169]. Friedler reviewed 25 reports, comprising 2665 ART cycles, and found that eight reports reported endometrial thickness to be a statistically significant factor in achieving conception, and 17 reports showed no significant difference in endometrial thickness [156]. A recent prospective study found that endometrial thickness was of limited value for clinical assessment to predict IVF outcome [170]. One explanation for the inconsistency of these reports is the difference in quality of IVF programs. When all other factors are optimized, endometrial thickness (or thinness) may not be such a barrier to implantation.

Endometrial characteristics by ultrasound also include examination of echogenic patterns. Smith et al. [171] proposed four types of endometrium. Gonen and Casper simplified this classification to three types [172]. Type "A" endometrium has an entirely homogeneous and hyperechogenic pattern without a central echogenic line (Figure 18.4C). Type "B" is classified as an intermediate isoechogenic pattern that has no echogenic line and more than 50% but less than 100% of the endometrium is hyperechoic. A third type "C," is a multi-layered triple ring endometrial pattern with a prominent outer hyperechoic line and an inner hypoechogenic black region (Figure 18.4B). The endometrial patterns have been further simplified into two types – multi-layered and non-multi-layered by Sher [173]. Several studies found that endometrial patterns were better at predicting pregnancy than endometrial thickness [163,174]. One large study reported that women with a trilaminar endometrial pattern had better pregnancy rates than subjects with a solid endometrial pattern [168]. Other studies showed no correlation between endometrial

pattern and pregnancy outcome [156]. Echogenic pattern may be a sign of hyperandrogenism or an indication of ovulation. It is likely that interpretation of echogenicity depends greatly on clinical context and should best be used in conjunction with other measures of endometrial response.

Doppler flow studies are non-invasive ultrasound methods used to evaluate the blood flow to the uterus and endometrium. The extent to which blood flow and Doppler findings predict the rate of implantation remains an active area of investigation. Blood flow changes during the menstrual cycle have been reported [175,176] and correlate with serum progesterone levels [177]. Uterine artery blood flow resistance has been reported to be predictive of implantation potential [178–181]. One report suggested that Doppler findings also correlated with immunohistochemical biomarkers of uterine receptivity [182]. Elevated uterine impedance was reported to be abnormal in recurrent pregnancy loss as well [177]. A recent report found that women with an end-diastolic blood flow, an endometrial–sub-endometrial blood flow and a multilayered endometrium were more likely to have a successful pregnancy than women without one or more of these signs [153]; Schild on the other hand found that blood flow in both the uterine and spiral arteries measured by power Doppler showed no correlation with implantation rates [183]. Although uterine Doppler remains an interesting parameter to evaluate, there is at present no consensus about the predictive potential of measurements of flow or resistance in the endometrial blood vessels [155].

Ultrasound is generally preferable to other imaging techniques such as magnetic resonance imaging (MRI). Magnetic resonance imaging has a high detection rate for uterine pathology, including submucosal, transmural fibroids, adenomyomas and uterine septa. The high cost, limited availability and paucity of good studies that support its use, limits the usefulness of MRI for routine evaluation of the endometrium.

### Sonohysterography

Two- and three-dimensional ultrasound are increasingly performed with fluid instillation into the uterine cavity (sonohysterography) to allow evaluation of the endometrium in women with infertility, recurrent pregnancy loss and abnormal uterine bleeding [184–188]. These techniques are highly sensitive at detecting intrauterine pathology [152,185,188–190]. Examples of the usefulness of sonohysterography are

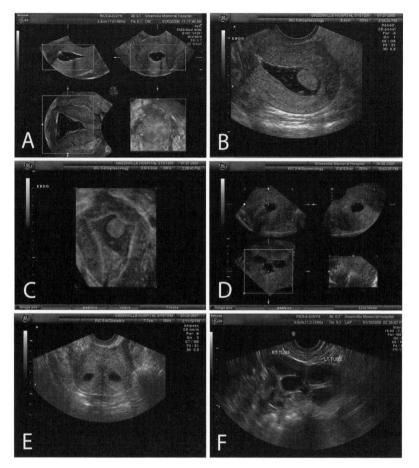

**Figure 18.5** Two- and three-dimensional ultrasound together with sonohysterography can be useful for the assessment of the endometrium. A normal sonohysterogram is shown (A). This technique can be used to detect endometrial polyps (B) that are well visualized using three-dimensional rendering (C). Ultrasound is also useful for detecting other pathology that can alter endometrial receptivity, including uterine adhesions (D), a uterine septum (E), or hydrosalpinges (F).

shown in Figure 18.5A–D. Compared with normal sonohysterograms (Figure 18.5A), polyps are easily detected when saline is introduced into the cavity and can be displayed well using two- and three-dimensional technology (Figure 18.5B, C). Similarly intrauterine adhesions seen in Asherman's syndrome can be clearly outlined by sonohysterography (Figure 18.5D). A uterine septum may predispose to recurrent pregnancy loss, and can be routinely detected by sonohysterography (Figure 18.5E). Sonohysterography has become a standard for evaluating the endometrial cavity, particularly in women who present for infertility, or to triage women who present with abnormal uterine bleeding. Although patients with significant pathology will ultimately undergo more invasive procedures such as hysteroscopy and/or endometrial dilation and curettage to diagnose and remove the abnormality, sonohystogram is an essential screening tool to assess the uterine cavity and aid in the clinical assessment of the endometrium.

Other pelvic pathology can also be readily detected at the time of gynecological ultrasound, including endometriomas or hydrosalpinges (Figure 18.5F).

## Biomarkers of endometrial receptivity

The NIH definition of a biomarker is a "characteristic that is objectively measured and evaluated as an indicator of normal biological processes, pathogenic processes, or pharmacologic responses to a therapeutic intervention." There are several excellent reviews of the use of biomarkers for the assessment of uterine receptivity [10,69,191–194]. Early strategies used to identify endometrial biomarkers included the incorporation of a radioactive label followed by two-dimensional electrophoresis [195–197]. Major endometrial secretory proteins were identified in the 1980s using this approach, including glycodelin (PP14) and IGFBP1 (a.k.a. PP12). Analysis of patterns of secreted proteins on thin layer chromatography included

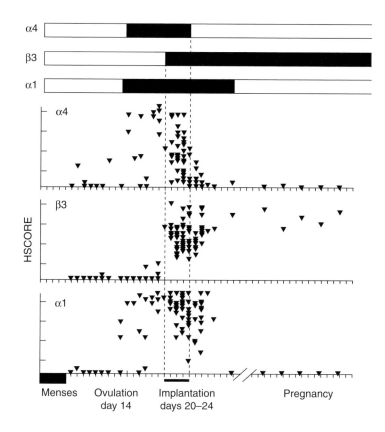

**Figure 18.6** Endometrial integrins have been shown to undergo changes in expression throughout the menstrual cycle. The expression pattern of three integrins, including α1β1, αvβ3 and α4β1 appear to frame the window of implantation, that was later defined by Wilcox and colleagues [14]. The αvβ3 integrin is located on the endometrial luminal surface appearing at the time of implantation and is absent in some women with implantation defects. This protein has also been shown to predict IVF success and can be used to identify women with endometriosis who have otherwise unexplained infertility. Used with permission from Elsevier (Lessey et al., 1994 [214]).

identification of histones as potential markers of receptive endometrium [198,199]. Ultimately, electrophoresis gave way to immunohistochemistry with the advent of specific monoclonal and polyclonal antibodies [20] and to more sophisticated methods involving differential display and DNA microarray, each of which has greatly expanded the number of biomarkers for consideration [24–26,193,194,200–206].

## Integrins and cell adhesion molecules

Cell adhesion molecules (CAMs) and the extracellular matrix (ECM) maintain tissue integrity and hormonal responsiveness within the endometrium [207]. Changes in the ECM have been described throughout the menstrual cycle [208] and into pregnancy [209] suggesting important roles for CAMS in embryo–endometrial interactions [210,211]. Integrins are cell-adhesion molecules that serve as receptors for the extracellular matrix [212]. Dynamic changes in integrin expression have also been described during the menstrual cycle and into pregnancy [209,213–216]. The 3-amino acid motif arg-gly-asp (RGD) was implicated in the process of implantation by several investigators [217–219]; RGD is present on many

extracellular matrix ligands in the receptive endometrium, including osteopontin, tenascin, IGF-BP1 and fibronectin [220–223]. RGD peptides and anti-RGD snake venom components were shown to effectively block implantation or attachment of embryos, suggesting a critical role of integrins and related ligands to endometrial–embryo interactions [218,222,224,225].

Integrins are arguably the best characterized markers of receptive endometrium. First studied in 1992, constitutive and cycle-dependent patterns of integrin expression were described [213,226]. Three integrins were noted to be co-expressed on receptive endometrium only during the putative window of implantation (Figure 18.6) [214]. The αvβ3 integrin appears on endometrial epithelium at the opening of the window of implantation around cycle day 20 or 21 and is present on the apical pole of the lumen corresponding to the site of pinopod expression. This integrin is regulated by EGF and EGF-related molecules and by Hoxa10 [227,228]. Integrins are also well-recognized on the placenta and invading cytotrophoblast [216,229–231], and disorders of placentation have been linked to aberrant integrin expression [232,233]. Such coordinated expression of integrins

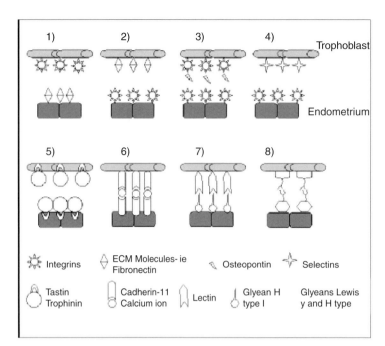

**Figure 18.7** Adhesion molecules serve many functions throughout the body. Endometrial-embryo interactions likely involve one or more of these mechanisms. As shown, many different combinations of ligands and receptors have been proposed, as outlined in the text. Interactions can involve integrins, extracellular matrix molecules such as fibronectin, tastin and trophinin, lectins and selectins. Although not mutually exclusive, the primary receptor for the embryo is likely a loose attachment as proposed for L-selectin and its ligand that allows a transient attachment phase that precedes invasion. Other mechanisms as depicted may have other roles including immune modulation and cell signaling at the time of implantation. Used with permission from Thieme Medical Publishers, Inc. (Donaghay & Lessey, 2007 [10])

on both the embryo and endometrium suggests a critical role during attachment and invasion [234,235]. Recent data also suggest that the αvβ3 integrin associates with osteopontin and decay accelerating factor (DAF) might inactivate the immune system and complement activation during implantation [144,236,237].

### Selectins/cadherins

The search for a true receptor that mediates embryo attachment is a goal for many implantation researchers [33,34]. Candidates for this receptor have been suggested [213,236,238–240], including growth factor/receptor pairs, CAMS, and extracellular matrix and members of the cell adhesion families (Figure 18.7). Recent evidence supports L-selectin, a member of the selectin family, as a key adhesion molecule during the initial attachment of the human embryo [241]. The presumed endometrial ligand for L-selectin appears to be a sialyl glycoprotein associated with the Lewis-X family that is recognized by the monoclonal antibody MECA-79. The interaction between L-selectin and this carbohydrate moiety on the endometrial surface may serve as a bridge to bring the embryo into intimate contact with the endometrium, prior to firm attachment. The mechanism of cell adhesion is thought to be similar to the rolling actions of leukocytes on vascular endothelium as they first become tethered prior to more robust adhesion and invasion that involves integrin binding [242,243].

If L-selectin is critical to early embryo–endometrial interaction, the absence of its cognate ligand could have profound effects, possibly leading to infertility or pregnancy loss. The distribution of this antigen, recognized by MECA79, has now been studied in normal cycling women during the menstrual cycle [244] and has been suggested to be a clinically useful marker of endometrial receptivity [148].

### Cytokines

The pattern of expression of cytokines and growth factors and their receptors during the menstrual cycle suggests a role in both endometrial development and implantation. One of the first proteins that was demonstrated to be critical for implantation was leukemia-inhibitory factor (LIF). Null mutation of the LIF gene in female mice resulted in complete lack of implantation and exhibited decidualization failure [245–247]. This phenotype could be rescued by administration of exogenous LIF. IL-11, another member of this IL-6 family, was implicated in decidualization as well, based on gene knock-out studies. Both LIF and IL-11 signal through the gp130 receptor. Leukemia-inhibitory factor and related proteins have been reported to be reduced in women with implantation failure and infertility [248–252].

The epidermal growth factor (EGF) family of growth factors and receptors also play a role in implantation [9]. Extensive work in the mouse uterus has demonstrated the importance of HB-EGF in blastocyst implantation. HB-EGF is produced as both a soluble and transmembrane form by the luminal epithelium at the time of implantation [253](Birdsall et al., 1996). HB-EGF as a transmembrane "receptor" could serve as an embryonic receptor through the EGF receptor on the embryonic epithelium (Figure 18.7) [254]. As a soluble factor, HB-EGF significantly improves embryonic development [255]. HB-EGF has also been implicated in the regulation of other key endometrial receptivity proteins [144,256,257]. The clinical use of HB-EGF as a marker in reproduction has been limited but intriguing [258–261]. For further information on cytokines during the implantation window see a recent review by Achahe and Revel [69].

### DNA microarray

The process of biomarker discovery has been dramatically accelerated by high-throughput techniques including DNA microarray, using both normal and pathological endometrium [24–26,194,200–204,262–269]. Identification of new pathways, signaling paradigms and metabolic processes have evolved rapidly as a result. The characterization of the endometrium throughout the normal menstrual cycle [26], sets the stage for a much better understanding of the factors involved in endometrial development and menstruation [201]. While known biomarkers are being rediscovered using this technique, new pathways and unsuspected proteins are also being reported [25,193,201]. Through the use of bioinformatics and in conjunction with proteomics these techniques promise that this field will remain active for years to come.

## Clinical perspective

The efficiency of implantation in the human is poor compared with most mammals. One in five couples experience infertility and it is estimated that 10 million couples will seek medical assistance for infertility and recurrent pregnancy loss this year. Up to one third of IVF failures are thought due to poor embryo quality, while it is estimated that up to 60% result from implantation defects. It is safe to say that most women with compromised endometrial receptivity go unrecognized. The large proportion of couples with unexplained loss reflects a lack of attention to endometrial assessment. On the other hand, widespread use of biomarkers has been limited by a paucity of

clinical studies that validate their usefulness. A marked heterogeneity in endometrial response to various conditions such as endometriosis, have also created a diversity of reports that questions the usefulness of any marker of endometrial function. The lack of a good understanding about how endometriosis or hydrosalpinges degrades endometrial receptivity also contributes to the confusion. Nevertheless, data now exist to suggest that there are common themes involved and therefore common strategies available for correcting implantation defects. The remainder of this chapter will review the available evidence for the clinical assessment of the endometrium with a focus on endometrial receptivity in the setting of infertility and pregnancy loss.

## Infertility

### Unexplained infertility

The endometrium serves as a bioassay for the cumulative effects of steroid hormones, growth factors and cytokines. The endometrial biopsy has been regarded as a good method for endometrial assessment and prediction of pregnancy potential [64,270–272]. Endometrium in women with unexplained infertility (UI) is different from that found in normal fertile controls, based on examination of many different biomarkers [10,22,148,249,251,252,258,273–283]. Many of these differences can be accounted for simply by delayed histological development (LPD) that is more common in unexplained infertility and pregnancy loss [73,104,273,284–286]. Other studies found no differences in histological delay between normal and infertile women, or reported that histological variability was too great to be clinically useful [60,61,287]. Biochemical differences in the endometrium of infertile women occur that cannot be explained by histological delay [22,52,53,57,67,68,283]. The application of biomarkers for clinical assessment appears to be a promising approach, but one that has yet to be widely adopted.

While unexplained infertility accounts for 10–15% of cases in a typical practice [288,289], a large proportion of these patients will ultimately be found to harbor endometriosis [284,290,291]. The movement away from laparoscopy and toward IVF has highlighted this problem and accounts for many unexplained failures during IVF [292,293].

If endometriosis accounts for most of these cases of unexplained infertility, why is it not actively being diagnosed and treated? Controversy surrounding the relationship between implantation defects and mild forms of endometriosis persist because of the lack of efficacy of medical treatments on cycle fecundity in women with this disorder [294]. Animal models of endometriosis have demonstrated an implantation defect exists [295–298] and confirmed that similar endometrial changes occur in response to induction of endometriosis [299–302]. Many clinical studies have shown adverse effects of endometriosis on pregnancy rates [47,303,304], but others fail to find this association [305]. Since many patients with minimal or mild endometriosis do conceive without therapy [306], many researchers in the field have concluded that endometriosis either does not cause infertility or that treatment is not beneficial. A large prospective surgical treatment study from Canada demonstrated benefit from surgical ablation of mild endometriosis [307]. Recently, GnRH analog (Lupron® TAP Pharmaceuticals, Chicago, IL) was shown to improve pregnancy rates in women undergoing IVF [308]. Given the heterogeneity observed in implantation defects in women with endometriosis, GnRH analogs cannot be used on everyone; pregnancy may be fostered in some women, but prevented in others. This fact alone could explain the lack of efficacy of medical therapy for infertility associated with endometriosis, described by many previous studies [309].

### In-vitro fertilization (IVF) and implantation

Ovarian hyperstimulation used during the typical IVF cycle likely has adverse effects on the endometrium [310,311], though not all studies agree [312]. The average implantation rate for IVF centers in the USA is only 29% (www.sart.org). Patients can be easily identified who do not achieve pregnancy even in repeat IVF cycles. The term repeated implantation failure (RIF) has been defined as failure to achieve pregnancy following 2–6 IVF cycles in which more than 10 embryos of good quality have been transferred [313]. The use of biomarkers to study implantation in assisted reproductive technology (ART) appears promising [314].

Causes of repeat IVF failure that are related to endometrial receptivity defects have recently been reviewed [56]. Obvious causes such as thin endometrium or mechanical disruption (e.g. uterine fibroids) must be ruled out prior to starting IVF. Alterations in endometrial function have been described in women with RIF, including elevated concentrations of natural killer (NK) cells [315,316,317], increased cytokine production [318,319] and alterations in cell adhesion molecule expression [23,293,320,321]. Pinopod expression is also altered in women with RIF [322,323] and changes in global gene expression changes have also been reported in this setting [11].

These observations surrounding RIF are likely to be related. Many cases could be a consequence of progesterone resistance or alterations in immunity associated with endometriosis [53,56,67,68,324–327]. Hoxa10, a transcription factor that directly regulates the αvβ3 integrin [328] is reduced, similar to the αvβ3 integrin in the endometrium of women with hydrosalpinges [48,329]. Both biomarkers are expressed normally after salpingectomy. Alteration in αvβ3 integrin expression may be related to high levels of aromatase P450 expression in these women [330], as local production of endometrial estrogen has a negative effect on endometrial integrin expression [102,227]. Other factors are affected as well, including endometrial bleeding associated factor (ebaf) [54,331,332]. Inappropriate or premature expression of this TGF-β inhibitor likely accounts for endometrial dysfunction and early bleeding noted in women with endometriosis leading to decreased implantation potential.

Aberrant patterns of gene expression in the endometrium of women with RIF point toward a contribution by endometriosis, which is known to reduce IVF success [47,304]. Diagnosis of even mild forms of this disease should be sought in women experiencing RIF [292]. While not enough studies exist on which to confidently base treatment decisions, suppression of endometriosis with surgical ablation [292], danazol [320,333] or GnRH agonists [308,334] all appear to have benefit. In addition, the use of aromatase inhibitors could also improve IVF success, especially in women with documented lack of normal integrin expression [293].

## Recurrent pregnancy loss

Pregnancy loss is common, occurring in up to 37% of pregnancies in any given cycle [335]. Recurrent pregnancy loss (RPL), on the other hand, affects only 5% of women attempting to conceive [336]. Factors that increase the risk for RPL include a loss of a chromosomally normal pregnancy, pregnancy loss after the first trimester, and difficulty conceiving. Up to half of all miscarriages in the general population can be assigned a cause, including chromosomal abnormalities, immunological, endocrine (luteal phase defect), anatomic, thrombophilic, infectious or environmental causes (smoking and caffeine) [336,337]. Loss of uterine receptivity leading to implantation failure has been suggested as a contributing factor, but remains poorly defined [336,338,339]; in up to half of cases a firm diagnosis is never established [336, 340].

Unexplained RPL (uRPL), like unexplained infertility (UI), can be caused by endometriosis [340,341]. Since the link between endometriosis and infertility is well established [291,342], it is reasonable to consider an association exists between endometriosis and RPL as well. Recurrent pregnancy loss may be part of a continuum of the population of women with infertility, as delay in implantation leading to asynchrony and implantation failure could apply to both. As outlined in the previous section, endometriosis causes biochemical changes in the endometrium including progesterone resistance and delayed expression of proteins essential for normal uterine receptivity [67,68]. While studies are ongoing to address this association between infertility and RPL, the choice of the appropriate biomarker for endometrial assessment continues to be a matter for debate.

## Summary and concluding thoughts

### Diagnostic dilemmas

Based on conservative estimates, implantation failure and endometrial receptivity defects account for up to one third of infertility and recurrent pregnancy loss cases. The clinical assessment of the endometrium includes many well-established methods that have been reviewed in this chapter. The use of biomarkers for endometrial assessment is also gaining acceptance and applications for their use are expanding. Studies to establish the usefulness and reliability of biomarkers are few and in many cases flaws in study design or implementation have been cited. As new biomarkers arise, efforts will need to focus on establishing common pathways of regulation. Efforts should be made to determine how endometrial patterns of expression are altered in common conditions. Recognition of protein biochemical defects may define an endometrial fingerprint to help identify the likelihood presence of gynecologic pathology that alters the endometrial phenotype. As outlined above, endometriosis and tubal disease both appear to reduce IVF success rates yet we do not yet know the similarities

and differences in the endometrium in each condition. All women with either condition are not affected equally, making it difficult to establish firm guidelines or recommendations about the prognosis or treatment.

To establish how endometrial assessment can best be approached, divergent views and dogmatic beliefs will need to be presented, evaluated and reconciled. Recognition of the heterogeneity in the population will need to be addressed. Endometrial assessment will likely require many markers that together predict endometrial health or disease. Variability in endometrial histology must be taken into account since the endometrial phenotype even in its normal state, is a moving target; analyses on endometrium must be standardized with respect to a defined period of time during the window of implantation. Women with infertility or pregnancy loss frequently have more than one disorder that can confuse or obscure our understanding of the underlying problem. Women with PCOS, for example, can have concomitant endometriosis that frequently goes unrecognized [343,344]. In many reports on the subject of endometrial assessment, these factors are not considered.

## Future directions

The endometrium provides a window into the endocrine milieu that can provide clues regarding the presence or absence of disorders associated with infertility or pregnancy loss. As DNA microarray and proteomic techniques mature, convergence of information will likely clarify how the endometrium changes in both health and disease. Discovery of underlying and unifying concepts that account for the many observations made so far, will likely determine the approach we adopt for the assessment of endometrial receptivity. As pathways of gene regulation are better established, dysregulation of those pathways can also be dissected and used to understand the mechanisms of disease. Diagnostics based on this understanding will lead to better and a more timely recognition of the ontogeny and pathophysiology of various conditions affecting women. Therapeutics directed at an underlying dysfunction will result in better treatment options that rely less on empiricism. Cost and side effects of treatments will be reduced as clinical assessment of the endometrium yields more information about the causes of infertility or pregnancy loss. All of these advances will require the contribution of basic and translational scientists, clinical investigators, statisticians and epidemiologists to discover, validate and verify these assessment tools of the future, as we move further from the bench top and closer to the bedside.

# References

1. Strauss JF III, Lessey BA. The structure, function and evaluation of the female reproductive tract. In JF Strauss III, RL Barbieri (eds), *Reproductive Endocrinology:Physiology, Pathophysiology and Clinical Management*. 5th edition. New York: W. B. Saunders, 2006.

2. Okulicz WC. Cellular and molecular regulation of the primate endometrium: a perspective. *Reprod Biol Endocrinol* 2006; **4**(Suppl. 1): S3.

3. Brenner RM, West NB. Hormonal regulation of the reproductive tract in female mammals. *Ann Rev Physiol* 1975; **37**: 273–302.

4. Markee JE. Menstruation in intraocular endometrial transplants in the rhesus monkey. *Am J Obstet Gynecol* 1978; **131**: 558–9.

5. Wentz AC. Physiologic and clinical considerations in luteal phase defects. *Clin Obstet Gynecol* 1979; **22**: 169.

6. Wentz AC. Diagnosing luteal phase inadequacy. *Fertil Steril* 1982; **37**: 334–5.

7. Castelbaum AJ, Lessey BA. Insights into the evaluation of the luteal phase. In MP Diamond (ed), *Infertility and Reproductive Medicine*. New York: Springer-Verlag, 1995.

8. Usadi RS, Groll JM, Lessey BA et al. Endometrial development and function in experimentally induced luteal phase deficiency. *J Clin Endocrinol Metab* 2008; **93**: 4058–64.

9. Dey SK., Lim H, Das SK et al. Molecular cues to implantation. *Endocr Rev* 2004; **25**: 341–73.

10. Donaghay M, Lessey BA. Uterine receptivity: alterations associated with benign gynecological disease. *Semin Reprod Med* 2007; **25**: 461–75.

11. Tapia A, Gangi LM, Zegers-Hochschild F et al. Differences in the endometrial transcript profile during the receptive period between women who were refractory to implantation and those who achieved pregnancy. *Hum Reprod* 2008; **23**: 340–51.

12. De Los Santos MJ, Mercader A, Galan A et al. Implantation rates after two, three, or five days of embryo culture. *Placenta* 2003; **24**(Suppl. B): S13–19.

13. Pope WF. Uterine asynchrony: a cause of embryonic loss. *Biol Reprod* 1988; **39**: 999–1003.

14. Wilcox AJ, Baird DD, Weinberg CR. Time of implantation of the conceptus and loss of pregnancy. *New Engl J Med* 1999; **340**: 1796–9.

15. Navot D, Bergh PA, Williams MA et al. Poor oocyte quality rather than implantation failure as a cause of age-related decline in female infertility. *Lancet* 1991b; **337**: 1375–7.

16. Hertig AT, Rock J, Adams EC. A description of 34 human ova within the first 17 days of development. *Am J Anat* 1956; **98**: 435–93.

17. Navot D, Bergh P. Preparation of the human endometrium for implantation. *Ann N Y Acad Sci* 1991; **622**: 212–19.

18. Navot D, Bergh PA, Williams M et al. An insight into early reproductive processes through the in vivo model of ovum donation. *J Clin Endocrinol Metab* 1991; **72**: 408–14.

19. Navot D, Scott RT, Droesch K et al. The window of embryo transfer and the efficiency of human conception in vitro. *Fertil Steril* 1991; **55**: 114–18.

20. Ilesanmi AO, Hawkins DA, Lessey BA. Immunohistochemical markers of uterine receptivity in the human endometrium. *Microsc Res Tech* 1993; **25**: 208–22.

21. Lessey BA, Castelbaum AJ, Guzick D, Sun J, Fritz M. The use of integrins as markers of uterine receptivity to date the endometrial biopsy. *Am Fertil Soc Annu Mtg* 1994; Abstr.

22. Kliman HJ, Honig S, Walls D et al. Optimization of endometrial preparation results in a normal endometrial function test (EFT) and good reproductive outcome in donor ovum recipients. *J Assist Reprod Genet* 2006; **23**, 299–303.

23. Wang B, Sheng JZ, He RH et al. High expression of L-selectin ligand in secretory endometrium is associated with better endometrial receptivity and facilitates embryo implantation in human being. *Am J Reprod Immunol* 2008; **60**: 127–34.

24. Dominguez F, Remohi J, Pellicer A, Simon C. Human endometrial receptivity: a genomic approach. *Reprod Biomed Online* 2003; **6**: 332–8.

25. Horcajadas JA, Pellicer A, Simon C. Wide genomic analysis of human endometrial receptivity: new times, new opportunities. *Hum Reprod Update* 2007; **13**: 77–86.

26. Talbi S, Hamilton AE, Vo KC et al. Molecular phenotyping of human endometrium distinguishes menstrual cycle phases and underlying biological processes in normo-ovulatory women. *Endocrinology* 2006; **147**: 1097–121.

27. Carter AM, Croy BA, Dantzer V et al. Comparative aspects of placental evolution: a workshop report. *Placenta* 2007; **28**(Suppl. A): S129–32.

28. Enders AC, Schlafke S. Comparative aspects of blastocyst-endometrial interactions at implantation. *Ciba Found Symp* 1978; 3–32.

29. Enders AC. Current topic: structural responses of the primate endometrium to implantation. *Placenta* 1991; **12**: 309–25.

30. Enders AC. Implantation (Embryology). *Encyclopedia Hum Biol* 1991; **4**: 423–35.

31. Aplin JD. Embryo implantation: the molecular mechanism remains elusive. *Reprod Biomed Online* 2006; **13**: 833–9.

32. Aplin JD, Kimber SJ. Trophoblast-uterine interactions at implantation. *Reprod Biol Endocrinol* 2004; **2**: 48.

33. Carson DD, Bagchi I, Dey SK et al. Embryo implantation. *Dev Biol* 2000; **223**: 217–37.

34. Yoshinaga K, Yoshinaga K, Mori T. Receptor concept in implantation research. In K Yoshinaga, T Mori (eds), *Development of Preimplantation Embryos and their Environment*. New York: Alan Liss, 1989, pp. 397–87.

35. Rogers PAW, Murphy CR, Yoshinaga K. Uterine receptivity for implantation: human studies. In *Blastocyst Implantation*. Serono Symposia, 1989.

36. Yoshinaga K. Uterine receptivity for blastocyst implantation. *Ann N Y Acad Sci* 1988; **541**: 424–31.

37. Denker HW. Implantation: A cell biological paradox. *J Exp Zool* 1993; **266**: 541–58.

38. Sutherland A. Mechanisms of implantation in the mouse: differentiation and functional importance of trophoblast giant cell behavior. *Dev Biol* 2003; **258**: 241–51.

39. Murphy CR, Rogers PA, Hosie MJ, Leeton J, Beaton L. Tight junctions of human uterine epithelial cells change during the menstrual cycle: a morphometric study. *Acta Anat (Basel)* 1992; **144**: 36–8.

40. Rogers PA, Murphy CR. Morphometric and freeze fracture studies of human endometrium during the peri-implantation period. *Reprod Fertil Dev* 1992; **4**: 265–9.

41. Jones GS. Some newer aspects of management of infertility. *J Am Med Assoc* 1949; **141**: 1123–9.

42. Andersen AN, Yue Z, Meng FJ, Petersen K. Low implantation rate after in-vitro fertilization in patients with hydrosalpinges diagnosed by ultrasonography. *Hum Reprod* 1994; **9**: 1935–8.

43. Lessey BA, Castelbaum AJ, Riben M et al. Effect of hydrosalpinges on markers of uterine receptivity and success in IVF. *Am Fertil Soc Annu Mtg* 1994; Abstr.

44. Strandell A, Waldenstrîm U, Nilsson L, Hamberger L. Hydrosalpinx reduces in-vitro fertilization/embryo transfer pregnancy rates. *Hum Reprod* 1994; **9**: 861–3.

45. Strandell A, Lindhard A, Waldenstrîm U et al. Hydrosalpinx and IVF outcome: a prospective, randomized multicentre trial in Scandinavia on salpingectomy prior to IVF. *Hum Reprod* 1999; **14**: 2762–9.

46. Strandell A, Lindhard A. Hydrosalpinx and ART – Salpingectomy prior to IVF can be recommended to a well-defined subgroup of patients. *Hum Reprod* 2000; **15**: 2072–4.

47. Barnhart KT, Dunsmoor R, Coutifaris C. The effect of endometriosis on IVF outcome. *Am Soc Reprod Med Annual Mtg* 2000; Abstract.

48. Meyer WR, Castelbaum AJ, Somkuti S et al. Hydrosalpinges adversely affect markers of endometrial receptivity. *Hum Reprod* 1997; **12**: 1393–8.

49. Bildirici I, Bukulmez O, Ensari A, Yarali H, Gurgan T. A prospective evaluation of the effect of salpingectomy on endometrial receptivity in cases of women with communicating hydrosalpinges. *Hum Reprod* 2001; **16**: 2422–6.

50. Savaris RF, Pedrini JL, Flores R, Fabris G, Zettler CG. Expression of alpha 1 and beta 3 integrins subunits in the endometrium of patients with tubal phimosis or hydrosalpinx. *Fertil Steril* 2006; **85**: 188–92.

51. Seli E, Kayisli UA, Cakmak H et al. Removal of hydrosalpinges increases endometrial leukaemia inhibitory factor (LIF) expression at the time of the implantation window. *Hum Reprod* 2005; **20**: 3012–17.

52. Lessey BA, Castelbaum AJ, Sawin SW et al. Aberrant integrin expression in the endometrium of women with endometriosis. *J Clin Endocrinol Metab* 1994; **79**: 643–9.

53. Selam B, Arici A. Implantation defect in endometriosis: endometrium or peritoneal fluid. *J Reprod Fertil* 2000; Suppl. **55**: 121–8.

54. Tabibzadeh S, Mason JM, Shea W et al. Dysregulated expression of ebaf, a novel molecular defect in the endometria of patients with infertility. *J Clin Endocrinol Metab* 2000; **85**: 2526–36.

55. Lessey BA. Two pathways of progesterone action in the human endometrium: implications for implantation and contraception. *Steroids* 2003; **68**: 809–15.

56. Margalioth EJ, Ben-Chetrit A, Gal M, Eldar-Geva T. Investigation and treatment of repeated implantation failure following IVF-ET. *Hum Reprod* 2006; **21**: 3036–43.

57. Minici F, Tiberi F, Tropea A et al. Endometriosis and human infertility: a new investigation into the role of eutopic endometrium. *Hum Reprod* 2008; **23**: 530–7.

58. Noyes RW, Hertig AI, Rock J. Dating the endometrial biopsy. *Fertil Steril* 1950; **1**: 3–25.

59. Key JD, Kempers RD. Citation classics: most-cited articles from *Fertil Steril*. *Fertil Steril* 1987; **47**: 910–15.

60. Coutifaris C, Myers ER, Guzick DS et al. Histological dating of timed endometrial biopsy tissue is not related to fertility status. *Fertil Steril* 2004; **82**: 1264–72.

61. Murray MJ., Meyer WR, Zaino RJ et al. A critical analysis of the accuracy, reproducibility, and clinical utility of histologic endometrial dating in fertile women. *Fertil Steril* 2004; **81**: 1333–43.

62. Hague WE, Maier DB, Schmidt CL, Randolph JF. An evaluation of late luteal phase endometrium in women requesting reversal of tubal ligation. *Obstet Gynecol* 1987; **69**: 926–8.

63. Li TC, Dockery P, Cooke ID. Endometrial development in the luteal phase of women with various types of infertility: comparison with women of normal fertility. *Hum Reprod* 1991; **6**: 325–30.

64. Li TC, Cooke ID. Evaluation of the luteal phase. *Hum Reprod* 1991; **6**: 484–99.

65. Castelbaum AJ, Wheeler J, Coutifaris CB, Mastroianni L, Jr, Lessey BA. Timing of the endometrial biopsy may be critical for the accurate diagnosis of luteal phase deficiency. *Fertil Steril* 1994; **61**: 443–7.

66. Davis OK, Berkeley AS, Naus GJ, Cholst IN, Freedman KS. The incidence of luteal phase defect in normal, fertile women, determined by serial endometrial biopsies. *Fertil Steril* 1989; **51**: 582–6.

67. Burney RO, Talbi S, Hamilton AE *et al.* Gene expression analysis of endometrium reveals progesterone resistance and candidate susceptibility genes in women with endometriosis. *Endocrinology* 2007; **148**: 3814–26.

68. Kao LC, Germeyer A, Tulac S *et al.* Expression profiling of endometrium from women with endometriosis reveals candidate genes for disease-based implantation failure and infertility. *Endocrinology* 2003; **144**: 2870–81.

69. Achache H, Revel A. Endometrial receptivity markers, the journey to successful embryo implantation. *Hum Reprod Update* 2006; **12**: 731–46.

70. Cumming DC, Honore LH, Scott JZ, Williams KP. The late luteal phase in infertile women: comparison of simultaneous endometrial biopsy and progesterone levels. *Fertil Steril* 1985; **43**: 715–19.

71. Daya S, Ward S, Burrows E. Progesterone profiles in luteal phase defect cycles and outcome of progesterone treatment in patients with recurrent spontaneous abortion. *Am J Obstet Gynecol* 1988; **158**: 225–32.

72. Hecht BR, Bardawil WA, Khan-Dawood FS, Dawood MY. Luteal insufficiency: Correlation between endometrial dating and integrated progesterone output in clomiphene citrate-induced cycles. *Am J Obstet Gyn* 1990; **163**: 1986–91.

73. Fritz MA, Lessey BA. Defective luteal function. In IS Fraser, RPS Jansen, RA Lobo, MI Whitehead (eds), *Estrogens and Progestogens in Clinical Practice*. London: Churchill Livingstone, 1998.

74. Strott CA, Cargille CM, Ross GT, Lipsett MB. The short luteal phase. *J Clin Endocrinol Metab* 1970; **30**: 246–51.

75. Groff TR, Raj HG, Talbert LM, Willis DL. Effects of neutralization of luteinizing hormone on corpus luteum function and cyclicity in *Macaca fascicularis*. *J Clin Endocrinol Metab* 1984; **59**: 1054–7.

76. Filicori M, Flamigni C. GnRH agonists and antagonists. Current clinical status. *Drugs* 1988; **35**: 63–82.

77. Ellinwood WE, Norman RL, Spies HG. Changing frequency of pulsatile luteinizing hormone and progesterone secretion during the luteal phase of the menstrual cycle of rhesus monkeys. *Biol Reprod* 1984; **31**: 714–22.

78. Soules MR, Mclachlan RI, Ek M *et al.* Luteal phase deficiency: characterization of reproductive hormones over the menstrual cycle. *J Clin Endocrinol Metab* 1989; **69**: 804–12.

80. Maclaughlan SD, Palomino WA, Mo B *et al.* Endometrial expression of Cyr61: a marker of estrogenic activity in normal and abnormal endometrium. *Obstet Gynecol* 2007; **110**: 146–54.

80. Cermik D, Selam B, Taylor HS. Regulation of HOXA-10 expression by testosterone in vitro and in the endometrium of patients with polycystic ovary syndrome. *J Clin Endocrinol Metab* 2003; **88**: 238–43.

81. Avellaira C, Villavicencio A, Bacallao K *et al.* Expression of molecules associated with tissue homeostasis in secretory endometria from untreated women with polycystic ovary syndrome. *Hum Reprod* 2006; **21**: 3116–21.

82. Dor J, Itzkowic DJ, Mashiach S, Lunenfeld B, Serr DM. Cumulative conception rates following gonadotropin therapy. *Am J Obstet Gynecol* 1980; **136**: 102–5.

83. Duquesnay R, Wright C, Aziz AA *et al.* Infertile women with isolated polycystic ovaries are deficient in endometrial expression of osteopontin but not alphavbeta3 integrin during the implantation window. *Fertil Steril* 2009; **91**: 489–99.

84. Apparao KB, Lovely LP, Gui Y, Lininger RA, Lessey BA. Elevated endometrial androgen receptor expression in women with polycystic ovarian syndrome. *Biol Reprod* 2002; **66**: 297–304.

85. Gregory CW, Wilson EM, Apparao KB *et al.* Steroid receptor coactivator expression throughout the menstrual cycle in normal and abnormal endometrium. *J Clin Endocrinol Metab* 2002; **87**: 2960–6.

86. Daly DC. The endometrium and luteal phase defect. *Semin Reprod Med* 1983; **1**: 237–47.

87. Homburg R., Giudice LC, Chang RJ. Polycystic ovary syndrome. *Hum Reprod* 1996; **11**: 465–6.

88. Liddell HS, Sowden K, Farquhar CM. Recurrent miscarriage: screening for polycystic ovaries and subsequent pregnancy outcome. *Aust N Z J Obstet Gynaecol* 1997; **37**: 402–6.

89. Rai R, Backos M, Rushworth F, Regan L. Polycystic ovaries and recurrent miscarriage – a reappraisal. *Hum Reprod* 2000; **15**: 612–15.

90. Tulppala M, Stenman UH, Cacciatore B, Ylikorkala O. Polycystic ovaries and levels of gonadotrophins and androgens in recurrent miscarriage: prospective study in 50 women. *Br J Obstet Gynecol* 1993; **100**: 348–52.

91. Baulieu EE. Contragestion and other clinical applications of RU-486, an antiprogesterone at the receptor. *Science* 1989; **245**: 1351–7.

92. Good RG, Moyer DL. Estrogen-progesterone relationships in the development of secretory endometrium. *Fertil Steril* 1968; **19**: 37–49.

93. Joshi SG, Ebert KM, Smith RA. Properties of the progestagen-dependent protein of the endometrium. *Journal of Reproduction and Fertiliy* 1980; **59**: 287–96.

94. Strinden ST, Shapiro SS. Progesterone-altered secretory proteins from cultured human endometrium. *Endocrinology* 1983; **112**: 862–70.

95. Ding YQ., Zhu LJ, Bagchi MK, Bagchi IC. Progesterone stimulates calcitonin gene expression in the uterus during implantation. *Endocrinology* 1994; **135**: 2265–74.

96. Lessey BA, Yeh I, Castelbaum AJ et al. Endometrial progesterone receptors and markers of uterine receptivity in the window of implantation. *Fertil Steril* 1996; **65**: 477–83.

97. Aplin JD, Jones CJP, McGinlay PB, Croxatto HB, Fazleabas AT. Progesterone regulates glycosylation in endometrium. *Biochem Soc Trans* 1997; **25**: 1184–7.

98. Lalitkumar PGL, Sengupta J, Karande AA, Ghosh D. Placental protein 14 in endometrium during menstrual cycle and effect of early luteal phase mifepristone administration on its expression in implantation stage endometrium in the rhesus monkey. *Hum Reprod* 1998; **13**: 3478–86.

99. Lessey BA. Endometrial integrins and the establishment of uterine receptivity. *Hum Reprod* 1998; **13**(Suppl. 3): 247–58.

100. Giudice LC. Genes associated with embryonic attachment and implantation and the role of progesterone. *J Reprod Med* 1999; **44**: 165–71.

101. Bulun SE, Cheng YH, Yin P et al. Progesterone resistance in endometriosis: link to failure to metabolize estradiol. *Mol Cell Endocrinol* 2006; **248**: 94–103.

102. Lessey BA, Palomino WA, Apparao KB, Young SL, Lininger RA. Estrogen receptor-alpha (ER-alpha) and defects in uterine receptivity in women. *Reprod Biol Endocrinol* 2006; **4**(Suppl. 1): S9.

103. Kitawaki J, Kusuki I, Koshiba H, Tsukamoto K, Honjo H. Detection of aromatase cytochrome P-450 in endometrial biopsy specimens as a diagnostic test for endometriosis. *Fertil Steril* 1999; **72**: 1100–6.

104. Klentzeris LD, Bulmer JN, Seppala M et al. Placental protein 14 in cycles with normal and retarded endometrial differentiation. *Hum Reprod* 1994; **9**: 394–8.

105. Anderson TL, Olson GE, Hoffman LH. Stage specific alterations in the apical membrane glycoproteins of endometrial epithelial cells related to implantation in rabbits. *Biol Reprod* 1986; **34**: 701–20.

106. Aplin JD, Seif MW, Behzad F et al. The endometrial cell surface and implantation. *Second Annual Meeting on Endometrium*. Bologna, Italy, 1993.

107. Anderson TL, Hoffman LH. Alterations in epithelial glycocalyx of rabbit uteri during early pseudopregnancy and pregnancy and following ovariectomy. *Am J Anat* 1984; **171**: 321–34.

108. Hewitt K, Beer AE, Grinnell F. Disappearance of anionic sites from the surface of the rat endometrial epithelium at the time of blastocyst implantation. *Biol Reprod* 1979; **21**: 691–707.

109. Pinsker MC, Mintz B. Change in cell-surface glycoproteins of mouse embryos before implantation. *Proc Natl Acad Sci USA* 1973; **70**: 1645–8.

110. Chavez DJ, Enders AC. Lectin binding of mouse blastocysts: appearance of *Dolichos biflorus* binding sites on the trophoblast during delayed implantation and their subsequent disappearance during implantation. *Biol Reprod* 1982; **26**: 545–52.

111. Chavez DJ, Enders AC. Temporal changes in lectin binding of peri-implantation mouse blastocysts. *Dev Biol* 1981; **87**: 267–76.

112. Hey NA, Graham RA, Seif MW, Aplin JD. The polymorphic epithelial mucin MUC1 in human endometrium is regulated with maximal expression in the implantation phase. *J Clin Endocrinol Metab* 1994; **78**: 337–42.

113. Hoffman LH, Olson GE, Carson DD, Chilton BS. Progesterone and implanting blastocysts regulate Muc1 expression in rabbit uterine epithelium. *Endocrinology* 1998; **139**: 266–71.

114. Surveyor GA, Gendler SJ, Pemberton L, Spicer AP, Carson DD. Differential expression of Muc-1 at the apical cell surface of mouse uterine epithelial cells. *FASEB J* 1993; **7**: 1151a.

115. Desouza MM, Mani SK, Julian J, Carson DD. Reduction of mucin-1 expression during the receptive phase in the rat uterus. *Biol Reprod* 1998; **58**: 1503–7.

116. Carson DD, Julian J, Lessey BA, Prakobphol A, Fisher SJ. MUC1 is a scaffold for selectin ligands in the human uterus. *Front Biosci* 2006; **11**: 2903–8.

117. Enders AC, Nelson DM. Pinocytotic activity of the uterus of the rat. *Am J Anat* 1973; **138**: 277–99.

118. Psychoyos A, Mandon P. Etude de la surface de l'epithelium uterin au microscope electronique a balayage. *C R Hebd Seances Acad Sci Paris* 1971; **272**: 2723–5.

119. Ciocca DR, Asch RS, Adams DJ, Mcguire WL. Evidence for the modulation of a 24K protein in human endometrium during the menstrual cycle. *J Clin Endocrinol Metab* 1983; **57**: 496–9.

120. Psychoyos A, Martel D. Embryo–endometrial interactions at implantation. *J Reprod Fertil* 1985; **41**: 195–218.

121. Frydman MR, Glissant M, Maggioni C, Roche D, Psychoyos A. Scanning electron microscopy of postovulatory human endometrium in spontaneous cycles and cycles stimulated by hormone treatment. *J Endocrinol* 1987; **114**: 319–24.

122. Martel D, Frydman R, Glissant M *et al.* Scanning electron microscopy of postovulatory human endometrium in spontaneous cycles and cycles stimulated by hormone treatment. *J Endocrinol* 1987; **114**: 319–24.

123. Martel D, Frydman R, Sarantis L *et al.* Scanning electron microscopy of the uterine luminal epithelium as a marker of the implantation window. In *Blastocyst Implantation*. Boston: Adams Publishing Group, 1993.

124. Psychoyos A, Nikas G. Uterine pinopodes as markers of uterine receptivity. *Assist Reprod Rev* 1994; **4**: 26–31.

125. Nikas G, Drakakis P, Loutradis D *et al.* Uterine pinopodes as markers of the 'nidation window' in cycling women receiving exogenous oestradiol and progesterone. *Hum Reprod* 1995; **10**: 1208–13.

126. Adams SM, Gayer N, Hosie MJ, Murphy CR. Human uterodomes (pinopods) do not display pinocytotic function. *Hum Reprod* 2002; **17**: 1980–6.

127. Develioglu OH, Nikas G, Hsiu JG, Toner JP, Jones HW Jr. Detection of endometrial pinopodes by light microscopy. *Fertil Steril* 2000; **74**: 767–70.

128. Bentin-Ley U. Relevance of endometrial pinopodes for human blastocyst implantation. *Hum Reprod* 2000; **15**(Suppl. 6): 67–73.

129. Bulletti C, Flamigni C, De Ziegler D. Implantation markers and endometriosis. *Reprod Biomed Online* 2005; **11**: 464–8.

130. Nardo LG, Nikas G, Makrigiannakis A, Sinatra F, Nardo F. Synchronous expression of pinopodes and alpha v beta 3 and alpha 4 beta 1 integrins in the endometrial surface epithelium of normally menstruating women during the implantation window. *J Reprod Med* 2003; **48**: 355–61.

131. Nikas G. Cell-surface morphological events relevant to human implantation. *Hum Reprod* 1999; **14**(Suppl. 2): 37–44.

132. Nikas G. Pinopodes as markers of endometrial receptivity in clinical practice. *Hum Reprod* 1999; **14**(Suppl. 2): 99–106.

133. Nikas G, Psychoyos A. Uterine pinopodes in peri-implantation human endometrium – clinical relevance. *Ann N Y Acad Sci* 1997; **816**: 129–42.

134. Stavreus-Evers A, Nikas G, Sahlin L, Eriksson H, Landgren BM. Formation of pinopodes in human endometrium is associated with the concentrations of progesterone and progesterone receptors. *Fertil Steril* 2001; **76**: 782–91.

135. Martel D, Monier MN, Roche D, Psychoyos A. Hormonal dependence of pinopode formation at the uterine luminal surface. *Hum Reprod* 1991; **6**: 597–603.

136. Bentin-Ley U, Pedersen B, Lindenberg S *et al.* Isolation and culture of human endometrial cells in a three-dimensional culture system. *J Reprod Fert* 1994; **101**: 327–32.

137. Bentin-Ley U, Sjigren A, Nilsson L *et al.* Presence of uterine pinopodes at the embryo-endometrial interface during human implantation in vitro *Hum Reprod* 1999; **14**: 515–20.

138. Acosta AA, Elberger L, Borghi M *et al.* Endometrial dating and determination of the window of implantation in healthy fertile women. *Fertil Steril* 2000; **73**: 788–98.

139. Usadi RS, Murray MJ, Bagnell RC *et al.* Temporal and morphologic characteristics of pinopod expression across the secretory phase of the endometrial cycle in normally cycling women with proven fertility. *Fertil Steril* 2003; **79**: 970–4.

140. Quinn C, Ryan E, Claessens EA *et al.* The presence of pinopodes in the human endometrium does not delineate the implantation window. *Fertil Steril* 2007; **87**: 1015–21.

141. Usadi RS, Lessey BA, Bagnell RC, Meyer WR, Fritz MA. Distribution of pinopods in the secretory phase: a prospective, randomized assessment in healthy, fertile women. *Fertil Steril* 2001; **76**: S39.

142. Murphy CR. Understanding the apical surface markers of uterine receptivity. Pinopods or uterodomes? *Hum Reprod* 2000; **15**: 2451–4.

143. Von Wolff M, Strowitzki T, Becker V *et al.* Endometrial osteopontin, a ligand of β3-integrin, is maximally expressed around the time of the "implantation" window. *Fertil Steril* 2001; **76**: 775–81.

144. Young SL, Lessey BA, Fritz MA *et al.* In vivo and in vitro evidence suggest that HB-EGF regulates endometrial expression of human decay-accelerating factor. *J Clin Endocrinol Metab* 2002; **87**: 1368–75.

145. Aghajanova L, Stavreus-Evers A, Nikas Y, Hovatta O, Landgren BM. Coexpression of pinopodes and leukemia inhibitory factor, as well as its receptor, in human endometrium. *Fertil Steril* 2003; **79** (Suppl. 1): 808–14.

146. Lai TH, Shih IeM, Vlahos N *et al.* Differential expression of L-selectin ligand in the endometrium during the menstrual cycle. *Fertil Steril* 2005; **83**(Suppl. 1): 1297–302.

147. Stavreus-Evers A, Mandelin E, Koistinen R *et al.* Glycodelin is present in pinopodes of receptive-phase human endometrium and is associated with down-regulation of progesterone receptor B. *Fertil Steril* 2006; **85**: 1803–11.

148. Foulk RA, Zdravkovic T, Genbacev O, Prakobphol A. Expression of L-selectin ligand MECA-79 as a predictive marker of human uterine receptivity. *J Assist Reprod Genet* 2007; **24**: 316–21.

149. Shimizu Y, Kabir-Salmani M, Azadbakht M, Sugihara K, Sakai K, Iwashita M. Expression and localization of galectin-9 in the human uterodome. *Endocr J* 2008; **55**: 879–87.

150. Dubrauszky V, Pohmann G. Strukturveränderungen am nukleolus von korpusendometriumzellen während der sekretionsphase. *Naturewissenschaften* 1960; **47**: 523–4.

151. Guffanti E, Kittur N, Brodt ZN et al. Nuclear pore complex proteins mark the implantation window in human endometrium. *J Cell Sci* 2008; **121**: 2037–45.

152. Alcazar JL. Three-dimensional ultrasound assessment of endometrial receptivity: a review. *Reprod Biol Endocrinol* 2006; **4**: 56.

153. Dechaud H, Bessueille E, Bousquet PJ et al. Optimal timing of ultrasonographic and Doppler evaluation of uterine receptivity to implantation. *Reprod Biomed Online* 2008; **16**: 368–75.

154. Smith P. Evaluation of endometrium with transvaginal ultrasound. *Acta Obstet Gynecol Scand* 1993; **72**: 686–7.

155. Friedler S, Schenker JG, Herman A, Lewin A. The role of ultrasonography in the evaluation of endometrial receptivity following assisted reproductive treatments: a critical review. *Hum Reprod Update* 1996; **2**: 323–35.

156. Van Voorhis BJ. Ultrasound assessment of the uterus and fallopian tube in infertile women. *Semin Reprod Med* 2008; **26**: 232–40.

157. De Geyter C, Schmitter M, De Geyter M et al. Prospective evaluation of the ultrasound appearance of the endometrium in a cohort of 1,186 infertile women. *Fertil Steril* 2000; **73**: 106–13.

158. Rabinowitz R, Laufer N, Lewin A et al. The value of ultrasonographic endometrial measurement in the prediction of pregnancy following in vitro fertilization. *Fertil Steril* 1986; **45**: 824–8.

159. Sterzik K, Grab D, Schneider V et al. Lack of correlation between ultrasonography and histologic staging of the endometrium in in vitro fertilization (IVF) patients. *Ultrasound Med Biol* 1997; **23**: 165–70.

160. Abdalla HI, Brooks AA, Johnson MR et al. Endometrial thickness: A predictor of implantation in ovum recipients? *Hum Reprod* 1994; **9**: 363–5.

161. El-Toukhy T, Coomarasamy A, Khairy M et al. The relationship between endometrial thickness and outcome of medicated frozen embryo replacement cycles. *Fertil Steril* 2008; **89**: 832–9.

162. Isaacs JD Jr, Wells CS, Williams DB et al. Endometrial thickness is a valid monitoring parameter in cycles of ovulation induction with menotropins alone. *Fertil Steril* 1996; **65**: 262–6.

163. Oliveira JBA, Baruffi RLR, Mauri AL et al. Endometrial ultrasonography as a predictor of pregnancy in an in-vitro fertilization programme after ovarian stimulation and gonadotrophin-releasing hormone and gonadotrophins. *Hum Reprod* 1997; **12**: 2515–18.

164. Bassil S. Changes in endometrial thickness, width, length and pattern in predicting pregnancy outcome during ovarian stimulation in in vitro fertilization. *Ultrasound Obstet Gynecol* 2001; **18**: 258–63.

165. Coulam CB, Bustillo M, Soenksen DM, Britten S. Ultrasonographic predictors of implantation after assisted reproduction. *Fertil Steril* 1994; **62**: 1004–10.

166. Glissant A, De Mouzon J, Frydman R. Ultrasound study of the endometrium during in vitro fertilization cycles. *Fertil Steril* 1985; **44**: 786–90.

167. Gonen Y, Casper RF, Jacobson W, Blankier J. Endometrial thickness and growth during ovarian stimulation: a possible predictor of implantation in in vitro fertilization. *Fertil Steril* 1989; **52**: 446–50.

168. Noyes N, Liu HC, Sultan K, Schattman G, Rosenwaks Z. Endometrial thickness appears to be a significant factor in embryo implantation in in-vitro fertilization. *Hum Reprod* 1995; **10**: 919–22.

169. Imoedemhe DA, Shaw RW, Kirkland A. Ultrasound measurement of endometrium: the predictive value for the outcome of in-vitro fertilization in stimulated cycles. *Hum Reprod* 1987; **2**: 545–7.

170. Puerto B, Creus M, Carmona F et al. Ultrasonography as a predictor of embryo implantation after in vitro fertilization: a controlled study. *Fertil Steril* 2003; **79**: 1015–22.

171. Smith B, Porter R, Ahuja K, Craft I. Ultrasonic assessment of endometrial changes in stimulated cycles in an in vitro fertilization and embryo transfer program. *J In Vitro Fert Embryo Transf* 1984; **1**: 233–8.

172. Gonen Y, Casper RF. Prediction of implantation by the sonographic appearance of the endometrium during controlled ovarian stimulation for in vitro fertilization (IVF). *J In Vitro Fert Embryo Transf* 1990; **7**: 146–52.

173. Sher G, Herbert C, Maassarani G, Jacobs MH. Assessment of the late proliferative phase endometrium by ultrasonography in patients undergoing in-vitro fertilization and embryo transfer (IVF/ET). *Hum Reprod* 1991; **6**: 232–7.

174. Sharara FI, Lim J, McClamrock HD. Endometrial pattern on the day of oocyte retrieval is more predictive of implantation success than the pattern or thickness on the day of hCG administration. *J Assist Reprod Genet* 1999; **16**: 523–8.

175. Scholtes MC, Wladimiroff JW, Van Rijen HJ, Hop WC. Uterine and ovarian flow velocity waveforms in the

normal menstrual cycle: a transvaginal Doppler study. *Fertil Steril* 1989; **52**: 981–5.

176. Goswamy RK, Steptoe PC. Doppler ultrasound studies of the uterine artery in spontaneous ovarian cycles. *Hum Reprod* 1988; **3**: 721–6.

177. Habara T, Nakatsuka M, Konishi H *et al*. Elevated blood flow resistance in uterine ateries of women with unexplained recurrent pregnancy loss. *Hum Reprod* 2002; **17**: 190–4.

178. Sterzik K, Grab D, Sasse V. Doppler sonographic findings and their correlation with implantation in an in vitro fertilization program. *Fertil Steril* 1989; **52**: 825–8.

179. Steer CV, Tan SL, Mason BA, Campbell S. Midluteal-phase vaginal color doppler assessment of uterine artery impedance in a subfertile population. *Fertil Steril* 1994; **61**: 53–8.

180. Yaron Y, Botchan A, Amit A *et al*. Endometrial receptivity in the light of modern assisted reproductive technologies. *Fertil Steril* 1994; **62**: 225–32.

181. Cacciatore B, Simberg N, Fusaro P, Tiitinen A. Transvaginal Doppler study of uterine artery blood flow in in vitro fertilization-embryo transfer cycles. *Fertil Steril* 1996; **66**: 130–4.

182. Steer CV, Tan SL, Dillon D, Mason BA, Campbell S. Vaginal color Doppler assessment of uterine artery impedance correlates with immunohistochemical markers of endometrial receptivity required for the implantation of an embryo. *Fertil Steril* 1995; **63**: 101–8.

183. Schild RL, Indefrei D, Eschweiler S *et al*. Three-dimensional endometrial volume calculation and pregnancy rate in an in-vitro fertilization programme. *Hum Reprod* 1999; **14**: 1255–8.

184. Alatas C, Aksoy E, Akarsu C *et al*. Evaluation of intrauterine abnormalities in infertile patients by sonohysterography. *Hum Reprod* 1997; **12**: 487–90.

185. Goldstein SR. Use of ultrasonohysterography for triage of perimenopausal patients with unexplained uterine bleeding. *Am J Obstet Gynecol* 1994; **170**: 565–70.

186. Keltz MD., Olive DL, Kim AH, Arici A. Sonohysterography for screening in recurrent pregnancy loss. *Fertil Steril* 1997; **67**: 670–4.

187. Parsons AK, Lense JJ. Sonohysterography for endometrial abnormalities: preliminary results. *J Clin Ultras* 1993; **21**: 87–95.

188. Burke C, Kelehan P, Wingfield M. Unsuspected endometrial pathology in the subfertile woman. *Ir Med J* 2007; **100**: 466–9.

189. Goldberg JM, Falcone T, Attaran M. Sonohysterographic evaluation of uterine abnormalities noted on hysterosalpingography. *Hum Reprod* 1997; **12**: 2151–3.

190. Hamilton JA, Larson AJ, Lower AM, Hasnain S, Grudzinskas JG. Routine use of saline hysterosonography in 500 consecutive, unselected, infertile women. *Hum Reprod* 1998; **13**: 2463–73.

191. Cavagna M, Mantese JC. Biomarkers of endometrial receptivity – a review. *Placenta* 2003; **24**(Suppl. B): S39–47.

192. Campbell KL, Rockett JC. Biomarkers of ovulation, endometrial receptivity, fertilisation, implantation and early pregnancy progression. *Paediatr Perinat Epidemiol* 2006; **20**(Suppl. 1): 13–25.

193. Aghajanova L, Hamilton AE, Giudice LC. Uterine receptivity to human embryonic implantation: histology, biomarkers, and transcriptomics. *Semin Cell Dev Biol* 2008; **19**: 204–11.

194. Haouzi D, Mahmoud K, Fourar M *et al*. Identification of new biomarkers of human endometrial receptivity in the natural cycle. *Hum Reprod* 2008; **24**: 19–25.

195. Bell SC. Secretory endometrial/decidual proteins and their function in early pregnancy. *J Reprod Fert Suppl* 1988; **36**: 109–25.

196. Heffner LJ, Iddenden DA, Lyttle CR. Electrophoretic analyses of secreted human endometrial proteins: identification and characterization of luteal phase prolactin. *J Clin Endocrinol Metab* 1986; **62**: 1288–95.

197. Santoro N, Maclaughlin DT, Bauer HH *et al*. In vitro protein production by the human endometrium. *Biol Reprod* 1989; **40**: 1047–55.

198. Beier HM, Beier-Hellwig K, Sterzik S *et al*. The significance of endometrial secretion proteins and their determination in human uterine secretions. In AR Genazzani, F Petraglia (eds), *Frontiers in Gynecologic and Obstetric Investigation*. Carnforth: Parthenon Publishing Group, 1993.

199. Beier-Hellwig K, Bonn B, Sterzik K *et al*. Uterine receptivity and endometrial secretory protein patterns. In SK Dey (ed), *Molecular and Cellular Aspects of Preimplantation Processes*. New York: Springer-Verlag, 1995.

200. Carson DD, Lagow E, Thathiah A *et al*. Changes in gene expression during the early to mid-luteal (receptive phase) transition in human endometrium detected by high-density microarray screening. *Mol Hum Reprod* 2002; **8**: 871–9.

201. Catalano RD, Critchley HO, Heikinheimo O *et al*. Mifepristone induced progesterone withdrawal reveals novel regulatory pathways in human endometrium. *Mol Hum Reprod* 2007; **13**: 641–54.

202. Kao LC, Yang J, Lessey BA, Giudice LC. Gene expression profiles in human endometrium during the implantation window from subjects with endometriosis, using Genechip' microarray technology. *Endocrine Soc Annu Mtg*, 2001, submitted.

203. Riesewijk A, Martin J, Van Os R *et al*. Gene expression profiling of human endometrial receptivity on days LH+2 versus LH+7 by microarray technology. *Mol Hum Reprod* 2003; **9**: 253–64.

204. Schmidt A, Groth P, Haendler B *et al*. Gene expression during the implantation window: microarray analysis of human endometrial samples. *Ernst Schering Res Found Workshop* 2005; 139–57.

205. Cowan BD, Hines RS, Brackin MN, Case ST. Temporal and cell-specific gene expression by human endometrium after coculture with trophoblast. *Am J Obstet Gynecol* 1999; **180**: 806–14.

206. Haendler B, Yamanouchi H, Lessey BA, Chwalisz K, Hess-Stumpp H. Cycle-dependent endometrial expression and hormonal regulation of the fibulin-1 gene. *Mol Reprod Dev* 2004; **68**: 279–87.

207. Getzenberg RH, Pienta KJ, Coffey DS. The tissue matrix: Cell dynamics and hormone action. *Endocrine Rev* 1990; **11**: 399–417.

208. Aplin JD, Charlton AK, Ayad S. An immunohistochemical study of human endometrial extracellular matrix during the menstrual cycle and first trimester of pregnancy. *Cell Tissue Res* 1988; **253**: 231–40.

209. Ruck P, Marzusch K, Kaiserling E *et al*. Distribution of cell adhesion molecules in decidua of early human pregnancy: an immunohistochemical study. *Lab.Invest* 1994; **71**: 94–101.

210. Feinberg RF, Kliman HJ. Tropho-uteronectin (TUN): A unique oncofetal fibronectin deposited in the extracellular matrix of the tropho-uterine junction and regulated in vitro by cultured human trophoblast cells. *Trophoblast Res* 1993; **7**: 167–73.

211. Turpeenniemi-Hujanen T, Feinberg RF, Kauppila A, Puistola U. Extracellular matrix interactions in early human embryos: implications for normal implantation events. *Fertil Steril* 1995; **64**: 132–8.

212. Albelda SM, Buck CA. Integrins and other cell adhesion molecules. *FASEB J* 1990; **4**: 2868–80.

213. Lessey BA, Damjanovich L, Coutifaris C *et al*. Integrin adhesion molecules in the human endometrium. Correlation with the normal and abnormal menstrual cycle. *J Clin Invest* 1992; **90**: 188–95.

214. Lessey BA, Castelbaum AJ, Buck CA *et al*. Further characterization of endometrial integrins during the menstrual cycle and in pregnancy. *Fertil Steril* 1994; **62**: 497–506.

215. Tabibzadeh S. Patterns of expression of integrin molecules in human endometrium throughout the menstrual cycle. *Hum Reprod* 1992; **7**: 876–82.

216. Damsky C, Sutherland A, Fisher S. Extracellular matrix 5: Adhesive interactions in early mammalian embryogenesis, implantation, and placentation. *FASEB J* 1993; **7**: 1320–9.

217. Armant DR, Kaplan HA, Mover H, Lennarz WJ. The effect of hexapeptides on attachment and outgrowth of mouse blastocysts cultured in vitro: evidence for the involvement of the cell recognition tripeptide Arg-Gly-Asp. *Proc Natl Acad Sci USA* 1986; **83**: 6751–5.

218. Illera MJ, Cullinan E, Gui Y *et al*. Blockade of the alpha(v)beta(3) integrin adversely affects implantation in the mouse. *Biol Reprod* 2000; **62**: 1285–90.

219. Illera MJ., Gui YT, Mohammand A, Lessey BA. Perturbation of implantation rate by neutralization of the alphavbeta3 vitronectin receptor in rabbits. *Ann Mtg Soc Gynecol Invest* 1999; **379**: 143A.

220. Bronson RA, Fusi F. Evidence that an Arg-Gly-Asp adhesion sequence plays a role in mammalian fertilization. *Biol Reprod* 1990; **43**: 1019–25.

221. Bronson RA, Fusi FM. Integrins and human reproduction. *Mol Hum Reprod* 1996; **2**: 153–68.

222. Yelian FD, Yang Y, Hirata JD, Schultz JF, Armant DR. Molecular interactions between fibronectin and integrins during mouse blastocyst outgrowth. *Mol Reprod Dev* 1995; **41**: 435–48.

223. Jones JI, Gockerman A, Busby WH, Wright G, Clemmons DR. Insulin-like growth factor binding protein 1 stimulates cell migration and binds to the alpha 5/1 integrin by means of its ARG-GLY-ASP sequence. *Proc Natl Acad Sci USA* 1993; **90**: 10553–7.

224. Illera MJ, Lorenzo PL, Gui YT *et al*. A role for alphavbeta3 integrin during implantation in the rabbit model. *Biol Reprod* 2003; **68**: 766–71.

225. Sutherland AE, Calarco PG, Damsky CH. Developmental regulation of integrin expression at the time of implantation in the mouse embryo. *Development* 1993; **119**: 1175–86.

226. Tabibzadeh S, Sun XZ. Cytokine expression in human endometrium throughout the menstrual cycle. *Hum Reprod* 7: 1214–21.

227. Somkuti SG, Yuan L, Fritz MA, Lessey BA. Epidermal growth factor and sex steroids dynamically regulate a marker of endometrial receptivity in Ishikawa cells. *J Clin Endocrinol Metab* 1997; **82**: 2192–7.

228. Daftary GS, Troy PJ, Bagot CN, Young SL, Taylor HS. Direct regulation of beta3-integrin subunit gene expression by HOXA10 in endometrial cells. *Mol Endocrinol* 2002; **16**: 571–9.

229. Damsky CH, Fitzgerald ML, Fisher SJ. Distribution patterns of extracellular matrix components and adhesion receptors are intricately modulated during first trimester cytotrophoblast differentiation along the invasive pathway, in vivo. *J Clin Invest* 1992; **89**: 210–22.

230. Damsky CH., Librach C, Lim KH *et al*. Integrin switching regulates normal trophoblast invasion. *Development* 1994; **120**: 3657–66.

**193**

231. Zhou Y, Fisher SJ, Janatpour M *et al.* Human cytotrophoblasts adopt a vascular phenotype as they differentiate – a strategy for successful endovascular invasion? *J Clin Invest* 1997; **99**: 2139–51.

232. Genbacev O, Joslin R, Damsky CH., Polliotti BM, Fisher SJ. Hypoxia alters early gestation human cytotrophoblast differentiation invasion in vitro and models the placental defects that occur in preeclampsia. *J Clin Invest* 1996; **97**: 540–50.

233. Zhou Y, Damsky CH, Fisher SJ. Preeclampsia is associated with failure of human cytotrophoblasts to mimic a vascular adhesion phenotype – One cause of defective endovascular invasion in this syndrome? *J Clin Invest* 1997; **99**: 2152–64.

234. Lessey BA. Endometrial receptivity and the window of implantation. *Bailliére's Clin Obstet Gynecol* 2000; **14**: 775–88.

235. Lessey BA. Adhesion molecules and implantation. *J Reprod Immunol* 2002; **55**: 101–12.

236. Apparao KB, Murray MJ, Fritz MA *et al.* Osteopontin and its receptor alphavbeta(3) integrin are coexpressed in the human endometrium during the menstrual cycle but regulated differentially. *J Clin Endocrinol Metab* 2001; **86**: 4991–5000.

237. Fisher LW, Torchia DA, Fohr B, Young MF, Fedarko NS. Flexible structures of SIBLING proteins, bone sialoprotein, and osteopontin. *Biochem Biophys Res Comm* 2001; **280**: 460–5.

238. Fukuda MN, Sato T, Nakayama J *et al.* Trophinin and tastin, a novel cell adhesion molecule complex with potential involvement in embryo implantation. *Genes Dev* 1995; **9**: 1199–210.

239. Paria BC, Zhao XM, Das SK, Dey SK, Yoshinaga K. Zonula occludens-1 and E-cadherin are coordinately expressed in the mouse uterus with the initiation of implantation and decidualization. *Dev Biol* 1999; **208**: 488–501.

240. Chobotova K, Spyropoulou I, Carver J *et al.* Heparin-binding epidermal growth factor and its receptor ErbB4 mediate implantation of the human blastocyst. *Mech Dev* 2002; **119**: 137–44.

241. Genbacev OD, Prakobphol A, Foulk RA *et al.* Trophoblast L-selectin-mediated adhesion at the maternal–fetal interface. *Science* 2003; **299**: 405–8.

242. Luscinskas FW, Kansas GS, Ding H *et al.* Monocyte rolling, arrest and spreading on IL-4-activated vascular endothelium under flow is mediated via sequential action of L-selectin, 1-integrins, and 2-integrins. *J Cell Biol* 1994; **125**: 1417–27.

243. Johnston B, Issekutz TB, Kubes P. The alpha 4 -integrin supports leukocyte rolling and adhesion in chronically inflamed postcapillary venules in vivo. *J Exp Med* 1996; **183**: 1995–2006.

244. Lai TH, Zhao Y, Shih IeM *et al.* Expression of L-selectin ligands in human endometrium during the implantation window after controlled ovarian stimulation for oocyte donation. *Fertil Steril* 2006; **85**: 761–3.

245. Bhatt H, Brunet LJ, Stewart CL. Uterine expression of leukemia inhibitory factor coincides with the onset of blastocyst implantation. *Proc Natl Acad Sci USA* 1991; **88**: 11408–12.

246. Stewart CL. Leukaemia inhibitory factor and the regulation of pre-implantation development of the mammalian embryo. *Mol Reprod Dev* 1994; **39**: 233–8.

247. Stewart CL, Kaspar P, Brunet LJ *et al.* Blastocyst implantation depends on maternal expression of leukaemia inhibitory factor. *Nature* 1992; **359**: 76–9.

248. Cullinan EB, Abbondanzo SJ, Anderson PS *et al.* Leukemia inhibitory factor (LIF) and LIF receptor expression in human endometrium suggests a potential autocrine/paracrine function in regulating embryo implantation. *Proc Natl Acad Sci USA* 1996; **93**: 3115–20.

249. Sherwin JR, Smith SK, Wilson A, Sharkey AM. Soluble gp130 is up-regulated in the implantation window and shows altered secretion in patients with primary unexplained infertility. *J Clin Endocrinol Metab* 2002; **87**: 3953–60.

250. Mikolajczyk M, Wirstlein P, Skrzypczak J. Leukaemia inhibitory factor and interleukin 11 levels in uterine flushings of infertile patients with endometriosis. *Hum Reprod* 2006; **21**: 3054–8.

251. Dimitriadis E, Sharkey AM, Tan YL, Salamonsen LA, Sherwin JR. Immunolocalisation of phosphorylated STAT3, interleukin 11 and leukaemia inhibitory factor in endometrium of women with unexplained infertility during the implantation window. *Reprod Biol Endocrinol* 2007; **5**: 44.

252. Aghajanova L, Altmae S, Bjuresten K *et al.* Disturbances in the LIF pathway in the endometrium among women with unexplained infertility. *Fertil Steril* 2008; **15**: 484–92.

253. Birdsall MA, Hopkisson JF, Grant KE, Barlow DH, Mardon HJ. Expression of heparin-binding epidermal growth factor messenger RNA in the human endometrium. *Mol Hum Reprod* 1996; **2**: 31–4.

254. Kimber SJ. Molecular interactions at the maternal-embryonic interface during the early phase of implantation. *Semin Reprod Med* 2000; **18**: 237–53.

255. Martin KL, Barlow DH, Sargent IL. Heparin-binding epidermal growth factor significantly improves human blastocyst development and hatching in serum-free medium. *Hum Reprod* 1998; **13**: 1645–52.

256. Lessey BA, Gui Y, Apparao KB, Young SL, Mulholland J. Regulated expression of heparin-binding EGF-like growth factor (HB-EGF) in the human endometrium: a

potential paracrine role during implantation. *Mol Reprod Dev* 2002; **62**: 446–55.

257. Yoo HJ, Barlow DH, Mardon HJ. Temporal and spatial regulation of expression of heparin-binding epidermal growth factor-like growth factor in the human endometrium: a possible role in blastocyst implantation. *Dev Genet* 1997; **21**: 102–8.

258. Aghajanova L, Bjuresten K, Altmae S, Landgren BM, Stavreus-Evers A. HB-EGF but not amphiregulin or their receptors HER1 and HER4 is altered in endometrium of women with unexplained infertility. *Reprod Sci* 2008; **15**: 484–92.

259. Stavreus-Evers A, Aghajanova L, Brismar H *et al.* Co-existence of heparin-binding epidermal growth factor-like growth factor and pinopodes in human endometrium at the time of implantation. *Mol Hum Reprod* 2002; **8**: 765–9.

260. Leach RE, Khalifa R, Ramirez ND *et al.* Multiple roles for heparin-binding epidermal growth factor-like growth factor are suggested by its cell-specific expression during the human endometrial cycle and early placentation. *J Clin Endocrinol Metab* 1999; **84**: 3355–63.

261. Leach RE, Romero R, Kim YM *et al.* Pre-eclampsia and expression of heparin-binding EGF-like growth factor. *Lancet* 2002; **360**: 1215–19.

262. Eyster KM, Boles AL, Brannian JD, Hansen KA. DNA microarray analysis of gene expression markers of endometriosis. *Fertil Steril* **77**: 38–42.

263. Kao LC, Yang J, Lessey BA, Giudice LC. Microarray expression profiling reveals candidate genes for human uterine receptivity. *Fertil Steril* 2001; **76**: S59.

264. Kao LC, Yang J, Lessey BA, Giudice LC. Discovery of candidate genes for human uterine receptivity by GeneChip' microarray expression profiling. *Am Soc Reprod Med Annual Mtg*, 2001.

265. Liu Y, Lee KF, Ng EH, Yeung WS, Ho PC. Gene expression profiling of human peri-implantation endometria between natural and stimulated cycles. *Fertil Steril* 2008; **90**: 2152–64.

266. Matsuzaki S, Canis M, Pouly JL *et al.* Differential expression of genes in eutopic and ectopic endometrium from patients with ovarian endometriosis. *Fertil Steril* 2006; **86**: 548–53.

267. Matsuzaki S, Canis M, Vaurs-Barriere C *et al.* DNA microarray analysis of gene expression in eutopic endometrium from patients with deep endometriosis using laser capture microdissection. *Fertil Steril* 2005; **84**(Suppl. 2): 1180–90.

268. Mettler L, Salmassi A, Schollmeyer T *et al.* Comparison of c-DNA microarray analysis of gene expression between eutopic endometrium and ectopic endometrium (endometriosis). *J Assist Reprod Genet* 2007; **24**: 249–58.

269. Wu Y, Kajdacsy-Balla A, Strawn E *et al.* Transcriptional characterizations of differences between eutopic and ectopic endometrium. *Endocrinology* 2006; **147**: 232–46.

270. Klentzeris LD, Li TC, Dockery P, Cooke ID. The endometrial biopsy as a predictive factor of pregnancy rate in women with unexplained infertility. *Eur J Obstet Gynecol Reprod Biol* 1992; **45**: 119–24.

271. Balasch J, Fabregues F, Creus M, Vanrell JA. The usefulness of endometrial biopsy for luteal phase evaluation in infertility. *Hum Reprod* 1992; **7**: 973–7.

272. Balasch J, Vanrell JA, Creus M, Marquez M, Gonzalez Merlo J. The endometrial biopsy for diagnosis of luteal phase deficiency. *Fertil Steril* 1985; **44**: 699–701.

273. Graham RA, Seif MW, Aplin JD *et al.* An endometrial factor in unexplained infertility. *Br Med J* 1990; **300**: 1428–31.

274. Fedele L, Acaia B, Ricciardiello O, Marchini M, Benzi-Cipelli R. Recovery of *Chlamydia trachomatis* from the endometria of women with unexplained infertility. *J Reprod Med* 1989; **34**: 393–6.

275. Klentzeris LD, Bulmer JN, Li TC *et al.* Lectin binding of endometrium in women with unexplained infertility. *Fertil Steril* 1991; **56**: 660–7.

276. Klentzeris LD, Bulmer JN, Warren MA *et al.* Lymphoid tissue in the endometrium of women with unexplained infertility: morphometric and immunohistochemical aspects. *Hum Reprod* 1994; **9**: 646–52.

277. Dockery P, Pritchard K, Taylor A *et al.* The fine structure of the human endometrial glandular epithelium in cases of unexplained infertility: a morphometric study. *Hum Reprod* 1993; **8**: 667–73.

278. Bilalis DA, Klentzeris LD, Fleming S. Immunohistochemical localization of extracellular matrix proteins in luteal phase endometrium of fertile and infertile patients. *Hum Reprod* 1996; **11**: 2713–18.

279. Kilic S, Hatipoglu T, Erdogan D *et al.* Impact of high levels of progesterone on alpha(1)-integrin distribution in the endometrium of patients with unexplained infertility. *Acta Histochem* 2008; **110**: 363–70.

280. Gonzalez RR, Palomino A, Boric A, Vega M, Devoto L. A quantitative evaluation of α1, α4, αV and 3 endometrial integrins of fertile and unexplained infertile women during the menstrual cycle. A flow cytometric appraisal. *Hum Reprod* 1999; **14**: 2485–92.

281. Nip MMC, Miller D, Taylor PV, Gannon MJ, Hancock KW. Expression of heat shock protein 70 kDa in human endometrium of normal and infertile women. *Hum Reprod* 1994; **9**: 1253–6.

282. Quenby S, Bates M, Doig T *et al.* Pre-implantation endometrial leukocytes in women with recurrent miscarriage. *Hum Reprod* 1999; **14**: 2386–91.

283. Tulppala M, Julkunen M, Tiitinen A, Stenman UH, Seppala M. Habitual abortion is accompanied by low serum levels of placental protein 14 in the luteal phase of the fertile cycle. *Fertil Steril* 1995; **63**: 792–5.

284. Lessey BA, Castelbaum AJ, Sawin SW, Sun J. Integrins as markers of uterine receptivity in women with primary unexplained infertility. *Fertil Steril* 1995; **63**: 535–42.

285. Serle E, Aplin JD, Li TC et al. Endometrial differentiation in the peri-implantation phase of women with recurrent miscarriage: a morphological and immunohistochemical study. *Fertil Steril* 1994; **62**: 989–96.

286. Creus M, Balasch J, Ordi J et al. Integrin expression in normal and out-of-phase endometria. *Hum Reprod* 1998; **13**: 3460–8.

287. Blacker CM, Ginsburg KA, Leach RE, Randolph J, Moghissi KS. Unexplained infertility: Evaluation of the luteal phase. Results of the National Center for Infertility Research at Michigan. *Fertil Steril* 1997; **67**: 437–42.

288. Crosignani PG, Collins J, Cooke ID, Diczfalusy E, Rubin B. Unexplained infertility. *Hum Reprod* 1993; **8**: 977–80.

289. Collins JA, Crosignani PG. Unexplained infertility: a review of diagnosis, prognosis, treatment efficacy and management. *Int J Gynaecol Obstet* 1992; **39**: 267–75.

290. Bancroft K, Vaughan Williams CA, Elstein M. Minimal/mild endometriosis and infertility. A review. *Br J Obstet Gynaecol* 1989; **96**, 454–60.

291. Verkauf BS. Incidence, symptoms, and signs of endometriosis in fertile and infertile women. *J Fla Med Assoc* 1987; **74**: 671–5.

292. Littman E, Giudice L, Lathi R et al. Role of laparoscopic treatment of endometriosis in patients with failed in vitro fertilization cycles. *Fertil Steril* 2005; **84**: 1574–8.

293. Lessey BA, Parnell B, Forstein DA et al. Endometrial integrin testing prior to In Vitro Fertilization and Embryo Transfer (IVF-ET) detects endometriosis and improves outcome. *Fertil Steril* 2008; Submitted.

294. Hughes EG, Fedorkow DM, Collins JA. A quantitative overview of controlled trials in endometriosis-associated infertility. *Fertil Steril* 1993; **59**: 963.

295. Hahn DW, Carraher RP, Foldesy RG, Mcguire JL. Experimental evidence for failure to implant as a mechanism of infertility associated with endometriosis. *Am J Obstet Gynecol* 1986; **155**: 1109–13.

296. Schenken RS, Asch RH. Surgical induction of endometriosis in the rabbit: effects on fertility and concentration of peritoneal fluid prostaglandins. *Fertil Steril* 1980; **34**: 581–7.

297. Vernon MW, Wilson EA. Studies on the surgical induction of endometriosis in the rat. *Fertil Steril* 1985; **44**: 684–94.

298. Illera MJ, Juan L, Stewart CL et al. Effect of peritoneal fluid from women with endometriosis on implantation in the mouse model. *Fertil Steril* 2000; **74**: 41–8.

299. Fazleabas AT, Brudney A, Chai D, Langoi D, Bulun SE. Steroid receptor and aromatase expression in baboon endometriotic lesions. *Fertil Steril* 2003; **80**(Suppl. 2): 820–7.

300. Gashaw I, Hastings JM, Jackson KS, Winterhager E, Fazleabas AT. Induced endometriosis in the baboon (*Papio anubis*) increases the expression of the proangiogenic factor CYR61 (CCN1) in eutopic and ectopic endometria. *Biol Reprod* 2006; **74**: 1060–6.

301. Jackson KS, Brudney A, Hastings JM et al. The altered distribution of the steroid hormone receptors and the chaperone immunophilin FKBP52 in a baboon model of endometriosis is associated with progesterone resistance during the window of uterine receptivity. *Reprod Sci* 2007; **14**: 137–50.

302. Kim JJ, Taylor HS, Lu Z et al. Altered expression of HOXA10 in endometriosis: potential role in decidualization. *Mol Hum Reprod* 2007; **13**: 323–32.

303. Jansen RP. Minimal endometriosis and reduced fecundability: prospective evidence from an artificial insemination by donor program. *Fertil Steril* 1986; **46**: 141–3.

304. Arici A, Oral E, Bukulmez O et al. The effect of endometriosis on implantation: Results from the Yale University in vitro fertilization and embryo transfer program. *Fertil Steril* 1996; **65**: 603–7.

305. Olivennes F, Feldberg D, Liu HC et al. Endometriosis: a stage by stage analysis – the role of in vitro fertilization. *Fertil Steril* 1995; **64**: 392–8.

306. Evers JL. The pregnancy rate of the no-treatment group in randomized clinical trials of endometriosis therapy. *Fertil Steril* 1989; **52**: 906–7.

307. Marcoux S, Maheux R, Bçrubç S et al. Laparoscopic surgery in infertile, women with minimal or mild endometriosis. *New Engl J Med* 1997; **337**: 217–22.

308. Surrey ES, Silverberg KM, Surrey MW, Schoolcraft WB. Effect of prolonged gonadotropin-releasing hormone agonist therapy on the outcome of in vitro fertilization-embryo transfer in patients with endometriosis. *Fertil Steril* 2002; **78**: 699–704.

309. Lessey BA. Implantation defects in infertile women with endometriosis. *Ann N Y Acad Sci* 2002; **955**: 265–80; discussion 293–5, 396–406.

310. Macklon NS, Fauser BC. Impact of ovarian hyperstimulation on the luteal phase. *J Reprod Fertil Suppl* 2000; **55**: 101–8.

311. Paulson RJ, Sauer MV, Lobo RA. Potential enhancement of endometrial receptivity in cycles using controlled ovarian hyperstimulation with antiprogestins: a hypothesis. *Fertil Steril* 1997; **67**: 321–5.

312. Van Der Gaast MH, Classen-Linke I, Krusche CA *et al.* Impact of ovarian stimulation on mid-luteal endometrial tissue and secretion markers of receptivity. *Reprod Biomed Online* 2008; **17**: 553–63.

313. Tan BK, Vandekerckhove P, Kennedy R, Keay SD. Investigation and current management of recurrent IVF treatment failure in the UK. *BJOG* 2005; **112**: 773–80.

314. Hoozemans DA, Schats R, Lambalk CB, Homburg R, Hompes PG. Human embryo implantation: current knowledge and clinical implications in assisted reproductive technology. *Reprod Biomed Online* 2004; **9**: 692–715.

315. Vaquero E, Lazzarin N, Caserta D *et al.* Diagnostic evaluation of women experiencing repeated in vitro fertilization failure. *Eur J Obstet Gynecol Reprod Biol* 2006; **125**: 79–84.

316. Ledee-Bataille N, Dubanchet S, Coulomb-L'hermine A *et al.* A new role for natural killer cells, interleukin (IL)-12, and IL-18 in repeated implantation failure after in vitro fertilization. *Fertil Steril* 2004; **81**: 59–65.

317. Coulam CB, Roussev RG. Increasing circulating T-cell activation markers are linked to subsequent implantation failure after transfer of in vitro fertilized embryos. *Am J Reprod Immunol* 2003; **50**: 340–5.

318. Ledee-Bataille N, Bonnet-Chea K, Hosny G *et al.* Role of the endometrial tripod interleukin-18, -15, and -12 in inadequate uterine receptivity in patients with a history of repeated in vitro fertilization-embryo transfer failure. *Fertil Steril* 2005; **83**: 598–605.

319. Inagaki N, Stern C, McBain J *et al.* Analysis of intra-uterine cytokine concentration and matrix-metalloproteinase activity in women with recurrent failed embryo transfer. *Hum Reprod* 2003; **18**: 608–15.

320. Tei C, Maruyama T, Kuji N *et al.* Reduced expression of alphavbeta3 integrin in the endometrium of unexplained infertility patients with recurrent IVF-ET failures: improvement by danazol treatment. *J Assist Reprod Genet* 2003; **20**: 13–20.

321. Revel A. Implementation of integrin β3 as a predictor of implantation in an IVF program. *ASRM//CFAS Annual Meeting*. Montreal, 2005.

322. Nikas G, Develioglu OH, Toner JP, Jones HW Jr. Endometrial pinopodes indicate a shift in the window of receptivity in IVF cycles. *Hum Reprod* 1999; **14**: 787–92.

323. Pantos K, Nikas G, Makrakis E *et al.* Clinical value of endometrial pinopodes detection in artificial donation cycles. *Reprod Biomed Online* 2004; **9**: 86–90.

324. Gleicher N. The role of humoral immunity in endometriosis. *Acta Obstet Gynecol Scand Suppl* 1994; **159**: 15–17.

325. Gleicher N. Immune dysfunction – a potential target for treatment in endometriosis. *Br J Obstet Gynaecol* 1995; (Suppl. 12): 4–7.

326. Bukulmez O, Hardy DB, Carr BR, Word RA, Mendelson CR. (2008) Inflammatory status influences aromatase and steroid receptor expression in endometriosis. *Endocrinology* 2008; **149**: 1190–204.

327. Klentzeris LD, Bulmer JN, Liu DT, Morrison L. Endometrial leukocyte subpopulations in women with endometriosis. *Eur J Obstet Gynecol Reprod Biol* 1995; **63**: 41–7.

328. Daftary G, Troy P, Bagot C, Pando S, Taylor HS. b3 integrin is directly regulated by HOXA10. *J Soc Gynecol Invest* 2000; **7**(Suppl.): 55A.

329. Daftary GS, Kayisli U, Seli E, Bukulmez O, Arici A, Taylor HS. Salpingectomy increases peri-implantation endometrial HOXA10 expression in women with hydrosalpinx. *Fertil Steril* 2007; **87**: 367–72.

330. Brosens J, Verhoeven H, Campo R *et al.* High endometrial aromatase P450 mRNA expression is associated with poor IVF outcome. *Hum Reprod* 2004; **19**: 352–6.

331. Tabizadeh S, Lessey B, Satyaswaroop PG. Temporal and site-specific expression of transforming growth factor-beta4 in human endometrium. *Mol Hum Reprod* 1998; **4**: 595–602.

332. Tabizadeh S, Shea W, Lessey BA, Broome J. From endometrial receptivity to infertility. *Semin Reprod Endocrinol* 1999; **17**: 197–203.

333. Tei CS, Miyazaki T, Kuji N *et al.* Effect of danazol on the pregnancy rate in patients with unsuccessful in vitro fertilization-embryo transfer. *J Reprod Med* 1998; **43**: 541.

334. Lessey BA. Medical management of endometriosis and infertility. *Fertil Steril* 2000; **73**: 1089–96.

335. Gilchrist DM, Livingston JE, Hurlburt JA, Wilson RD. Recurrent spontaneous pregnancy loss. Investigation and reproductive follow-up. *J Reprod Med* 1991; **36**: 184–8.

336. Stephenson M, Kutteh W. Evaluation and management of recurrent early pregnancy loss. *Clin Obstet Gynecol* 2007; **50**: 132–45.

337. Stephenson MD, Awartani KA, Robinson WP. Cytogenetic analysis of miscarriages from couples with recurrent miscarriage: a case-control study. *Hum Reprod* 2002; **17**: 446–51.

338. Li TC, Tuckerman EM, Laird SM. Endometrial factors in recurrent miscarriage. *Hum Reprod Update* 2002; **8**: 43–52.

339. Tomassetti C, Meuleman C, Pexsters A *et al.* Endometriosis, recurrent miscarriage and implantation failure: is there an immunological link? *Reprod Biomed Online* 2006; **13**: 58–64.

340. Vercammen EE, D'hooghe TM. Endometriosis and recurrent pregnancy loss. *Semin Reprod Med* 2000; **18**: 363–8.

341. Daya S. Endometriosis and spontaneous abortion. In *Infertility and Reproductive Medicine Clinics of North America*. Philadelphia: W. B. Saunders, 1996.

342. Strathy JH, Molgaard CA, Coulam CB, Melton LJ. Endometriosis and infertility: A laparoscopic study of endometriosis among fertile and infertile women. *Fertil Steril* 1982; **38**: 667–72.

343. Singh KB, Patel YC, Wortsman J. Coexistence of polycystic ovary sydrome and pelvic endometriosis. *Obstet Gynecol* 74, 650–2.

344. Brincat M, Galea R, Buhagiar A. Polycystic ovaries and endometriosis: a possible connection. *Br J Obstet Gynaecol* 1994; **101**: 346–8.

# Chapter 19

# Implantation events

Isaac E. Sasson and Errol R. Norwitz

## Introduction

Implantation is a critical step in the establishment of a successful pregnancy supported by a healthy placenta, and requires meticulous synchronization between the developing embryo and the cycling endometrium. Numerous endocrine, paracrine and autocrine signals mediate the complex, bidirectional communication between the endometrium and the blastocyst. Very few specimens exist that document the first weeks of embryonic development in humans. In some cases, information about a particular stage of development comes from a single specimen. Other crucial events, such as initial adhesion of the blastocyst to the uterine epithelium, have never been observed in vivo. Therefore, much of our understanding of early human development is inferred from animal studies. Given that the cellular interactions culminating in implantation and placentation vary greatly, even among primates, the relevance of this information is unclear [1]. This chapter aims to describe the biological processes and some of the molecular mediators required during early implantation events and to illustrate the clinical consequences when these processes are perturbed.

## Biological processes required for early implantation events

The interaction between an activated blastocyst and a receptive uterus is part of a continuum that leads to implantation and the early stages of placental development. Many of the regulatory mechanisms identified govern important transitions along this continuum. As such, considering their functions in the context of any single event draws an arbitrary distinction that does not exist in vivo. Nonetheless, analogous to events in several primate species, implantation in humans probably includes three stages: (i) *apposition*

of a competent blastocyst and a receptive endometrium, (ii) *adhesion* of the embryo to the epithelium and (iii) penetration of the embryo through epithelium and basal lamina with *invasion* of the uterine vasculature [2]. Establishment of a receptive endometrium and a competent blastocyst are addressed in detail elsewhere in this text.

## Pre-implantation blastocyst

Fertilization occurs in the fallopian tube within 24 to 48 hours of ovulation. The initial stages of development, from fertilized ovum (zygote) to a mass of 12 to 16 cells (morula), occur as the embryo passes through the fallopian tube encased within a non-adhesive protective coating known as the zona pellucida. The morula enters the uterine cavity approximately 2–3 days after fertilization and 4 days after ovulation (Figure 19.1). Five days after ovulation, the appearance of a fluid-filled inner cavity within the mass of cells marks the transition from morula to blastocyst, and is accompanied by cellular differentiation: the surface cells become the trophectoderm, which gives rise to extra-embryonic structures including the placenta, and the inner cell mass, which gives rise to the fetus. Within 72 hours of entering the uterine cavity (6 days post-fertilization), the embryo containing 100–200 cells hatches from the zona pellucida, exposing its outer covering of syncytial trophoblasts to the adjacent luminal epithelium of the endometrium.

It is during this period of time that numerous processes occur to generate a competent blastocyst capable of implanting in a receptive endometrium. Maternally derived RNA transcripts that drive protein synthesis within the early embryo are degraded with the concomitant transcription of the embryonic genome in a process termed *zygotic genome activation*. Extensive epigenetic modifications reprogram the

*Early Pregnancy*, ed. Roy G. Farquharson and Mary D. Stephenson. Published by Cambridge University Press.
© Cambridge University Press 2010.

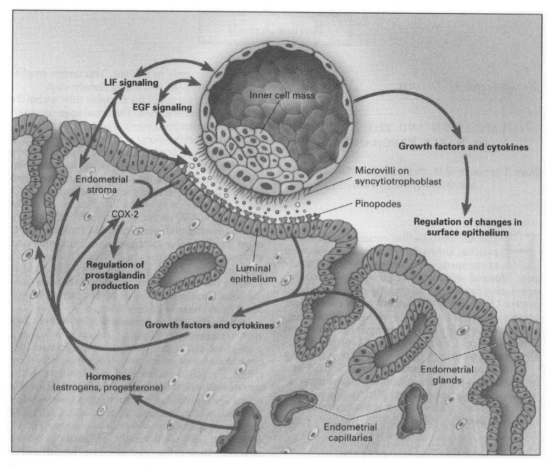

**Figure 19.1** Apposition and stable adhesion. Six days post-fertilization, the embryo containing hatches from the zona pellucida exposing its outer covering of syncytial trophoblasts to the adjacent luminal epithelium of the endometrium. Microvilli on the apical surface of syncytiotrophoblasts interdigitate with pinopodes on the apical surface of the uterine epithelium. Stable adhesion produces a functional relationship between the cell membranes of the endometrium and trophoblast. COX-2, cyclooxygenase-2; EGF, epidermal growth factor; LIF, leukemia inhibitory factor.

embryonic genome to restrict the totipotency of the zygote while maintaining the pleuripotency of the inner cell mass. Other epigenetic modifications are required for erasure and reestablishment of the imprinting pattern on the paternal chromosomes and for X-chromosome inactivation. At the same time, signals from within the dividing embryo trigger cell fate specification cues to differentiate the putative germline from cells that will become the somatic tissues.

## Apposition and adhesion

Implantation occurs at approximately 6–7 days after fertilization. Initial adhesion of the blastocyst to the uterine wall, termed *apposition*, is unstable. Microvilli on the apical surface of syncytiotrophoblasts interdigitate

with microprotrusions from the apical surface of the uterine epithelium, known as pinopodes (Figure 19.1). The formation of pinopodes is associated with increased endometrial receptivity [3]. While their function remains unclear, their postulated functions are transport of macromolecules, absorption of fluid from the uterine cavity, and facilitating adhesion of the blastocyst to the uterine epithelium.

*Stable adhesion* is characterized by increased physical interaction between the blastocyst and the luminal uterine epithelium. This process is transient and not easily explored, but likely represents a period when the cell membranes of the uterine epithelium and trophoblasts develop a functional relationship. There are likely several post-translational mechanisms that mediate this process including redistribution of cell surface molecules, activation of signaling cascades and remodeling of cytoskeleton within the uterine epithelium. Transmission electron microscopy has demonstrated an interaction between the trophoblasts and, specifically, the lateral aspects of the endometrial cells. Here, disruption of the junctional complexes between endometrial cells and invasion of trophectodermal processes project into these spaces [4,5].

## Invasion

With *invasion*, the syncytiotrophoblasts penetrate through the uterine epithelium and, by 10 days after fertilization, the blastocyst is completely embedded in stromal tissue of the uterus. The uterine epithelium re-grows over the implantation site [Figure 19.2]. Eventually, cytotrophoblasts invade the entire endometrium and the inner third of the myometrium, known as *interstitial invasion*, and penetrate the uterine vasculature, known as *endovascular invasion*. This process establishes the uteroplacental circulation and marks the transition from *histiotrophic* support of the embryo, where the embryo obtains metabolic support from maternal extracellular fluid coming primarily from the endometrial glands, to a *hematrophic* system,

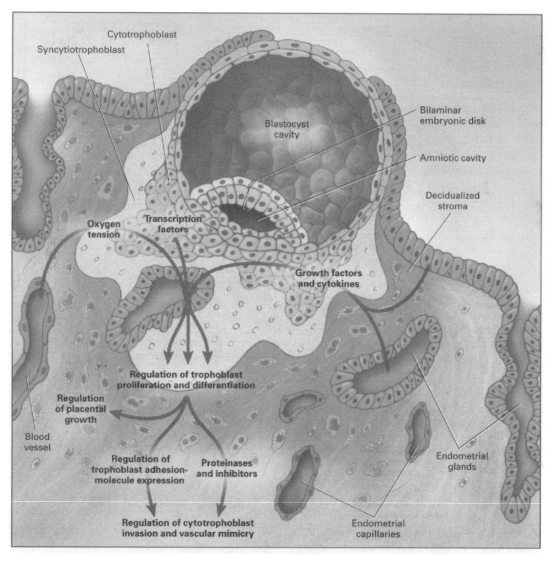

**Figure 19.2** Invasion. Ten days after fertilization, the syncytiotrophoblasts penetrate through the uterine epithelium and the blastocyst is completely embedded in stromal tissue of the uterus.

where the maternal and fetal circulation lie in close proximity to rapidly exchange nutrients and waste.

During endovascular invasion, invasive cytotrophoblast cells breach the termini of spiral arterioles. As these fetal cells move in a retrograde direction, they entirely replace the resident maternal endothelium and a portion of the muscular tunica media. This mechanism appears to be driven by oxygen tension, since the invasive cytotrophoblast cells target spiral arterioles and not veins [6]. The result is uterine arterioles that are hybrid structures composed of fetal and maternal cells. With regards to physiology, cytotrophoblast invasion transforms the maternal arterioles from small-bore, high-resistance vessels to large-bore, low-resistance vessels capable of meeting the fetal demands for maternal blood flow.

# Molecular mediators of implantation

The molecular mechanisms that regulate early implantation events in humans are not well understood. The temporal and spatial expression of several growth factors, cytokines and adhesion molecules within the uterus and pre-implantation blastocyst suggests that they may play important roles [Figure 19.3] [7]. Additionally, targeted disruption of genes in mouse studies have provided some data on the function of these genes in mediating early implantation events [8]. However, the extent to which human embryos utilize the same signaling components needs to be determined, and caution should be used in extending observations made in model systems to normal human physiology. Finally, gene expression analysis of signaling molecules in patients with specific reproductive phenotypes (so-called genotype–phenotype studies) also provide some associative information between particular proteins and their role in maintaining fertility [Tables 19.1 and 19.2]

## Steroid hormones

Estrogen and progesterone act primarily through their nuclear receptors, the estrogen receptor (ER) and progesterone receptor (PR), respectively [9]. Ligand binding to the receptor results in dimerization and subsequent binding to response elements on DNA that result in activation or repression of downstream target genes. Several isoforms of each receptor exist, and the best characterized isoforms include the estrogen receptors, ER-α and ER-β, and the progesterone

**Table 19.1** Uterine (maternal) factors associated with implantation.

| Cytokines/Growth factors | Facilitate cross-talk between the blastocyst and uterus |
|---|---|
| Interleukin-1<br>Interleukin-2<br>Interleukin-11 and IL-11 receptor<br>Leukemia inhibitory factor and LIF receptor<br>Insulin growth factor-1 and -2<br>Insulin growth factor binding proteins<br>Colony stimulating factor-1<br>Transforming growth factor-α and -β<br>Hepatocyte growth factor<br>Fibroblast growth factor<br>Heparin binding – Epidermal growth factor<br>Hypoxia inhibitory factor-1<br>Vascular endothelial growth factor<br>Indian hedgehog | |
| Steroid hormones | Preparation of a receptive endometrium and competent blastocyst |
| Estradiol-17β<br>Progesterone<br>Catecholestrogens | |
| Immunological factors | Immunosuppression |
| Interleukin-10<br>Indoleamine 2,3-dioxygenase<br>Crry (complement regulator) | |
| Changes in luminal epithelium | Facilitate blastocyst recognition and attachment |
| Pinopodes<br>MUC-1<br>Glycodelin<br>Integrin-αvβ3<br>Calcitonin | |
| Transcription factors | Effect changes in gene expression as a result of upstream signaling pathways |
| Estrogen receptor<br>Progesterone receptor<br>MASH-2<br>HAND-1<br>Ids<br>PPARδ | |
| Other factors | |
| HoxA-10 and -11 | Homeobox genes expressed in endometrial stromal cells during implantation |
| COX-2 | Regulates prostaglandin production |
| Oxygen tension | Facilitates trophoblast vascular mimicry |

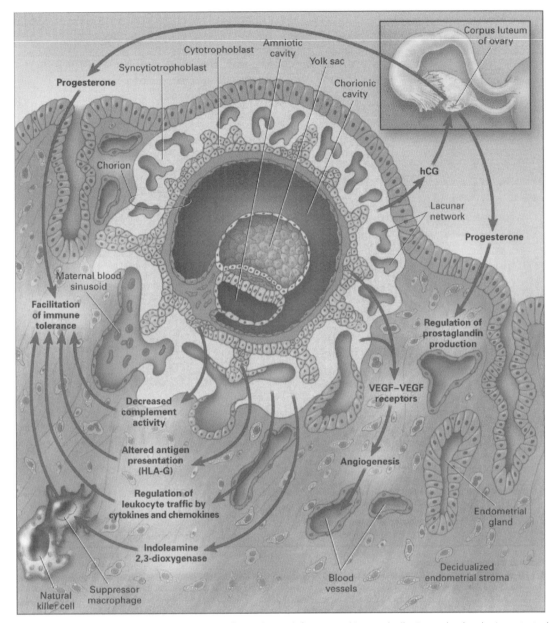

**Figure 19.3** The temporal and spatial expression of several growth factors, cytokines, and adhesion molecules play important roles in mediating blastocyst invasion and the survival of the early pregnancy. VEGF, vascular endothelial growth factor; hCG, human chorionic gonadotropin.

receptors, PR-A and PR-B [10]. The specific biological response of a cell to hormonal stimulation is dependent on the relative abundance of the receptor subtypes and the co-activators/co-repressors expressed within the cell.

Steroid hormones are required to coordinate the development of the conceptus with the receptivity of the endometrium, and the regulation of the hypothalamic–pituitary–ovarian axis in the event of an implantation failure. Progesterone expression is essential for implantation and maintenance of early pregnancy in all mammals. By contrast, estrogen requirement during implantation is species dependent [7]. Nonetheless, both estrogen and progesterone are required for endometrial receptivity. Interestingly, however, ER and PR are absent from the endometrial

**Table 19.2** Blastocyst factors associated with implantation.

| Cytokines/Growth factors | Facilitate cross-talk between the blastocyst and uterus |
|---|---|
| Interleukin-1<br>Interleukin-6<br>Leukemia inhibitory factor and LIF receptor<br>Insulin growth factor-2<br>Colony stimulating factor-1<br>Transforming growth factor-α and -β | |
| Proteinases/Inhibitors | |
| MMP-9/TIMP-3 | Regulates trophoblast invasion |
| uPA/ PAI-4 | Facilitates trophoblast vascular mimicry |
| Cathepsin B and L | Regulates trophoblast invasion |
| Immunological factors | |
| HLA-G | Prevents immune rejection of the fetal hemi-allograft |
| Adhesion molecule expression | Promotes trophoblast differentiation and invasion |
| Integrin-α6β4, E-cadherin<br>Integrin-α1β1 and αvβ3, VE-cadherin | |

glandular epithelium at the mid-late luteal phase during the implantation window, suggesting that these genes are not directly required for implantation but rather required to generate the molecular profile essential for embryo attachment and implantation [11].

Targeted gene disruption of the estrogen receptor indicates that ER-α is the primary mediator of estrogen signaling in the uterus [12]. ER-α knockout mice are infertile as a result of pleiotropic effects on the female reproductive tract [13]. These mice display small, hypoplastic uteri that are unable to support implantation. By contrast, ER-β knock-out mice remain fertile despite a decrease in ovarian function [14].

Knock-out studies in the mouse demonstrate that the PR isoforms have discrete, non-overlapping functions in the female reproductive system. PR knock-out (PRKO) mice demonstrate behavioral defects, failure to ovulate, defective uterine implantation, lack of decidualization, and defects in mammary gland morphogenesis and development [15]. PR-A knockout results in diminished ovarian function and a failure of decidualization leading to female infertility. These data suggest that PR-A is the major mediator of progesterone signaling in the female reproductive tract.

Furthermore, these animals demonstrate increased uterine epithelial proliferation suggesting that PR-A inhibits the mitogenic effects of PR-B. Conversely, animals with a selective elimination of PR-B do not demonstrate a uterine phenotype, but rather display abnormal mammary gland development [16].

## Integrins

Integrins are a large family of cell adhesion molecules. These transmembrane proteins are formed by heterodimerization of α and β subunits, and function as receptors for the extracellular matrix components laminin, fibronectin, perlecan, thrombospondin and osteopontin. Multiple combinations of integrin heterodimers are expressed on both the endometrium and the embryo. Several studies suggest that integrin signaling is functionally important during apposition, attachment and invasion of the embryo [7].

The cohort of integrins expressed in the uterus has been well described, and they appear to be critical markers for determining endometrial receptivity [17,18]. Alpha-4 and β3 integrins exhibit cycle-dependent changes in expression with an increase in β3 and a decrease in α4 levels during the implantation window. The apical localization of αvβ3 and αvβ5 integrins in the luminal epithelium is critical for mediating the interaction between endometrium and the trophoblast [19]. In humans, integrin expression is altered in patients with impaired fertility. Patients with endometriosis, hydrosalpinges and unexplained infertility demonstrate decreased β3 expression in the endometrium [20–22].

To complement the expression pattern of integrins in the endometrium, the pre-implantation blastocyst expresses several integrin heterodimers, including αvβ3 and α5β1. α5β1 is expressed on trophoblast cells and is translocated to their apical surface upon blastocyst activation, suggesting a role for initial attachment after hatching from the zona pellucida [23]. Mice treated with competitive inhibitors of αv demonstrate decreased implantation rates [24]. β3 null mutant mice demonstrate abnormal placentation, although they fail to demonstrate a fertility defect, likely due to functional redundancy within this gene family [25]. Analysis of the effects of adding function-perturbing antibodies to an in vitro model of cytotrophoblast invasion reveals a delicate balance between members of this gene family. For example, integrins αvβ3 and α1β1 promote invasion, whereas α5β1 restrains it [26].

Invading cytotrophoblasts modulate their adhesion molecule expression in a stepwise fashion to a profile similar to that of endothelial cells. This enables invading cytotrophoblasts to assume characteristics similar to those of maternal vascular cells. Particularly striking is the decrease in adhesion receptors characteristic of polarized cytotrophoblast stem cells (integrin α6β4 and epithelial cadherin) and increased expression of adhesion receptors characteristic of endothelium, including cadherins (vascular endothelial cadherin and cadherin-11), IgG-family receptors (vascular cell adhesion molecule-1, platelet-endothelial cell adhesion molecule-1 and Mel-CAM), and integrins αvβ3 and α1β1 [27].

## Growth factors

Many growth factors are expressed in the luminal epithelium during the window of differentiation and are often increased at the site of embryo apposition. These include several members of the epidermal growth factor (EGF) family, vascular endothelial growth factors (VEGF), transforming growth factor-beta (TGF-β), insulin-like growth factors (IGF), fibroblast growth factors (FGF) and platelet-derived growth factors (PDGF) [7].

### Epidermal growth factors

Epidermal growth factors are a family of extracellular signaling molecules that are characterized by a 40–60 amino acid structural domain. This family of growth factors includes EGF, TGF-α, HB-EGF, amphiregulin (Ar), epiregulin (Er), β-cellulin and neuregulins. EGFs signal through a family of receptor tyrosine kinases known as the ErbB family. This family is comprised of 4 members: EGFR/ErbB-1, HER2/ErbB-2, HER3/ErbB-3 and HER4/ErbB4. These receptors are composed of an extracellular ligand binding domain and a catalytically active cytoplasmic kinase. Ligand binding induces activation of the receptor and subsequent phosphorylation of downstream signaling components [28].

The expression patterns of EGF ligands and receptors within the endometrium suggest a local paracrine/autocrine signaling pathway necessary for embryo attachment. In the mouse, expression of the EGF ligands, HB-EGF and Ar, are regulated by estrogen and progesterone. Ar is expressed throughout the uterus during the implantation window, but its expression level is restricted to and increased specifically at the sites of blastocyst apposition [29]. HB-EGF is expressed in the luminal endometrium exclusively at sites adjacent to active blastocysts prior to attachment of the embryo [30]. Subsequently, the other EGF ligands (β-cellulin, neuregulin-1 and Er) are expressed in the luminal epithelium and stroma at the site of blastocyst attachment [7]. In a complementary fashion, blastocysts express the EGF receptors ErbB-1, ErbB-2 and ErbB-4 [31,32].

Similarly, in humans, HB-EGF is expressed in luminal endometrial cells and expression levels peak during the implantation window and ErbB4 is expressed in the trophectoderm of the peri-implantation blastocyst [33,34]. HB-EGF stimulates growth and development of blastocysts in vitro and may induce endometrial expression of integrin αvβ3 required for blastocyst attachment [35,36]. However, little is known about the function of EGFs in regulating implantation events. Beads saturated with HB-EGF are capable of inducing decidualization when implanted into the uterus of pseudo-pregnant mice [37]. By contrast, mice lacking EGF, Ar, or TGF-α, as well as compound null mutant for all three genes do not exhibit fertility defects, possibly due to the overlapping expression pattern of other EGF ligands [38].

### Insulin-like growth factors

Insulin-like growth factors signal through the insulin receptor to regulate cell growth, differentiation, and metabolism in multiple tissues. Ligand availability is modulated by IGF binding proteins (IGFBPs). The expression pattern of IGFBP-1 and IGF-II suggest autocrine/paracrine signaling between the decidua and trophoblast that is critical to regulating blastocyst invasion. IGFBP-1 is expressed in the secretory and decidualized endometrium, while IGF-I and IGF-II are highly expressed by invading cytotrophoblast [39]. In vitro experiments indicate that IGFBP-1 can alter the invasiveness of cytotrophoblast cells [40]. IGFBP-1 likely serves multiple functions, since it binds the integrin, αvβ1, which plays a role in embryo attachment [41].

### Vascular endothelial growth factors

Vascular endothelial growth factor was first described for its ability to induce endothelial cell proliferation and increase vascular permeability. Its functions have been well described and include angiogenesis, vascularization and vasodilatation. In humans, five isoforms of VEGF-A are generated from alternative splicing of a single gene. VEGF-A signals through two receptor tyrosine kinases: VEGFR-1/flt-1 and VEGFR-2/flk-1 (also known as KDR in the mouse).

Expression of VEGF-A in the reproductive tract has been well characterized in the human. Vascular endothelial growth factor is expressed throughout the menstrual cycle with peak levels in the glandular epithelium during the secretory phase. Expression of several VEGF isoforms is induced by estrogen treatment [42]. In the mouse, blastocyst attachment results in an increase in VEGF expression in the luminal epithelium and adjacent stroma at the implantation site [43].

## Leukemia-inhibitory factor

Leukemia-inhibitory factor (LIF) is a member of the IL-6 cytokine subfamily. This 180 amino acid protein is transcribed from a single gene, and highly conserved between species. It signals through the LIF receptor (LIF-R) and, upon binding, heterodimerizes with glycoprotein 130 (GP130) to activate an intracellular signaling cascade. Expression pattern analysis and targeted disruption of the LIF signaling pathway demonstrate that LIF has multiple functions in the female reproductive tract, and is important for both decidualization and implantation [44].

Leukemia-inhibitory factor expression displays a biphasic pattern and varies with the menstrual cycle [44]. In the proliferative phase, LIF expression is not detected. Leukemia-inhibitory factor mRNA and protein can be detected throughout the secretory phase in the glandular and luminal epithelium. Its expression peaks in the late secretory phase between cycle days 19 and 25, correlating with the ideal implantation window. By contrast, both LIF-R and GP130 are expressed in the proliferative and secretory phases on the luminal and glandular epithelium of the endometrium [44]. The responsiveness of LIF-R to the presence of LIF is dependent on estrogen and progesterone activity. Progesterone, HB-EGF and TGF-ß may all regulate LIF secretion [45].

Targeted disruption of the LIF gene indicates that maternal LIF expression is required for successful implantation. LIF null females ovulate and their oocytes are fertilized, but embryos are unable to implant due to a defect in decidualization [46]. GP130 hypomorphic alleles demonstrate a similar defect to LIF null mice [47]. By contrast, LIF-R null embryos are able to implant, suggesting that LIF may signal through an alternative pathway. Nonetheless, LIF-R null mice demonstrate defective placentation and display an early perinatal lethality consistent with its pleiotrophic effects [48]. Leukemia-inhibitory factor also appears to be necessary and sufficient to mediate the effects of estrogen on the endometrium during the period of implantation, suggesting that LIF is a target of estrogen in the endometrium [49].

Several clinical observations further suggest a critical role for LIF in human reproduction. Women with unexplained infertility or recurrent pregnancy loss have decreased levels of LIF expression in uterine lavage specimens [50]. Conditioned media collected from cultured endometrial explants derived from women with unexplained infertility have decreased levels of LIF as compared with fertile controls [51]. Women treated with antiprogestins display decreased LIF expression in the endometrium [52].

## Matrix metalloproteinases

Invading cytotrophoblasts extensively regulate their expression of matrix metalloproteinases (MMPs) and tissue inhibitors of metalloproteinases (TIMPs) [53]. Of particular functional importance is their ability to express and activate matrix metalloproteinase-9 (MMP-9), a major regulator of cytotrophoblast invasion in vitro [54]. The simultaneous upregulation of tissue inhibitor of metalloproteinase-3 (TIMP-3) expression provides a regulatory mechanism to restrict cytotrophoblast invasion [55]. An additional level of complexity in this pathway is illustrated by the complex expression pattern of MMPs and TIMPs in maternal decidual cells adjacent to the invading blastocyst [56].

## *Hox* genes

*Hox* genes are a highly conserved family of transcription factors characterized by a 183 base pair segment of DNA known as the *homeobox* that encodes a 61 amino acid segment, the *homeodomain*. These transcription factors are responsible for patterning the anterior-posterior axis during early embryonic development [57]. In the development of the female reproductive tract, *Hoxa-9* is expressed in the developing fallopian tube, *Hoxa-10* in the uterus, *Hoxa-11* in the lower uterine segment, and *Hoxa-13* in the primordial vagina [58].

Multiple gene targeting experiments in mice demonstrate important roles for *Hoxa-10* and *Hoxa-11* in implantation. *Hoxa-10* and *Hoxa-11* null mice demonstrate implantation failure likely secondary to the pleiotropic effects of these patterning genes during embryonic development [59–61]. To circumvent these confounding factors, modulation of *Hoxa-10* expression in the adult endometrium in the mouse has been shown to affect the number of implantation sites in otherwise wild-type animals [62]. When endogenous levels of *Hoxa-10* are reduced, the number of implantation sites and the litter size is reduced, while increased expression of *Hoxa-10* in the endometrium results in an increased number of implantation sites and larger litter sizes [62]. The effect of *Hoxa-10* on implantation is likely related to the effect of maternal *Hoxa-10* expression on pinopod formation. Decreased *Hoxa-10* expression results in a decreased pinopod formation, while overexpression of *Hoxa-10* results in increased pinopod formation [62]. By contrast, embryos derived from *Hoxa-10* or *Hoxa-11* null mutant mice are able to implant in wild-type surrogates [59–61].

Several clinical studies suggest that *Hoxa-10* and *Hoxa-11* play a critical role in human implantation. While the expression of most *Hox* genes in the female reproductive tract is limited to embryonic development, *Hoxa-10* and *Hoxa-11* are expressed also in adult endometrial glands and stroma [63]. Their regulated expression levels peak at the mid-secretory phase during the implantation window and remain elevated thereafter [64,65]. *Hoxa-10* and *Hoxa-11* are regulated by estrogen and progesterone through their cognate receptors by direct binding of the receptors to regulatory elements in the respective gene promoters [66]. Furthermore, a number of different clinical conditions associated with infertility appear to demonstrate alterations in *Hoxa-10* and *Hoxa-11* expression. For example, women with endometriosis fail to demonstrate a mid-luteal phase increase in *Hoxa-10* or *Hoxa-11* expression. Similarly, *Hoxa-10* levels are decreased in patients with polycystic ovarian syndrome, leiomyomas, and in the presence of hydrosalpinges [67–69]. Taken together, these data suggest that maternal *Hoxa-10* expression contributes to endometrial receptivity and is required for successful implantation.

## Prostaglandins

Implantation requires prostaglandin biosynthesis. Cyclooxygenase, the rate-limiting enzyme in conversion of arachidonic acid to prostaglandin $H_2$, exists in two isoforms: constitutive (COX-1) and inducible (COX-2). In the endometrium, COX-1 production decreases in response to progesterone and estradiol-17β, and the endometrial content of COX-1 falls

precipitously in the mid-luteal phase of the menstrual cycle in anticipation of implantation [70]. By contrast, COX-2 production, which is not affected by steroid hormones, is restricted to the implantation site and depends on the presence of a competent blastocyst [70,71]. Moreover, interleukin-1 (IL-1) detected in the conditioned medium of human embryos, induces COX-2 gene expression in cultured endometrial stromal cells [72]. Prostaglandin $I_2$ (prostacyclin), produced by the action of COX-2 on arachidonic precursor, is a ligand for the nuclear receptor, peroxisome proliferator-activated receptor-δ (PPARδ) [71]. This interaction is likely critical because mice lacking a related receptor (PPARγ) die at mid-gestation due to defective placentation [73].

## Immunological factors

One of the most interesting functions of the placenta is regulation of the maternal immune response such that the fetal hemi-allograft is tolerated during pregnancy. Trophoblasts are presumed to be essential to this allograft tolerance because they lie at the maternal–fetal interface where there is direct contact with cells of the maternal immune system. Several studies suggest that trophoblasts do not express classical major histocompatibility complex (MHC) class II molecules, but that cytotrophoblasts upregulate a non-classical MHC class Ib molecule, HLA-G, as they invade the uterus [74]. This observation, and the fact that HLA-G exhibits limited polymorphism, suggests functional importance. The exact mechanisms involved are not known, but may include upregulation of the inhibitory immunoglobulin-like transcript 4, a HLA-G receptor that is expressed on macrophages and a subset of natural killer lymphocytes [75].

Cytotrophoblasts that express HLA-G come in direct contact with maternal lymphocytes that are abundant in the uterus during early pregnancy. Although estimates vary, a minimum of 10–15% of all cells found in the decidua are lymphocytes [76]. These maternal lymphocytes have unusual properties in that most are CD56+ natural killer (NK) cells. However, compared with peripheral blood lymphocytes, decidual NK cells have low cytotoxic activity, and interestingly, are directly recruited by invading cytotrophoblasts via chemokine secretion [77,78].

Cytotoxicity against hemi-allogeneic trophoblasts must be selectively inhibited. The factors responsible for this localized immunosuppression are unclear, but likely include cytotrophoblast-derived interleukin-10, a cytokine that inhibits allo-responses in mixed lymphocyte reactions [79]. Steroid hormones, including progesterone, have similar effects. The complement system may also be involved, since deletion of the complement regulator, Crry, in mice leads to fetal loss secondary to placental inflammation [80]. Finally, pharmacological data from studies performed in mice, suggest that trophoblasts express an enzyme, indoleamine 2,3-dioxygenase, that rapidly degrades tryptophan, which is essential for T-cell activation [81]. Whether this mechanism occurs in humans is not known, although human syncytiotrophoblasts express indoleamine 2,3-dioxygenase and maternal serum tryptophan concentrations fall during pregnancy [82,83].

## Clinical implications

Reproductive pathologies resulting from implantation defects span a spectrum of clinical presentations ranging from infertility to recurrent pregnancy loss to pre-eclampsia. Infertility may result from failure of fertilization or from loss of the fertilized blastocyst prior to implantation. Both occur in the setting of a negative pregnancy test. Sporadic pregnancy loss occurs in 15–20% of women. Recurrent pregnancy loss, defined as spontaneous loss of three or more confirmed early intrauterine pregnancies, affects 0.3–1% of reproductive age women. These pathologies are examined elsewhere in this book.

The intriguing possibility exists that most complications that arise late in gestation (such as pre-eclampsia, pre-term labor and pre-term premature rupture of membranes) actually reflect aberrant biological processes that occurred much earlier in pregnancy, specifically during placental development [84]. Biopsy of the placenta and uterus at the time of delivery has allowed microscopic assessment of the maternal–fetal interface in a variety of pregnancy complications.

*Excessive invasion* of the cytotrophoblast with deficient development of the decidua may lead to abnormally firm attachment of the placenta directly onto the myometrium (placenta accreta), to extension into the myometrium (placenta increta) or to invasion through the myometrium into the uterine serosa and even into adjacent organs (placenta percreta). Despite improvements in diagnosis and clinical management, such disorders of placentation are still associated with significant intrapartum maternal morbidity and mortality, due primarily to excessive hemorrhage.

By contrast, *inadequate invasion* has been implicated in the pathophysiology of intrauterine growth restriction (IUGR) and pre-eclampsia. The placenta of the IUGR fetus demonstrates compromised syncytiotrophoblast function with fewer capillary loops and branches in the villus cores and with fibrin deposition on the syncytial surface. The mesenchymal cores of these villi also display increased density and areas of the syncytium thin dramatically, all of which likely contribute to the impaired fetal growth [85].

Pre-eclampsia, a clinical syndrome characterized by hypertension and proteinuria that develops after 20 weeks' gestation, is the leading cause of maternal mortality in the industrialized world and increases perinatal mortality five-fold. Although the etiology of pre-eclampsia is unknown, the condition appears to result from aberrant biological processes that occur shortly after implantation, weeks or months prior to the clinical manifestation of the disease. The characteristic pathological lesion found in the placentas of pre-eclamptic patients is shallow interstitial cytotrophoblast invasion and, more consistently, restricted endovascular invasion [86]. In pre-eclampsia, cytotrophoblasts that invade uterine vessels fail to switch their adhesion molecule repertoire to resemble that of vascular cells [87]. The uterine arterioles, rather than becoming large-bore, low-resistance vessels, therefore remain as small-bore, high-resistance vessels that cannot adequately respond to the ever-increasing fetal demands for blood flow. The maternal physiology responds with an elevation in blood pressure to maintain adequate placental perfusion, and consequently, the patient displays the clinical symptoms of pre-eclampsia.

## References

1. Lee KY, DeMayo FJ, Lee KY, DeMayo FJ. Animal models of implantation. *Reproduction* 2004; **128**(6): 679–95.

2. Norwitz ER, Schust DJ, Fisher SJ. Implantation and the survival of early pregnancy. *New Engl J Med* 2001; **345** (19): 1400–8.

3. Psychoyos A, Nikas G, Gravanis A. The role of prostaglandins in blastocyst implantation. *Hum Reprod* 1995; **10** (Suppl. 2): 30–42.

4. Bentin-Ley U. Relevance of endometrial pinopodes for human blastocyst implantation. *Hum Reprod* 2000; **15** (Suppl. 6): 67–73.

5. Lopata A, Bentin-Ley U, Enders A. "Pinopodes" and implantation. *Rev Endocr Metab Disord* 2002; **3**(2): 77–86.

6. Red-Horse K, Zhou Y, Genbacev O *et al.* Trophoblast differentiation during embryo implantation and formation of the maternal-fetal interface. *J Clin Invest* 2004; **114**(6): 744–54.

7. Dey SK, Lim H, Das SK *et al.* Molecular cues to implantation. *Endocr Rev* 2004; **25**(3): 341–73.

8. Lee KY, Jeong JW, Tsai SY *et al.* Mouse models of implantation. *Trends Endocrinol Metab* 2007; **18**(6): 234–9.

9. Carpenter KD, Korach KS. Potential biological functions emerging from the different estrogen receptors. *Ann N Y Acad Sci* 2006; **1092**: 361–73.

10. Kastner P, Krust A, Turcotte B *et al.* Two distinct estrogen-regulated promoters generate transcripts encoding the two functionally different human progesterone receptor forms A and B. *Embo J* 1990; **9**(5): 1603–14.

11. Lessey BA, Killam AP, Metzger DA *et al.* Immunohistochemical analysis of human uterine estrogen and progesterone receptors throughout the menstrual cycle. *J Clin Endocrinol Metab* 1988; **67**(2): 334–40.

12. Hewitt SC, Korach KS. Oestrogen receptor knockout mice: roles for oestrogen receptors alpha and beta in reproductive tissues. *Reproduction* 2003; **125**(2): 143–9.

13. Curtis SW, Clark J, Myers P, Korach KS. Disruption of estrogen signaling does not prevent progesterone action in the estrogen receptor alpha knockout mouse uterus. *Proc Natl Acad Sci USA* 1999; **96**(7): 3646–51.

14. Krege JH, Hodgin JB, Couse JF *et al.* Generation and reproductive phenotypes of mice lacking estrogen receptor beta. *Proc Natl Acad Sci USA* 1998; **95**(26): 15677–82.

15. Lydon JP, DeMayo FJ, Funk CR *et al.* Mice lacking progesterone receptor exhibit pleiotropic reproductive abnormalities. *Genes Dev* 1995; **9**(18): 2266–78.

16. Mulac-Jericevic B, Mullinax RA, DeMayo FJ, Lydon JP, Conneely OM. Subgroup of reproductive functions of progesterone mediated by progesterone receptor-B isoform. *Science* 2000; **289**(5485): 1751–4.

17. Lessey BA, Young SL. Integrins and other cell adhesion molecules in endometrium and endometriosis. *Semin Reprod Endocrinol* 1997; **15**(3): 291–9.

18. Lessey BA. The use of integrins for the assessment of uterine receptivity. *Fertil Steril* 1994; **61**(5): 812–14.

19. Aplin JD, Spanswick C, Behzad F, Kimber SJ, Vicovac L. Integrins beta 5, beta 3 and alpha v are apically distributed in endometrial epithelium. *Mol Hum Reprod* 1996; **2**(7): 527–34.

20. Lessey BA, Castelbaum AJ, Sawin SW *et al.* Aberrant integrin expression in the endometrium of women with endometriosis. *J Clin Endocrinol Metab* 1994; **79**(2): 643–9.

21. Lessey BA, Castelbaum AJ, Sawin SW, Sun J. Integrins as markers of uterine receptivity in women with primary unexplained infertility. *Fertil Steril* 1995; **63**(3): 535–42.

22. Meyer WR, Castelbaum AJ, Somkuti S *et al.* Hydrosalpinges adversely affect markers of endometrial receptivity. *Hum Reprod* 1997; **12**(7): 1393–8.

23. Aplin JD. Adhesion molecules in implantation. *Rev Reprod* 1997; **2**(2): 84–93.

24. Illera MJ, Cullinan E, Gui Y *et al.* Blockade of the alpha (v)beta(3) integrin adversely affects implantation in the mouse. *Biol Reprod* 2000; **62**(5): 1285–90.

25. Hodivala-Dilke KM, McHugh KP, Tsakiris DA *et al.* Beta3-integrin-deficient mice are a model for Glanzmann thrombasthenia showing placental defects and reduced survival. *J Clin Invest* 1999; **103**(2): 229–38.

26. Damsky CH, Librach C, Lim KH *et al.* Integrin switching regulates normal trophoblast invasion. *Development* 1994; **120**(12): 3657–66.

27. Damsky CH, Fisher SJ. Trophoblast pseudo-vasculogenesis: faking it with endothelial adhesion receptors. *Curr Opin Cell Biol* 1998; **10**(5): 660–6.

28. Yarden Y, Sliwkowski MX. Untangling the ErbB signalling network. *Nat Rev Mol Cell Biol* 2001; **2**(2): 127–37.

29. Das SK, Chakraborty I, Paria BC *et al.* Amphiregulin is an implantation-specific and progesterone-regulated gene in the mouse uterus. *Mol Endocrinol* 1995; **9**(6): 691–705.

30. Das SK, Wang XN, Paria BC *et al.* Heparin-binding EGF-like growth factor gene is induced in the mouse uterus temporally by the blastocyst solely at the site of its apposition: a possible ligand for interaction with blastocyst EGF-receptor in implantation. *Development* 1994; **120**(5): 1071–83.

31. Paria BC, Elenius K, Klagsbrun M, Dey SK. Heparin-binding EGF-like growth factor interacts with mouse blastocysts independently of ErbB1: a possible role for heparan sulfate proteoglycans and ErbB4 in blastocyst implantation. *Development* 1999; **126**(9): 1997–2005.

32. Paria BC, Das SK, Andrews GK, Dey SK. Expression of the epidermal growth factor receptor gene is regulated in mouse blastocysts during delayed implantation. *Proc Natl Acad Sci USA* 1993; **90**(1): 55–9.

33. Yoo HJ, Barlow DH, Mardon HJ. Temporal and spatial regulation of expression of heparin-binding epidermal growth factor-like growth factor in the human endometrium: a possible role in blastocyst implantation. *Dev Genet* 1997; **21**(1): 102–8.

34. Chobotova K, Spyropoulou I, Carver J *et al.* Heparin-binding epidermal growth factor and its receptor ErbB4 mediate implantation of the human blastocyst. *Mech Dev* 2002; **119**(2): 137–44.

35. Martin KL, Barlow DH, Sargent IL. Heparin-binding epidermal growth factor significantly improves human blastocyst development and hatching in serum-free medium. *Hum Reprod* 1998; **13**(6): 1645–52.

36. Lessey BA, Gui Y, Apparao KB, Young SL, Mulholland J. Regulated expression of heparin-binding EGF-like growth factor (HB-EGF) in the human endometrium: a potential paracrine role during implantation. *Mol Reprod Dev* 2002; **62**(4): 446–55.

37. Paria BC, Ma W, Tan J *et al.* Cellular and molecular responses of the uterus to embryo implantation can be elicited by locally applied growth factors. *Proc Natl Acad Sci USA* 2001; **98**(3): 1047–52.

38. Troyer KL, Luetteke NC, Saxon ML *et al.* Growth retardation, duodenal lesions, and aberrant ileum architecture in triple null mice lacking EGF, amphiregulin, and TGF-alpha. *Gastroenterology* 2001; **121**(1): 68–78.

39. Han VK, Bassett N, Walton J, Challis JR. The expression of insulin-like growth factor (IGF) and IGF-binding protein (IGFBP) genes in the human placenta and membranes: evidence for IGF-IGFBP interactions at the feto-maternal interface. *J Clin Endocrinol Metab* 1996; **81**(7): 2680–93.

40. Irwin JC, Suen LF, Martina NA, Mark SP, Giudice LC. Role of the IGF system in trophoblast invasion and pre-eclampsia. *Hum Reprod* 1999; **14** (Suppl. 2): 90–6.

41. Irving JA, Lysiak JJ, Graham CH *et al.* Characteristics of trophoblast cells migrating from first trimester chorionic villus explants and propagated in culture. *Placenta* 1995; **16**(5): 413–33.

42. Shifren JL, Tseng JF, Zaloudek CJ *et al.* Ovarian steroid regulation of vascular endothelial growth factor in the human endometrium: implications for angiogenesis during the menstrual cycle and in the pathogenesis of endometriosis. *J Clin Endocrinol Metab* 1996; **81**(8): 3112–18.

43. Chakraborty I, Das SK, Dey SK. Differential expression of vascular endothelial growth factor and its receptor mRNAs in the mouse uterus around the time of implantation. *J Endocrinol* 1995; **147**(2): 339–52.

44. Cullinan EB, Abbondanzo SJ, Anderson PS *et al.* Leukemia inhibitory factor (LIF) and LIF receptor expression in human endometrium suggests a potential autocrine/paracrine function in regulating embryo implantation. *Proc Natl Acad Sci USA* 1996; **93**(7): 3115–20.

45. Aghajanova L, Hamilton AE, Giudice LC. Uterine receptivity to human embryonic implantation: histology, biomarkers, and transcriptomics. *Sem Cell Dev Biol* 2008; **19**(2): 204–11.

46. Stewart CL, Kaspar P, Brunet LJ *et al.* Blastocyst implantation depends on maternal expression of leukaemia inhibitory factor. *Nature* 1992; **359**(6390): 76–9.

47. Ernst M, Inglese M, Waring P *et al.* Defective gp130-mediated signal transducer and activator of transcription (STAT) signaling results in degenerative joint disease, gastrointestinal ulceration, and failure of uterine implantation. *J Exp Med* 2001; **194**(2): 189–203.

48. Ware CB, Horowitz MC, Renshaw BR *et al.* Targeted disruption of the low-affinity leukemia inhibitory factor receptor gene causes placental, skeletal, neural and metabolic defects and results in perinatal death. *Development* 1995; **121**(5): 1283–99.

49. Chen JR, Cheng JG, Shatzer T *et al.* Leukemia inhibitory factor can substitute for nidatory estrogen and is essential to inducing a receptive uterus for implantation but is not essential for subsequent embryogenesis. *Endocrinology* 2000; **141**(12): 4365–72.

50. Laird SM, Tuckerman EM, Dalton CF *et al.* The production of leukaemia inhibitory factor by human endometrium: presence in uterine flushings and production by cells in culture. *Hum Reprod* 1997; **12**(3): 569–74.

51. Hambartsoumian E. Endometrial leukemia inhibitory factor (LIF) as a possible cause of unexplained infertility and multiple failures of implantation. *Am J Reprod Immunol* 1998; **39**(2): 137–43.

52. Danielsson KG, Swahn ML, Bygdeman M. The effect of various doses of mifepristone on endometrial leukaemia inhibitory factor expression in the midluteal phase – an immunohistochemical study. *Hum Reprod* 1997; **12**(6): 1293–7.

53. Huppertz B, Kertschanska S, Demir AY, Frank HG, Kaufmann P. Immunohistochemistry of matrix metalloproteinases (MMP), their substrates, and their inhibitors (TIMP) during trophoblast invasion in the human placenta. *Cell Tissue Res* 1998; **291**(1): 133–48.

54. Librach CL, Werb Z, Fitzgerald ML *et al.* 92-kD type IV collagenase mediates invasion of human cytotrophoblasts. *J Cell Biol* 1991; **113**(2): 437–49.

55. Bagot CN, Kliman HJ, Taylor HS. Maternal Hoxa10 is required for pinopod formation in the development of mouse uterine receptivity to embryo implantation. *Dev Dyn* 2001; **222**(3): 538–44.

56. Schatz F, Krikun G, Runic R *et al.* Implications of decidualization-associated protease expression in implantation and menstruation. *Semin Reprod Endocrinol* 1999; **17**(1): 3–12.

57. McGinnis W, Krumlauf R. Homeobox genes and axial patterning. *Cell* 1992; **68**(2): 283–302.

58. Taylor HS, Vanden Heuvel GB, Igarashi P. A conserved Hox axis in the mouse and human female reproductive system: late establishment and persistent adult expression of the Hoxa cluster genes. *Biol Reprod* 1997; **57**(6): 1338–45.

59. Satokata I, Benson G, Maas R. Sexually dimorphic sterility phenotypes in Hoxa10-deficient mice. *Nature* 1995; **374**(6521): 460–3.

60. Benson GV, Lim H, Paria BC *et al.* Mechanisms of reduced fertility in Hoxa-10 mutant mice: uterine homeosis and loss of maternal Hoxa-10 expression. *Development* 1996; **122**(9): 2687–96.

61. Hsieh-Li HM, Witte DP, Weinstein M *et al.* Hoxa 11 structure, extensive antisense transcription, and function in male and female fertility. *Development* 1995; **121**(5): 1373–85.

62. Bagot CN, Troy PJ, Taylor HS. Alteration of maternal Hoxa10 expression by in vivo gene transfection affects implantation. *Gene Ther* 2000; **7**(16): 1378–84.

63. Taylor AH, Ang C, Bell SC, Konje JC. The role of the endocannabinoid system in gametogenesis, implantation and early pregnancy. *Hum Reprod Update* 2007; **13**(5): 501–13.

64. Taylor HS, Arici A, Olive D, Igarashi P. HOXA10 is expressed in response to sex steroids at the time of implantation in the human endometrium. *J Clin Invest* 1998; **101**(7): 1379–84.

65. Taylor HS, Igarashi P, Olive DL, Arici A. Sex steroids mediate HOXA11 expression in the human peri-implantation endometrium. *J Clin Endocrinol Metab* 1999; **84**(3): 1129–35.

66. Ma L, Benson GV, Lim H, Dey SK, Maas RL. Abdominal B (AbdB) Hoxa genes: regulation in adult uterus by estrogen and progesterone and repression in mullerian duct by the synthetic estrogen diethylstilbestrol (DES). *Dev Biol* 1998; **197**(2): 141–54.

67. Cermik D, Selam B, Taylor HS. Regulation of HOXA-10 expression by testosterone in vitro and in the endometrium of patients with polycystic ovary syndrome. *J Clin Endocrinol Metab* 2003; **88**(1): 238s–43.

68. Cermik D, Arici A, Taylor HS. Coordinated regulation of HOX gene expression in myometrium and uterine leiomyoma. *Fertil Steril* 2002; **78**(5): 979–84.

69. Daftary GS, Taylor HS. Hydrosalpinx fluid diminishes endometrial cell HOXA10 expression. *Fertil Steril* 2002; **78**(3): 577–80.

70. Marions L, Danielsson KG. Expression of cyclo-oxygenase in human endometrium during the implantation period. *Mol Hum Reprod* 1999; **5**(10): 961–5.

71. Lim H, Gupta RA, Ma WG *et al.* Cyclo-oxygenase-2-derived prostacyclin mediates embryo implantation in the mouse via PPARdelta. *Genes Dev* 1999; **13**(12): 1561–74.

72. Huang JC, Liu DY, Yadollahi S, Wu KK, Dawood MY. Interleukin-1 beta induces cyclooxygenase-2 gene expression in cultured endometrial stromal cells. *J Clin Endocrinol Metab* 1998; **83**(2): 538–41.

73. Barak Y, Nelson MC, Ong ES *et al.* PPAR gamma is required for placental, cardiac, and adipose tissue development. *Mol Cell* 1999; **4**(4): 585–95.

74. Le Bouteiller P, Legrand-Abravanel F, Solier C. Soluble HLA-G1 at the materno-foetal interface – a review. *Placenta* 2003; **24** (Suppl. A): S10–15.

75. Allan DS, Colonna M, Lanier LL *et al.* Tetrameric complexes of human histocompatibility leukocyte antigen (HLA)-G bind to peripheral blood myelomonocytic cells. *J Exp Med* 1999; **189**(7): 1149–56.

76. King A, Burrows T, Verma S, Hiby S, Loke YW. Human uterine lymphocytes. *Hum Reprod Update* 1998; **4**(5): 480–5.

77. Deniz G, Christmas SE, Brew R, Johnson PM. Phenotypic and functional cellular differences between human CD3- decidual and peripheral blood leukocytes. *J Immunol* 1994; **152**(9): 4255–61.

78. Drake PM, Gunn MD, Charo if *et al.* Human placental cytotrophoblasts attract monocytes and CD56(bright) natural killer cells via the actions of monocyte inflammatory protein 1alpha. *J Exp Med* 2001; **193**(10): 1199–212.

79. Roth I, Corry DB, Locksley RM *et al.* Human placental cytotrophoblasts produce the immunosuppressive cytokine interleukin 10. *J Exp Med* 1996; **184**(2): 539–48.

80. Xu C, Mao D, Holers VM *et al.* A critical role for murine complement regulator crry in fetomaternal tolerance. *Science* 2000; **287**(5452): 498–501.

81. Munn DH, Zhou M, Attwood JT *et al.* Prevention of allogeneic fetal rejection by tryptophan catabolism. *Science* 1998; **281**(5380): 1191–3.

82. Kamimura S, Eguchi K, Yonezawa M, Sekiba K. Localization and developmental change of indoleamine 2,3-dioxygenase activity in the human placenta. *Acta Med Okayama* 1991; **45**(3): 135–9.

83. Schrocksnadel H, Baier-Bitterlich G, Dapunt O, Wachter H, Fuchs D. Decreased plasma tryptophan in pregnancy. *Obstet Gynecol* 1996; **88**(1): 47–50.

84. Norwitz ER. Defective implantation and placentation: laying the blueprint for pregnancy complications. *Reprod Biomed Online* 2006; **13**(4): 591–9.

85. Krebs C, Macara LM, Leiser R *et al.* Intrauterine growth restriction with absent end-diastolic flow velocity in the umbilical artery is associated with maldevelopment of the placental terminal villous tree. *Am J Obstet Gynecol* 1996; **175**(6): 1534–42.

86. Meekins JW, Pijnenborg R, Hanssens M, McFadyen IR, van Asshe A. A study of placental bed spiral arteries and trophoblast invasion in normal and severe pre-eclamptic pregnancies. *Br J Obstet Gynaecol* 1994; **101**(8): 669–74.

87. Zhou Y, Damsky CH, Fisher SJ. Preeclampsia is associated with failure of human cytotrophoblasts to mimic a vascular adhesion phenotype. One cause of defective endovascular invasion in this syndrome? *J Clin Invest* 1997; **99**(9): 2152–64.

# Chapter 20

# Recurrent implantation failure

Nick S. Macklon and Carolien M. Boomsma

## Introduction

In recent years, much progress has been made in improving embryo quality and selection for transfer after in-vitro fertilization (IVF). However, despite these advances, even when embryos are considered to be of high quality using morphological and chromosomal criteria, implantation rates remain around 25–35% per embryo transfer procedure [1]. Recently it has been demonstrated that around half of embryo transfer procedures result in implantation, but only half of these initiated implantations will result in an ongoing pregnancy [2]. In the same study, around two-thirds of pregnancy losses were shown to occur in the immediate post-implantation period, resulting in a negative clinical pregnancy test (Figure 20.1). When considering where the ceiling on improving IVF results may lie, it is important to realize that this apparently high rate of peri-implantation failure mirrors that reported in spontaneous conceptions (Figure 20.2) [3].

Nevertheless, when implantation failure after IVF occurs, it is a cause of considerable frustration and disappointment for all concerned. Recurrent implantation failure (RIF) has been defined as three or more unsuccessful IVF cycles or the failure of conception after the replacement of 10 or more good-quality embryos [4]. However in the age of single embryo transfer (SET), fewer patients will undergo this number of embryo transfer procedures and alternative definitions have therefore been proposed. The chance of pregnancy per cycle tends to remain stable in the first three attempts, but declines thereafter [5,6], suggesting an underlying cause for implantation failure in these patients rather than simple calculation of probability. Women who have undergone more than three high-quality embryo transfer procedures without achieving a positive pregnancy test may therefore be considered to have recurrent implantation failure [7].

Around 10% of women undergoing IVF will meet these criteria for diagnosis. Multiple etiologies for implantation failure have been proposed (Figure 20.3). They can be described in terms of maternal or embryo-related factors, and may in some cases be iatrogenic. In this chapter the principal putative causes of implantation failure are described, and therapeutic strategies are reviewed.

## Maternal factors

### Tubal disease

With regard to the impact of tubal disease on implantation, there is now convincing evidence that distal pathology associated with hydrosalpinx has a detrimental effect. A meta-analysis evaluating differences in pregnancy rates after IVF in tubal infertility with or without hydrosalpinx, showed an odds ratio (OR) 0.64 (95% confidence interval (CI) 0.56–0.74) [8]. Current evidence indicates that laparoscopic salpingectomy before IVF treatment should be advised for women with hydrosalpinges: a meta-analysis of three randomized controlled trials (RCT) comparing surgical intervention versus no intervention showed an OR 1.8 (95% CI 1.1–2.9) [9] (Johnson et al, 2002). The major study addressed in this meta-analysis demonstrated that this effect was entirely due to the positive effect among those with a hydrosalpinx visible on ultrasound [10,11]. A recent RCT compared the clinical impact of proximal tubal occlusion and salpingectomy prior to IVF in patients with hydrosalpinges. Proximal tubal occlusion was shown to be as effective as salpingectomy in improving implantation rates compared with no intervention [12].

### Fibroids

The relationship between fibroids and fertility remains controversial, but is generally considered to

---

*Early Pregnancy*, ed. Roy G. Farquharson and Mary D. Stephenson. Published by Cambridge University Press.
© Cambridge University Press 2010.

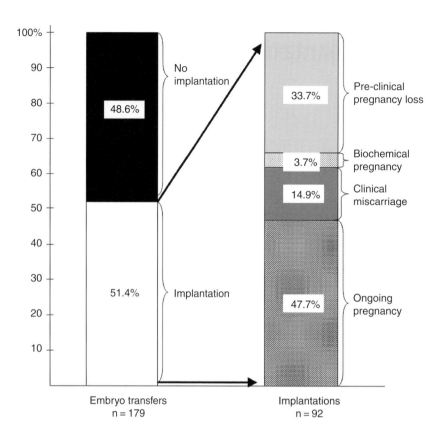

**Figure 20.1** Treatment outcome after embryo transfer (left bar) and subsequent implantation (right bar). From Boomsma *et al.* 2009 [2].

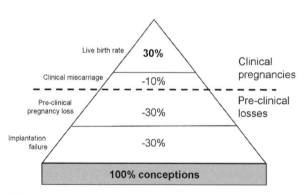

**Figure 20.2** An overview of the outcome of human conceptions. Adapted from Macklon *et al.* 2002 [3].

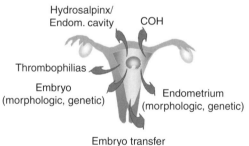

**Figure 20.3** Principal reported causes of recurrent implantation failure. Figure courtesy of J. Garcia-Velasco.

be related to the location, size and degree of associated distortion of the endometrial cavity. Unfortunately, no well-designed prospective studies are available to guide practice in this field, and current opinion is based primarily on data from retrospective studies. One of these reported a 50% decrease in implantation rate when intramural fibroids were present [13]. However, whether or not their removal improves outcomes has not yet been clarified by a prospective randomized study. A meta-analysis has suggested that removing submucosal fibroids may confer some benefit [14].

## Thrombophilias

The principal thrombophilias associated with poorer reproductive outcomes include the inherited thrombophilias caused by activated protein C resistance and the factor V Leiden mutation, and antithrombin III, protein C and S deficiencies. Acquired thrombophilias associated with miscarriage and intrauterine growth retardation include anticardiolipin antibodies and lupus anticoagulant. While the precise role of thrombophilias as a cause of RIF remains unclear, a number of studies suggest that they may be one of the contributing etiologies. In one study, thrombophilias were reported to be present in 44% of women presenting with RIF, compared with 18% in a control cohort. In a further study in which 10 thrombophilic genes were screened, three or more mutations were observed in 74% of women with RIF compared with just 20% in controls ($P < 0.005$) [15]. Combined thrombophilia was reported in 36% of women with RIF compared to 3% rate normally reported in the general population. Further data supporting the concept that combined thrombophilias may be associated with RIF come from a study in which 46% of affected women were observed to have at least one thrombophilia [16].

Screening for these disorders is not merited in routine practice, but may be indicated in recurrent implantation failure. Although aspirin and heparin offer a therapeutic strategy when combined thrombophilias are present, they have not been shown to improve outcomes in randomized studies.

## Endometrial abnormalities

The endometrium undergoes dramatic cyclical changes in response to changing sex steroids levels. In the mid-luteal phase, the endometrium becomes receptive to implantation from approximately cycle days 19 to 24 in a normal menstrual cycle, referred to as the window of implantation [17,18]. Although a multitude of complex molecular pathways modulate this process, no specific individual factor in the endometrium has been shown to be crucial for implantation in the human [19,20]. The development of DNA microarray gene expression profiling has made it possible to investigate the endometrium from a global genomic perspective. Altered expression of endometrial regulatory genes has been postulated as an underlying cause of infertility and implantation failure. A number of studies have demonstrated that endometrial gene expression profiles change throughout the menstrual cycle [21]. In addition, endometrial gene expression has been investigated under non-physiological and pathological conditions, such as ovarian stimulated cycles [22–24]. These studies have provided indirect evidence of genes involved in endometrial receptivity. However, many of the gene transcripts changing throughout the menstrual cycle may

not be involved in endometrial receptivity and many dysregulated genes observed in cycles stimulated with exogenous gonaodotropins, may represent different dysregulated pathways compared with those occurring in women with implantation failure after IVF treatment.

The molecular profile of the receptive endometrium can be described by analyzing endometrial secretions aspirated at the time of embryo transfer. Van der Gaast et al. recently showed a correlation between endometrial secretion glycodelin levels and endometrial maturity as assessed by modified Noyes criteria [25]. Moreover, Boomsma et al have recently shown that successful implantation is associated with increased levels of interferon inducible 10 kD protein, and lower levels of monocyte chemoattractant protein 1 [26]. Ongoing pregnancy was predicted by higher levels of tumor necrosis factor-alpha and lower levels of interleukin-1beta in endometrial secretions during the window of implantation. Aspirating endometrial secretions prior to embryo transfer has been shown not to disrupt implantation [25,26] and may offer the basis of an objective test of endometrial receptivity [26].

At present, the thickness of the endometrium when measured on ultrasound is considered by many to be an important determinant of implantation success. However, in a well-controlled study in donor oocyte recipients with similar embryo quality, endometrial thickness did not predict implantation. Many adjuvant therapies prescribed to improve implantation rates are aimed at modulating endometrial receptivity, and these are reviewed later in the chapter.

## The embryo factor

Human embryos are known to demonstrate high rates of aneuploidy, and this appears to be increased when ovarian stimulation with high-dose exogenous gonadotropins is employed [27]. A number of these may reflect maternal or paternal chromosomal abnormalities, and there is some evidence of increased rates of balanced translocations in women who have failed to conceive after the transfer of 15 embryos [28]. There may therefore be a place for karyotypic evaluation in couples with recurrent failure of this degree.

Since embryo aneuploidy has been reported to be present with higher frequency in women with recurrent implantation failure [29], there would appear to be an important role for pre-implantation genetic screening (PGS) in improving outcomes in RIF. By removing one or two blastomeres at the 3-day stage of development, and subjecting these to analysis by fluorescent in-situ hybridization (FISH), the presence of aneuploidy can be tested, and those embryos which meet both morphological criteria for selection, and in which no chromosomal abnormality is detected can be transferred. The theoretical benefits of PGS have resulted in a rapid growth in its application and it is now offered in many clinics to women with a history of RIF. However, although a large number of retrospective studies have encouraged the belief that PGS could revolutionize embryo selection and IVF outcomes, the few randomized trials thus far published have not been able to demonstrate a clear benefit.

There are a number of possible explanations for this. Protagonists suggest that poor results reflect poor individual technique in applying the tests, whereas skeptics point to the invasive nature of the test, the limited (and therefore insufficiently representative) number of chromosomes analyzed by current FISH techniques, and the phenomenon of chromosomal mosaicism. It is now clear that many developing embryos contain blastomeres of variable chromosomal constitution, and that the presence of aneuploidy in one cell does not necessarily reflect the situation in other cells. The risk of misdiagnosis is therefore considerable [30] .

A number of challenges therefore remain before the place of PGS in the armory of the embryologist can be confirmed. While technical improvements will be helpful, the developmental importance of mosaicism, and how it should be interpreted when selecting embryos needs to be more fully understood. Until then, PGS should only be offered to women with RIF in a research setting [31].

As an alternative strategy for overcoming the clinical problem of recurrent implantation failure, endometrial co-culture systems have been advocated as a means of improving the implantation potential of embryos generated by IVF. The rationale is based on the supposition that the embryo can benefit from exposure to factors such as cytokines, growth factors and nutrients secreted by the endometrium, which in theory can also remove potentially harmful metabolites from the culture medium. Most systems in current use involve co-culture of homologous endometrial epithelial cells with embryos. Using such a system, Mercader *et al.* reported high blastocyst formation rates [32] of up to 58%. In a study of 1030 women with RIF, Spandorfer *et al.* reported a

pregnancy rate of 49% [33]. Prospective randomized studies are however still required in order to clarify the role and value of this approach.

Another intervention aimed at facilitating contact between embryo and endometrium is assisted hatching. This technique involves the creation of a hole in the zona pellucida by chemical or mechanical means, and by doing so, facilitating the exit of the embryo from within the zona and improving contact with the endometrium. A number of indications for this technique have been suggested, such as in older women, RIF or when there is evidence of a thickened zona pellucida. While retrospective studies indicated a possible benefit in women with RIF [34,35], this has not been confirmed in prospective randomized studies. Currently available data, scrutinized by meta-analysis [36], reveal that there is insufficient evidence to support the use of assisted hatching outwith a research setting.

## The clinical approach

When faced with a patient presenting with recurrent implantation failure, a number of possible causes should be excluded before further management and support is instituted. Although data from randomized studies are not available to support routine hysteroscopy for the evaluation of the uterine cavity prior to IVF, it can be reassuring to both clinician and patient if structural intrauterine pathology, can be excluded. An endometrial biopsy taken during this procedure may identify the presence of an endometritis, which may respond to antibiotic treatment. Careful ultrasound assessment of the fallopian tubes may reveal a hydrosalpinx, which can vary in size with time, and which may have previously been missed.

The assessment of presence of autoantibodies and thrombophilia may be considered although as described earlier, the evidence for their role in RIF, and the impact of treatment on IVF outcomes is unclear.

In the majority of cases, no specific cause will be identified. There is however considerable pressure on clinicians to offer remedial therapies when recurrent implantation failure presents. A number of strategies are outlined below, and summarized in Table 20.1[37].

## Ovarian stimulation regimen

The contemporary approach to ovarian stimulation in IVF treatment is based on the perceived need to

**Table 20.1** What can the clinician do to improve embryo implantation? A summary.

| What can the clinician do to improve implantation? | (Presumed) method of action | Empirical use in non-selected IVF population |
| --- | --- | --- |
| Careful embryo transfer technique | Minimize trauma and cervical manipulation | Soft ET catheter: significantly higher pregnancy rates |
| Adjuvant pharmaceutical therapies | | |
| Aspirin | Vasodilatation and anticoagulant properties | No significant beneficial effect on pregnancy rates in a non-selected IVF population |
| Nitric oxide donors | Uterine vasodilatation | No significant beneficial effect on pregnancy rates. Possible detrimental effect on the embryo |
| Aromatase inhibitors | Reduction in estrogen synthesis: improving endometrial receptivity | No significant beneficial effect on pregnancy rates in a non-selected IVF population |
| Ascorbic acid | Anti-inflammatory and immunostimulant effects | No significant beneficial effect on pregnancy rates in a non-selected IVF population |
| Prolonged progesterone | Luteal phase supplementation in a downregulated cycle | No significant beneficial effect on pregnancy rates in a non-selected IVF population |
| Luteal E2 supplementation | Luteal phase supplementation in a downregulated cycle | Application of luteal E2 supplementation remains controversial |
| Glucocorticoids | Immunomodulatory effect reduction number NK cells | No significant beneficial effect on pregnancy rates in a non-selected IVF population |
| Insulin sensitizing drugs | Minimizing insulin resistance | No significant beneficial effect on pregnancy rates, may reduce miscarriage/OHSS rate in PCOS; empirical use in a non-selected IVF population has not been investigated |
| GnRH agonist | LH-releasing properties | Can possibly be exploited as luteal support: no beneficial effect on implantation rates described |
| Ovarian stimulation | | |
| Mild stimulation regimens | Improvement of endometrial receptivity and embryo quality | Comparable IVF outcomes, despite fewer oocytes |
| Prediction of optimal starting dose FSH in the patient | Optimal stimulation level | Prediction models may have a role. In the future, pharmacogenetics is likely to become important |
| Selecting optimal embryo, endometrium and patient | | |
| Pre-implantation genetic screening | Selection of euploid embryos | No RCTs in a non-selected IVF population have been published yet |
| Marker for endometrial receptivity | Correcting and optimizing receptivity prior to embryo transfer | A reliable test remains elusive |
| Selecting patients for single embryo transfer (SET) | Identification of patients in which SET does not reduce the pregnancy rate | No prospective analysis of prediction models has yet been performed. |
| Optimize lifestyle and nutrition | Optimizing oocyte and semen quality and implantation rates. Decrease rate pregnancy complications | Significantly higher pregnancy rates among women with a lower BMI, non-smokers. Higher miscarriage rate in women using caffeine or alcohol |

Adapted from Boomsma et al. [37].

maximize the number of oocytes available for fertilization, in order to generate multiple embryos for selection and transfer. Ovaries are stimulated with exogenous FSH in order to obtain multiple oocytes during IVF treatment. However, ovarian hyperstimulation and the resultant elevated estradiol levels have been shown to impact negatively on endometrial receptivity [38–40]). Endometrial receptivity may have declined due to advanced post-ovulatory endometrial maturation and defective induction of progesterone receptors. Supra-physiological estrogen concentrations may increase sensitivity to progesterone action and lead to secretory advancement. Studies of the impact of ovarian stimulation on endometrial maturation several days after ovulation have shown either no effect or endometrial delay. Additionally, a study on endometrial histology has shown that advancement on the day of oocyte retrieval exceeding 3 days, was associated with no subsequent pregnancies [41]. Moreover, the magnitude of estrogen dose to which the endometrium is exposed has been shown to affect the duration of the receptive phase [42]. Kolibianakis *et al.* have demonstrated the effect of prolongation of the follicular phase by delaying hCG administration by 2 days in a randomized controlled trial. They showed endometrial advancement on the day of oocyte retrieval of 2–3 days in all women when hCG was delayed versus no secretory changes in the control group [43].

Increasing awareness of the possible detrimental effects of standard ovarian stimulation regimens on endometrium and embryo has stimulated a reassessment of the optimal approach to ovarian stimulation for IVF [39,44] 2000). Increasing knowledge regarding the physiology of ovarian follicle development, together with the clinical availability of GnRH antagonists, which allows ovarian stimulation to be commenced in the undisturbed menstrual cycle, has presented the opportunity to develop novel, milder approaches for ovarian stimulation for IVF [40,45]. In an RCT, it has been shown that the initiation of exogenous FSH (fixed dose, 150 IU/day, GnRH antagonist co-treatment) as late as cycle day 5 results in a comparable clinical IVF outcome, despite a reduced duration of stimulation (and total dose of FSH given) and increased cancellation rates [46]. The quality of embryos obtained after mild stimulation was significantly greater compared with the conventional long protocol. Moreover, almost all the pregnancies after minimal stimulation were observed in patients with a relatively low oocyte yield, whereas no pregnancies were observed when a similar yield was obtained after conventional IVF.

In a recent randomized study, pre-implantation genetic screening (PGS) was employed to investigate the chromosomal constitution of embryos obtained after conventional ovarian stimulation compared with embryos obtained after mild ovarian stimulation [27] . Although more oocytes were obtained in the conventional ovarian stimulation group, the mild group demonstrated an increased percentage of euploid embryos per number of oocytes retrieved. These observations support the concept of a "natural" selection of oocytes during follicular development which may be overridden by conventional "maximal" stimulation protocols. Employing mild stimulation regimens may aid embryo selection by increasing the chance that the transferred embryo is euploid.

## Embryo transfer technique

The technique of embryo transfer (ET) has been shown to be an important factor in determining the outcome of assisted reproductive technology (ART) cycles. A number of studies have shown that significant improvements in clinical pregnancy rates can be achieved by giving due attention to the technique employed.

Stiff catheters make catheter placement easier when difficulty in passing the catheter through the cervix is experienced. These catheters are, however, associated with more bleeding and trauma. Additionally, cervical manipulation may result in an increase in uterine contractions, which have been observed to hinder IVF outcome [47]. A recent meta-analysis of seven RCTs, comparing stiff and soft ET catheters, showed significantly increased pregnancy rates when soft catheters were applied (OR 1.34, 95% CI 1.18–1.54) [48].

In current practice, embryo transfer during IVF treatment is usually performed "blindly," with the aim of placing the embryos 1 cm below the fundus of the uterus. However, transferring embryos lower in the uterine cavity has been suggested to improve implantation rates. In a prospective trial, the effects of both the distance from the fundus and the relative position in the uterus of the catheter tip were investigated. Significantly better results were obtained when the catheter tip was positioned close to the middle of the endometrial cavity [13] . In this study, the absolute distance from the fundus appeared less important.

However, another randomized study revealed significantly higher implantation rates when embryos were deposited 1.5 or 2 cm from the fundus compared with 1 cm [49]. As a result of these and other similar studies, many centers have adjusted their ET procedures. It has been recently postulated that embryo transfer in the lower uterine segment may result in an increased risk of placenta previa, since a six-fold higher risk of placenta previa in singleton pregnancies conceived by assisted fertilization compared with naturally conceived pregnancies has been reported [50].

The blind nature of traditional "clinical touch" embryo transfer had led to the suggestion of the use of ultrasound to improve IVF outcome. Following initial encouraging reports, there have been numerous studies evaluating the use of ultrasound-guided embryo transfer. A meta-analysis of four RCTs comparing ultrasound-guided embryo transfer versus clinical touch showed a significantly higher pregnancy rate and implantation rate after ultrasound-guided transfer (1.38, 95% CI 1.20–1.60) [51].

During embryo transfer it is likely that bacteria from the cervix may be introduced into the uterine cavity. Bacterial vaginosis (BV) is characterized by an overgrowth of anerobic organisms and the prevalence among women undergoing IVF is approximately 25% [52]. There is growing evidence that the pathogenic effects of bacterial vaginosis may not be confined to the lower genital tract. Histopathological evidence of plasma cell endometritis was seen in almost half of the women with symptomatic BV [53]. There is no consensus in the literature whether BV is associated with the success of embryo implantation. Salim et al. reported a significantly higher pregnancy rate among women without cervical colonization in the cervix versus women with bacterial colonization (30.7% versus 16.3%) [54]. However, other studies have not revealed this correlation [52]. At present, routine screening for bacterial vaginosis in the hope of improving the success of IVF treatment is not justified.

## Adjuvant medical therapies

Adjuvant medical therapies to those required for ovarian hyperstimulation are frequently applied in an empirical manner with the aim of improving embryo implantation and particularly when the clinician is faced with recurrent implantation failure. However, the evidence for their efficacy and safety does not always justify the enthusiasm with which they are prescribed.

### Aspirin

The rationale for the use of aspirin as an adjuvant drug in IVF is based on its vasodilatation and anticoagulant properties. The main method of action of aspirin is the inhibition of cyclo-oxygenase (the rate-limiting enzyme in the prostaglandin synthesis pathway) and subsequent reduction of platelet aggregation. As a result, blood perfusion to the ovaries and the endometrium are both presumed to be improved. Indeed, a significant improvement in the uterine blood perfusion (reduction of the pulsatility index of the uterine artery) in the peri-implantation period after aspirin supplementation has been shown [55].

Aspirin has been shown to be effective in combination with heparin, in the treatment of recurrent miscarriage in women with antiphospholipid antibody syndrome (APS) [56]. However, efficacy in recurrent miscarriage in women without APS has not been proven [57]. In the context of IVF treatment, a randomized controlled trial was performed comparing aspirin plus heparin treatment with placebo from embryo transfer onwards in 143 women with antiphospholipid or antinuclear antibodies with a history of embryo implantation failure [58]. No significant differences in implantation or pregnancy rates were observed.

Randomized controlled studies investigating the use of aspirin in a non-selected IVF population as an empirical therapy have shown conflicting results (Table 20.2). One study showed significantly improved ovarian response and implantation rates [59], all other studies showed no significant differences [60–63]. A meta-analysis of 10 RCTs showed no statistically significant improvement in clinical pregnancy rates with aspirin versus no or placebo treatment (OR 1.18, 95% CI 0.86–1.61) [64]. At present there is insufficient evidence to support the use of aspirin outwith the context of randomized controlled trials.

### Nitric oxide donors

Nitric oxide (NO) acts as a relaxant of arterial and smooth muscle, and inhibits platelet aggregation. On the day of either human chorionic gonadotropin (hCG) administration or embryo transfer, a high resistance to uterine blood flow is reported to be correlated with a poor clinical outcome for patients undergoing IVF [65]. These observations suggested that uterine vasodilatation induced by a NO donor might improve endometrial receptivity.

However, while initial studies suggested beneficial effects on ovarian response and implantation [66], more recent studies have suggested a detrimental effect of NO on implantation [67]. In addition, a recent prospective study of women undergoing IVF reported an association between high follicular NO levels and advanced embryo fragmentation and implantation failure [68]. Although subgroups of women may be identified who benefit from NO donor therapy, at present the available data demand caution in its use, which at present should be restricted to well-designed studies.

### Aromatase inhibitors

The conversion of androstenedione and testosterone to estriol and estradiol, respectively, is blocked by aromatase inhibitors [69]. This approach reduces the amount of estrogens synthesized, rather than antagonizing estrogen feedback activity at the hypothalamic-pituitary axis as with clomiphene citrate. As a result, gonadotropin secretion is increased and follicular growth is stimulated. Moreover, by preventing excessive estradiol synthesis, it has been hypothesized that adjuvant treatment with aromatase inhibitors during ovarian stimulation may result in less disruption of endometrial receptivity. One RCT has been performed on women with a poor ovarian response (defined by Goswami *et al.* [70] as less than two dominant follicles). Women using aromatase inhibitors required a significantly lower total dose of FSH, however, the pregnancy rates were comparable [71]. These results are in line with three non-randomized trials investigating aromatase inhibitors as an adjunct treatment in normal responders [71–73]. Only a subgroup of women with PCOS showed significantly higher pregnancy rates after addition of an aromatase inhibitor [73]. While of considerable potential value, further studies are required to confirm the value and safety of aromatase inhibitors in IVF.

### Ascorbic acid

Ascorbic acid (AA) appears to be involved in normal folliculogenesis [74] and luteal formation and regression [75] . Moreover, transient high plasma levels can be achieved by a high-dose intake of AA, which can exert anti-inflammatory and immunostimulant effects. These effects might benefit embryo implantation. An imbalance of oxidative stress and antioxidant defence has been implicated in the pathogenesis of several diseases, including recurrent abortion, unexplained infertility and defective embryo development. However, an RCT investigating the effect of 1, 5 or 10 mg of AA versus a placebo during the luteal phase in 620 women undergoing IVF showed no difference in implantation rates [76].

### Glucocorticoids

Locally-acting growth factors, cytokines and uterine natural killer (uNK) cells control uterine receptivity during the window of implantation [19]. Studies on murine knock-out models have shown the effect of NK cells on fertility and pregnancy outcome[77] . The uNK cells accumulate around arteries supplying the implantation site. A defect in the integrity of the number of uNK cells has also been implicated in implantation failure among women undergoing IVF. Higher numbers of NK cells in endometrial biopsies from women with implantation failure versus fertile controls have been reported [78]. In women with recurrent miscarriage prednisolone has been shown to reduce the expression of uNK cells in the endometrium [79]. There is therefore evidence to support a possible role for glucocorticoids in improving the intrauterine environment by acting as an immunomodulator.

A meta-analysis of 13 randomized controlled trials including a total of 1759 couples showed no evidence that glucocorticoids improved clinical outcome (OR 1.16, 95% CI 0.94–1.44). However, a subgroup analysis of 650 women undergoing IVF rather than ICSI (six RCTs) revealed an improvement in pregnancy rates of borderline statistical significance for women using glucocorticoids (OR 1.50, 95% CI 1.05–2.13) (Figure 20.4) [80]. Overall, there is at present insufficient evidence to support the empirical use of glucocorticoids to improve implantation in IVF. Moreover, the potential deleterious effects of prolonged glucocorticoid therapy on pregnancy with premature delivery should be considered [81]. However, there may be a specific role for this therapy in subgroups of patients, such as women with antiphospholipid syndrome. Two RCTs investigating implantation rates among women with positive anti-nuclear, anti-double-stranded DNA, anti-cardiolipin antibodies and lupus anticoagulant, reported significantly higher pregnancy rates after glucocorticoid administration [82,83]. Further research is necessary to clarify the role of glucocorticoid therapy as an aid to implantation in certain well-defined subgroups of patients.

Other immunosuppressive therapies which have been advocated include immunogammaglobulin infusions and recombinant anti-TNF-α. These treatments

Review:Peri-implantation glucocorticoid administration for assisted reproductive technology cycles
Comparison:01 Glucocorticoids versus no glucocorticoids/ placebo
Outcome:04 Pregnancy rate per couple: type of ART

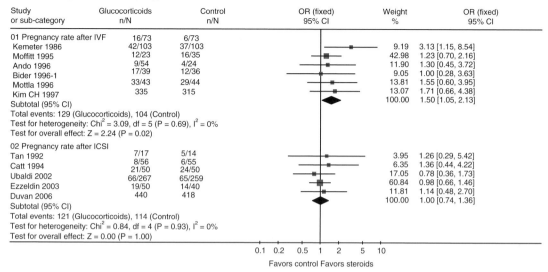

| Study or sub-category | Glucocorticoids n/N | Control n/N | OR (fixed) 95% CI | Weight % | OR (fixed) 95% CI |
|---|---|---|---|---|---|
| **01 Pregnancy rate after IVF** | 16/73 | 6/73 | | 9.19 | 3.13 [1.15, 8.54] |
| Kemeter 1986 | 42/103 | 37/103 | | 42.98 | 1.23 [0.70, 2.16] |
| Moffitt 1995 | 12/23 | 16/35 | | 11.90 | 1.30 [0.45, 3.72] |
| Ando 1996 | 9/54 | 4/24 | | 9.05 | 1.00 [0.28, 3.63] |
| Bider 1996-1 | 17/39 | 12/36 | | 13.81 | 1.55 [0.60, 3.95] |
| Mottla 1996 | 33/43 | 29/44 | | 13.07 | 1.71 [0.66, 4.38] |
| Kim CH 1997 | 335 | 315 | | 100.00 | 1.50 [1.05, 2.13] |
| Subtotal (95% CI) | | | | | |

Total events: 129 (Glucocorticoids), 104 (Control)
Test for heterogeneity: Chi² = 3.09, df = 5 (P = 0.69), I² = 0%
Test for overall effect: Z = 2.24 (P = 0.02)

| Study or sub-category | Glucocorticoids n/N | Control n/N | OR (fixed) 95% CI | Weight % | OR (fixed) 95% CI |
|---|---|---|---|---|---|
| **02 Pregnancy rate after ICSI** | 7/17 | 5/14 | | 3.95 | 1.26 [0.29, 5.42] |
| Tan 1992 | 8/56 | 6/55 | | 6.35 | 1.36 [0.44, 4.22] |
| Catt 1994 | 21/50 | 24/50 | | 17.05 | 0.78 [0.36, 1.73] |
| Ubaldi 2002 | 66/267 | 65/259 | | 60.84 | 0.98 [0.66, 1.46] |
| Ezzeldin 2003 | 19/50 | 14/40 | | 11.81 | 1.14 [0.48, 2.70] |
| Duvan 2006 | 440 | 418 | | 100.00 | 1.00 [0.74, 1.36] |
| Subtotal (95% CI) | | | | | |

Total events: 121 (Glucocorticoids), 114 (Control)
Test for heterogeneity: Chi² = 0.84, df = 4 (P = 0.93), I² = 0%
Test for overall effect: Z = 0.00 (P = 1.00)

0.1  0.2   0.5   1   2   5   10
Favors control  Favors steroids

**Figure 20.4** Adjuvant glucocorticoid administration and pregnancy outcome in IVF and ICSI. From Boomsma *et al.* 2009 [80].

should be subject to properly designed studies in order to confirm efficacy and safety before they are considered for use in clinical practice [84].

## What can the patient do?

There is now a substantial amount of evidence showing that environmental and lifestyle factors influence the success rates of ART [85,86], and it is therefore important that serious attempts are made to provide adequate preconceptional screening counseling and interventions in order to optimize health prior to starting IVF. The importance of full medical assessment prior to IVF treatment is increasing as the average age of our patients continues to rise. A greater proportion of infertility patients may now also present with concurrent medical conditions which may impact on the safety and management of the IVF treatment as well as pregnancy. The appropriate management of the medically complicated patient presenting for IVF can be complex and often requires an interdisciplinary approach. For further information in this field, the reader is referred to Macklon [87] .

The most important lifestyle factor impacting on fertility outcomes is tobacco smoking. Smoking during pregnancy has long been known to increase the risk of a number of adverse obstetric and fetal outcomes such as miscarriage, placenta previa, pre-term birth and low birthweight [86]. In recent years the association between smoking and infertility in women has become clear. Chemicals present in cigarette smoke can reach the developing egg in vivo, as both cotinine, the metabolite of nicotine, and cadmium and heavy metal in cigarette smoke are increased in the follicular fluid surrounding the egg [88] . It has also been demonstrated that active smoking increases oxidative stress in the growing follicle and cytotoxicity in the egg and surrounding granulosa cells [89]. Reports have appeared linking smoking to damage of the meiotic spindle in oocytes, increasing the risk of chromosomal errors [90]. In men who smoke, all parameters of sperm quality are reduced [86]. Smoking in men and passive smoking in women has been associated with a longer time to achieve a pregnancy [86].

The effects of smoking on live-birth rate among women who undergo IVF is similar in magnitude to the effect of an increase in female age of more than 10 years [85]. As a result, smokers require twice as many IVF cycles to become pregnant as non-smokers [85]. A recent ASRM Practice Committee publication on smoking and infertility has highlighted the considerable contribution of smoking to infertility and treatment outcomes and the need for a more proactive approach to stop smoking prior to fertility treatment [91].

Epidemiological evidence clearly shows that being overweight contributes to menstrual disorders, infertility, miscarriage, poor pregnancy outcome, impaired fetal wellbeing and diabetes mellitus [92]. Overweight women (BMI > 27 kg/m$^2$) have been shown to have a 33% reduced chance of a live-birth after their first IVF cycle compared with women with a body mass index 20–27 kg/m$^2$. The association was strongest in women with unexplained infertility [85]. In men a BMI <20 or >25 kg/m$^2$ is associated with reduced sperm quality [86].

A number of studies have shown that weight loss can improve fecundity in overweight women, and many centers include weight-loss programs as part of their fertility treatment. However, few data are available regarding the impact of type of diet on IVF outcomes. Recent studies have highlighted the importance of certain nutritional factors. Folic acid supplementation was shown to alter the vitamin microenvironment of the oocyte [93], while seminal plasma cobalamin levels were demonstrated to affect sperm concentration [94]. Moreover, intake of alcohol and caffeine are associated with the success rate of IVF. A high intake of caffeine has been linked to an increased risk of spontaneous abortions and lower live-birth rates after IVF treatment. Similarly, female alcohol consumption was associated with a decrease in pregnancy rates and an increase of spontaneous miscarriages. Male alcohol consumption up to one week before sperm collection may increase the risk of miscarriage [86]. While few data from lifestyle studies relate specifically to the process of implantation, patients with negative lifestyle factors who suffer recurrent implantation failure should be encouraged to optimize all amenable factors to improve the chance of success from further treatments.

## Conclusions

Recurrent implantation failure is a significant and distressing clinical problem. As this chapter shows, the number of evidence-based therapeutic options to manage this condition are limited. There are three main reasons for this. Firstly, the etiology of the condition is very heterogeneous. Prospective studies are therefore unlikely to reveal a benefit from specific therapies unless the included patients are carefully phenotyped to reduce the heterogeneity of the study cohorts. Secondly, the huge complexity of the processes which govern implantation failure mean that it is unlikely that the problem can be solved by addressing just one aspect. Thirdly, studying endometrial/

embryo interactions in the human is very challenging. In-vitro models are now providing a window on this process, and recently developed non-invasive tests of endometrial receptivity may increase our understanding of the molecular mechanisms disrupted in RIF, and those potentially amenable to therapeutic intervention.

At present however, our attention should be focused on optimizing those factors known to influence the chance of successful implantation. Increasing awareness of the possible detrimental effects of ovarian hyperstimulation and their burdens on the patient has stimulated development of milder ovarian stimulation regimens. Standard ovarian hyperstimulation and the resultant supraphysiological estradiol levels have been shown to impact negatively on endometrial receptivity and embryo quality. Studies of mild ovarian stimulation regimens have shown encouraging results. Although fewer embryos are obtained, an increased percentage of euploid embryos per number of oocytes retrieved has been reported. Therefore, in addition to causing less disruption of endometrial receptivity, mild ovarian stimulation may therefore also improve embryo quality.

Despite this, clinicians continue to strive to find adjuvant interventions, which can improve the chances of their patients to successfully conceive. However, the evidence for their efficacy and safety, supporting the application of the most commonly prescribed drug interventions during ART and subsequent pregnancies, is limited, therefore their use should be restricted to well-designed studies. Embryo implantation failure can be caused by multiple factors; as a result, no single additional treatment is likely to be the key solution. Until our understanding of the factors which determine the ability of an embryo to successfully implant are better understood, it is unlikely that additional medical interventions, such as those addressed in this chapter, will be shown to have anything but a marginal effect on IVF outcomes.

While much progress has been made in technical aspects of IVF treatment to optimize embryo quality and stimulation regimens, it is becoming increasingly clear that patient-related factors may be just as important or more important in determining the chance of success of treatment. Due attention to lifestyle factors may be as effective as more expensive and complex medical interventions for improving implantation rates.

In summary, many clinical interventions aimed at increasing the chance of implantation in IVF have

**Table 20.2** Summary table of studies on the effect of aspirin on IVF outcome.

| Study | n | Dose aspirin | Timing | Pregnancy rate | | P |
|---|---|---|---|---|---|---|
| | | | | Aspirin | Placebo | |
| Rubinstein et al. [59] | 298 | 100 mg | From cycle day 21 (preceding menstrual cycle) onwards | 45% | 28% | <.05 |
| Urman et al. [62] | 279 | 80 mg | From ovarian stimulation onwards | 40% | 43% | NS |
| Waldenström et al. [63] | 1380 | 75 mg | From ET onwards | 35% | 30% | NS |
| Pakilla et al. [61] | 374 | 100 mg | From ovarian stimulation onwards | 25% | 27% | NS |
| Duvan et al. [60] | 100 | 100 mg | From ET onwards | 29% | 40% | NS |

From Boomsma et al. [37].

been proposed but few have been shown to be effective in well-designed studies. Significant improvements in clinical pregnancy rates can be achieved by giving due attention to embryo transfer technique. However, the empirical use of adjuvant medical therapies during IVF treatment have not been shown to be effective, and may in some cases be detrimental. Subgroups of patients who may benefit from such therapies still need to be identified. In most cases, no clear cause for RIF will be found, and management should focus on optimizing all aspects of IVF therapy, preconceptional health and counseling the couple. With regard to the latter the chances of success achievable with IVF should be considered within the context of what nature can achieve following spontaneous conception (Figure 20.2).

# References

1. The European IVF-monitoring Program 2005 Assisted reproductive technology in Europe, 2001. Results generated from European registers by ESHRE. *Hum Reprod* 2005; **20**: 1158–76.

2. Boomsma CM, Kavelaars A, Eijkemans MJ *et al.* Endometrial secretion analysis identifies a cytokine profile predictive of pregnancy in IVF. *Hum Reprod* 2009; **24**: 1427–35.

3. Macklon NS, Geraedts JPM, Fauser BCJM. Conception to ongoing pregnancy: the 'black box' of early pregnancy loss. *Hum Reprod Update* 2002; **8**: 333–43.

4. Tan BK, Vandekerckhove P, Kennedy P, Keay SD. Investigation and current management of recurrent IVF treatment failure in the UK. *Br J Obstet Gynaecol* 2005; **112**: 773–80.

5. Templeton A, Morris JK, Parslow W. Factors that affect outcome of in-vitro fertilisation treatment. *Lancet* 1996; **348**: 1402–6.

6. Croucher CA, Lass A, Margara R, Winston RM. Predictive value of the results of a first in-vitro fertilization cycle on the outcome of subsequent cycles. *Hum Reprod* 1998; **13**: 403–8.

7. Garcia Velasco J, Sanchez E. Implantation failure. In NS Macklon, IA Greer, EAP Steegers (eds.), *Textbook of Periconceptional Medicine*. Informa, London: Informa Healthcare, 2009.

8. Aboulghar MA, Mansour RT, Serour GI. Controversies in the modern management of hydrosalpinx. *Hum Reprod Update* 1998; **4**: 882–90.

9. Johnson NP, Mak W, Sowter MC. Laparoscopic salpingectomy for women with hydrosalpinges enhances the success of IVF: a Cochrane review. *Hum Reprod* 2002; **17**: 543.

10. Strandell A, Lindhard A, Waldenstrom U, Thorburn J. Hydrosalpinx and IVF outcome: cumulative results after salpingectomy in a randomized controlled trial. *Human Reprod* 2001; **16**: 2403–10.

11. Strandell A. The patient with hydrosalpinx. In NS Macklon (ed.), *IVF in the Medically Complicated Patient: A Guide to Management*. London: Taylor and Francis.

12. Kontoravdis A, Makrakis E, Pantos K *et al.* Proximal tubal occlusion and salpingectomy result in similar improvement in in vitro fertilization outcome in patients with hydrosalpinx. *Fertil Steril* 2006; **86**: 1642–9.

13. Oliveira JB, Martins AM, Baruffi RL *et al.* Increased implantation and pregnancy rates obtained by placing the tip of the transfer catheter in the central area of the endometrial cavity. *Reprod Biomed Online* 2004; **9**: 435–41.

14. Pritts EA, Parker WH, Olive DL. Fibroids and infertility: an updated systematic review of the evidence. *Fertil Steril* 2009; **91**: 1215–23.

15. Coulam CB, Kay C, Jeyendran RS. Role of p53 codon 72 polymorphism in recurrent pregnancy loss. *Reprod Biomed Online* 2006; **12**: 378–82.

16. Bellver J, Soares SR, Alvarez C et al. The role of thrombophilia and thyroid autoimmunity in unexplained infertility, implantation failure and recurrent spontaneous abortion. Hum Reprod 2008; 23: 278–84.

17. Navot D, Scott RT, Droesch K et al. The window of embryo transfer and the efficiency of human conception in vitro. Fertil Steril 1991; 55: 114–18.

18. Wilcox AJ, Baird DD, Weinberg CR. Time of implantation of the conceptus and loss of pregnancy. New Engl J Med 1999; 340: 1796–9.

19. Dey SK, Lim H, Das SK et al. Molecular cues to implantation. Endocr Rev 2004; 25: 341–73.

20. Hoozemans DA, Schats R, Lambalk CB, Homburg R, Hompes PG. Human embryo implantation: current knowledge and clinical implications in assisted reproductive technology. Reprod Biomed Online 2004; 9: 692–715.

21. Talbi S, Hamilton AE, Vo KC et al. Molecular phenotyping of human endometrium distinguishes menstrual cycle phases and underlying biological processes in normo-ovulatory women. Endocrinology 2006; 147: 1097–121.

22. Mirkin S, Nikas G, Hsiu JG, Diaz J, Oehninger S. Gene expression profiles and structural/functional features of the peri-implantation endometrium in natural and gonadotropin-stimulated cycles. J Clin Endocrinol Metab 2004; 89: 5742–52.

23. Horcajadas JA, Riesewijk A, Polman J et al. Effect of controlled ovarian hyperstimulation in IVF on endometrial gene expression profiles. Mol Hum Reprod 2005; 11: 195–205.

24. Macklon NS, Van der Gaast MH, Hamilton AE et al. The effect of stimulation with recombinant FSH and GnRH antagonists on endometrial gene expression in the absence of luteal support. Reprod Sci 2008; 15: 357–65.

25. Van der Gaast MH, Macklon NS, Beier-Hellwig K et al. The feasibility of a less invasive method to assess endometrial maturation – comparison of simultaneously obtained uterine secretion and tissue biopsy. BJOG 2009; 116(2): 304–12.

26. Boomsma CM, Kavelaars A, Eijkemans MJC et al. 2009 Cytokine profiling in endometrial secretions: a non invasive window on endometrial receptivity. Reprod Biomed Online 2009; 18: 85–94.

27. Baart EB, Martini E, Eijkemans MJC et al. Milder ovarian stimulation for in vitro fertilization reduces aneuploidy in the human preimplantation embryo: a randomized controlled trial. Hum Reprod 2007; 22: 980–8.

28. Raziel A, Friedler S, Schachter M et al. Increased frequency of female partner chromosomal abnormalities in patients with high-order implantation failure after in vitro fertilization. Fertil Steril 2002; 78: 515–19.

29. Pehlivan T, Rubio C, Rodrigo L et al. Preimplantation genetic diagnosis by fluorescence in situ hybridization: clinical possibilities and pitfalls. J Soc Gynecol Investig 2003; 10: 315–22.

30. Los FJ, Van Opstal D, van den Berg C. The development of cytogenetically normal, abnormal and mosaic embryos: a theoretical model. Hum Reprod Update 2004; 10: 79–94.

31. Devroey P, Fauser BC. Preimplantation aneuploidy screening: a research tool for now. Lancet 2007; 370 (9604): 1985–6.

32. Mercader A, Garcia-Velasco JA, Escudero E et al. Clinical experience and perinatal outcome of blastocyst transfer after coculture of human embryos with human endometrial epithelial cells: a 5-year follow-up study. Fertil Steril 2003; 80: 1162–8.

33. Spandorfer SD, Pascal P, Parks J et al. Autologous endometrial coculture in patients with IVF failure: outcome of the first 1,030 cases. J Reprod Med 2004; 49: 463–7.

34. Sallam HN, Sadek SS, Agameya AF. Assisted hatching – a meta-analysis of randomized controlled trials. J Assist Reprod Genet 2003; 20: 332–42.

35. Dayal MB, Dubey A, Frankfurter D, Peak D, Gindoff PR. Second cycle: to hatch or not to hatch? Fertil Steril 2007; 88(3): 718–20.

36. Seif MM, Edi-Osagie EC, Farquhar C et al. Assisted hatching on assisted conception (IVF & ICSI). Cochrane Database Syst Rev 2006; 1: CD001894.

37. Boomsma CM, Macklon NS. What can the clinician do to improve implantation? Reprod Biomed Online 2006; 13: 845–55.

38. Simon C, Cano F, Valbuena D, Remohi J, Pellicer A. Clinical evidence for a detrimental effect on uterine receptivity of high serum oestradiol concentrations in high and normal responder patients. Hum Reprod 1995; 10: 2432–7.

39. Macklon NS, Fauser BC. Impact of ovarian hyperstimulation on the luteal phase. J Reprod Fertil 2000; 55: 101–8.

40. Macklon NS, Stouffer RL, Giudice LC, Fauser BC. The science behind 25 years of ovarian stimulation for in vitro fertilization. Endocr Rev 2006; 27: 170–207.

41. Devroey P, Bourgain C, Macklon NS, Fauser BC. Reproductive biology and IVF: ovarian stimulation and endometrial receptivity. Trends Endocrinol Metab 2004; 15: 84–90.

42. Ma Wg, Song H, Das SK, Paria BC, Dey SK. Estrogen is a critical determinant that specifies the duration of the window of uterine receptivity for implantation. Proc Natl Acad Sci USA 2003; 100: 2963–8.

43. Kolibianakis EM, Bourgain C, Papanikolaou EG et al. Prolongation of follicular phase by delaying hCG administration results in a higher incidence of endometrial advancement on the day of oocyte retrieval in GnRH antagonist cycles. Hum Reprod 2005; 20: 2453–6.

44. Fauser BC, Devroey P, Yen SS et al. Minimal ovarian stimulation for IVF: appraisal of potential benefits and drawbacks. Hum Reprod 1999; 14: 2681–6.

45. Fauser BC, Macklon NS. Medical approaches to ovarian stimulation for infertility. In JF Strauss, RL Barbieri (eds.), Yen and Jaffe's Reproductive Endocrinology. 5th edition. Philadelphia: Elsevier Saunders, 2004, pp. 965–1012.

46. Hohmann FP, Macklon NS, Fauser BC. A randomized comparison of two ovarian stimulation protocols with gonadotropin-releasing hormone (GnRH) antagonist cotreatment for in vitro fertilization commencing recombinant follicle-stimulating hormone on cycle day 2 or 5 with the standard long GnRH agonist protocol. J Clin Endocrinol Metab 2003; 88: 166–73.

47. Fanchin R, Righini C, Olivennes F et al. Uterine contractions at the time of embryo transfer alter pregnancy rates after in-vitro fertilization. Hum Reprod 1998; 13: 1968–74.

48. Buckett WM. A review and meta-analysis of prospective trials comparing different catheters used for embryo transfer. Fertil Steril 2006; 85: 728–34.

49. Coroleu B, Barri PN, Carreras O et al. The influence of the depth of embryo replacement into the uterine cavity on implantation rates after IVF: a controlled, ultrasound-guided study. Hum Reprod 2002; 17: 341–6.

50. Romundstad LB, Romundstad PR, Sunde A et al. Increased risk of placenta previa in pregnancies following IVF/ICSI; a comparison of ART and non-ART pregnancies in the same mother. Hum Reprod 2006; 21: 2353–8.

51. Buckett WM. A meta-analysis of ultrasound-guided versus clinical touch embryo transfer. Fertil Steril 2003; 80: 1037–41.

52. Liversedge NH, Turner A, Horner PJ et al. The influence of bacterial vaginosis on in-vitro fertilization and embryo implantation during assisted reproduction treatment. Hum Reprod 1999; 14: 2411–15.

53. Korn AP, Bolan G, Padian N et al. Plasma cell endometritis in women with symptomatic bacterial vaginosis. Obstet Gynecol 1995; 85: 387–90.

54. Salim R, Ben Shlomo I, Colodner R, Keness Y, Shalev E. Bacterial colonization of the uterine cervix and success rate in assisted reproduction: results of a prospective survey. Hum Reprod 2002; 17: 337–40.

55. Kuo HC, Hsu CC, Wang ST, Huang KE. Aspirin improves uterine blood flow in the peri-implantation period. J Formosan Med Assoc 1997; 96: 253–7.

56. Empson M, Lassere M, Craig J, Scott J. Prevention of recurrent miscarriage for women with antiphospholipid antibody or lupus anticoagulant. Cochrane Database System Rev 2005; 2: CD002859.

57. Di Nisio M, Peters L, Middeldorp S. Anticoagulants for the treatment of recurrent pregnancy loss in women without antiphospholipid syndrome. Cochrane Database System Rev 2005; 2: CD004734.

58. Stern C, Chamley L, Norris H, Hale L, Baker HW. A randomized, double-blind, placebo-controlled trial of heparin and aspirin for women with in vitro fertilization implantation failure and antiphospholipid or antinuclear antibodies. Fertil Steril 2003; 80: 376–83.

59. Rubinstein M, Marazzi A, Polak DF. Low-dose aspirin treatment improves ovarian responsiveness, uterine and ovarian blood flow velocity, implantation, and pregnancy rates in patients undergoing in vitro fertilization: a prospective, randomized, double-blind placebo-controlled assay. Fertil Steril 1999; 71: 825–9.

60. Duvan CI, Ozmen B, Satiroglu H, Atabekoglu CS, Berker B. Does addition of low-dose aspirin and/or steroid as a standard treatment in nonselected intracytoplasmic sperm injection cycles improve in vitro fertilization success? A randomized, prospective, placebo-controlled study. J Assist Reprod Genet 2006; 23: 15–21.

61. Pakkila M, Rasanen J, Heinonen S et al. Low-dose aspirin does not improve ovarian responsiveness or pregnancy rate in IVF and ICSI patients: a randomized, placebo-controlled double-blind study. Hum Reprod 2005; 20: 2211–14.

62. Urman B, Mercan R, Alatas C et al. Low-dose aspirin does not increase implantation rates in patients undergoing intracytoplasmic sperm injection: a prospective randomized study. J Assist Reprod Genet 2000; 17: 586–90.

63. Waldenstrom U, Hellberg D, Nilsson S. Low-dose aspirin in a short regimen as standard treatment in in vitro fertilization: a randomized, prospective study. Fertil Steril 2004; 81: 1560–4.

64. Daya S. Is there a benefit of low-dose aspirin in assisted reproduction? Curr Opin Obstet Gynecol 2006; 18: 313–18.

65. Coulam CB, Stern JJ, Soenksen DM, Britten S, Bustillo M. Comparison of pulsatility indices on the day of oocyte retrieval and embryo transfer. Hum Reprod 1995; 10: 82–4.

66. Battaglia C, Salvatori M, Maxia N et al. Adjuvant L-arginine treatment for in-vitro fertilization in poor responder patients. Hum Reprod 1999; 14: 1690–7.

67. Battaglia C, Regnani G, Marsella T et al. Adjuvant L-arginine treatment in controlled ovarian hyperstimulation: a double-blind, randomized study. Hum Reprod 2002; 17: 659–65.

68. Lee TH, Wu MY, Chen MJ *et al*. Nitric oxide is associated with poor embryo quality and pregnancy outcome in in vitro fertilization cycles. *Fertil Steril* 2004; **82**: 126–31.

69. Cole PA, Robinson CH. Mechanism and inhibition of cytochrome P-450 aromatase. *J Med Chemistry* 1990; **33**: 2933–42.

70. Goswami SK, Das T, Chattopadhyay R *et al*. A randomized single-blind controlled trial of letrozole as a low-cost IVF protocol in women with poor ovarian response: a preliminary report. *Hum Reprod* 2004; **19**: 2031–5.

71. Healey S, Tan SL, Tulandi T, Biljan MM. Effects of letrozole on superovulation with gonadotropins in women undergoing intrauterine insemination. *Fertil Steril* 2003; **80**: 1325–9.

72. Mitwally MF, Casper RF. Aromatase inhibition reduces gonadotrophin dose required for controlled ovarian stimulation in women with unexplained infertility. *Hum Reprod* 2003; **18**: 1588–97.

73. Mitwally MF, Casper RF. Aromatase inhibition reduces the dose of gonadotropin required for controlled ovarian hyperstimulation. *J Social Gynecol Invest* 2004; **11**: 406–15.

74. Luck MR, Jeyaseelan I, Scholes RA. Ascorbic acid and fertility. *Biol Reprod* 1995; **52**: 262–6.

75. Luck MR, Zhao Y. Identification and measurement of collagen in the bovine corpus luteum and its relationship with ascorbic acid and tissue development. *J Reprod Fertil* 1993; **99**: 647–52.

76. Griesinger G, Franke K, Kinast C *et al*. Ascorbic acid supplement during luteal phase in IVF. *J Assist Reprod Genet* 2002; **19**: 164–8.

77. Miyazaki S, Tanebe K, Sakai M *et al*. Interleukin 2 receptor gamma chain (gamma(c)) knockout mice show less regularity in estrous cycle but achieve normal pregnancy without fetal compromise. *Am J Reprod Immunol* 2002; **47**: 222–30.

78. Ledee-Bataille N, Bonnet-Chea K, Hosny G *et al*. Role of the endometrial tripod interleukin-18, -15, and -12 in inadequate uterine receptivity in patients with a history of repeated in vitro fertilization-embryo transfer failure. *Fertil Steril* 2005; **83**: 598–605.

79. Quenby S, Kalumbi C, Bates M, Farquharson R, Vince G. Prednisolone reduces preconceptual endometrial natural killer cells in women with recurrent miscarriage. *Fertil Steril* 2005; **84**: 980–4.

80. Boomsma CM, Eijkemans MJ, Keay SD, Macklon NS. Peri-implantation glucocorticoid administration for assisted reproductive technology cycles. *Cochrane Database System Rev* 2007; **1**: CD005996.

81. Empson M, Lassere M, Craig JC, Scott JR. Recurrent pregnancy loss with antiphospholipid antibody: a systematic review of therapeutic trials. *Obstetrics Gynecol* 2002; **99**: 135–44.

82. Geva E, Amit A, Lerner-Geva L *et al*. Prednisone and aspirin improve pregnancy rate in patients with reproductive failure and autoimmune antibodies: a prospective study. *Am J Reprod Immunol* 2000; **43**: 36–40.

83. Ando T, Suganuma N, Furuhashi M *et al*. Successful glucocorticoid treatment for patients with abnormal autoimmunity on in vitro fertilization and embryo transfer. *J Assist Reprod Genet* 1996; **13**: 776–81.

84. Rai R, Sacks G, Trew G. Natural killer cells and reproductive failure – theory, practice and prejudice. *Hum Reprod* 2005; **20**: 1123–6.

85. Lintsen AM, Pasker-de Jong PC, de Boer EJ *et al*. Effects of subfertility cause, smoking and body weight on the success rate of IVF. *Hum Reprod* 2005; **20**: 1867–75.

86. Younglai EV, Holloway AC, Foster WG. Environmental and occupational factors affecting fertility and IVF success. *Hum Reprod Update* 2005; **11**: 43–57.

87. Macklon NS (ed.) *IVF in the Medically Complicated Patient*. London: Taylor and Francis, 2005.

88. Zenzes MT, Krishnan S, Krishnan B, Zhang H, Casper RF. Cadmium accumulation in follicular fluid of women in in vitro fertilization-embryo transfer is higher in smokers. *Fertil Steril* 1995; **64**: 599–603.

89. Paszkowski T, Clarke RN, Hornstein MD. Smoking induces oxidative stress inside the Graafian follicle. *Hum Reprod* 2002; **17**: 921–5.

90. Zenzes MT, Wang P, Casper RF. Cigarette smoking may affect meiotic maturation of human oocytes. *Hum Reprod* 1995; **10**: 3213–17.

91. The Practice Committee of the American Society for Reproductive Medicine Smoking and Infertility. *Fertil Steril* 2006; **86**: S172–7.

92. Norman RJ, Clark AM. Obesity and reproductive disorders: a review. *Reprod Fertil Dev* 1998; **10**: 55–63.

93. Boxmeer JC, Brouns MM, Lindemans J *et al*. Folic acid treatment affects oocyte environment. *J Social Gynecol Invest* 2005; **12**: 24A.

94. Boxmeer JC, Smit M, Weber RFA *et al*. Seminal plasma cobalamin significantly correlates with sperm concentration. *J Social Gynecol Invest* 2006; **11**: 406–15.

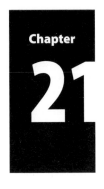

Chapter

21

# Trophoblast biology and early pregnancy

Peter R. Stone and Larry W. Chamley

## Introduction

Implantation of the embryo and establishment of the placenta takes place during the first trimester of pregnancy and placentation is tightly regulated, although we do not as yet have a full understanding of the relevant controls. Failure to establish normal placentation may result not only in embryonic/fetal compromise in early gestation but may also lead to poor outcomes later in gestation if the fetus is not provided with an adequate maternal blood supply. In addition, abnormal placentation may include excessive invasion into the myometrium. This chapter briefly examines the role of the unique cells of the placenta, the trophoblast, in the establishment of the placenta and the changes trophoblasts induce in the uterine environment.

## Implantation overview

The very earliest stages of human implantation are poorly documented due to lack of specimens and both ethical and practical constraints that prevent in vitro study of the first few days of implantation. Much of what we do know about early implantation is derived from the studies of early implantation sites that are mostly found in historical collections such as the Boyd collection, held in Cambridge, UK, and from analogy with other primate species [1]. Indeed, pre-eclampsia, a disease at least in part associated with abnormal placentation occurs in women and few non-human primates [2] and only studies in such species with hemochorial placentae are relevant to the human situation. For those interested in studying in greater detail early human implantation the outstanding monograph reporting the findings from the Boyd collection, despite its age, is still singularly useful [1].

Implantation commences with the hatched blastocyst attaching to the uterine wall at approximately 6 days post-conception. The blastocyst then burrows into the receptive uterine decidua and the uterine luminal epithelium heals over the implanted embryo. The trophectoderm of the blastocyst, now referred to as the trophoblast is thought to form a primary syncytiotrophoblast layer by fusion of adjacent cytotrophoblast cells at the pole of the blastocyst in direct contact with the decidua. This syncytiotrophoblast layer is non-proliferative and is expanded and regenerated by fusion of additional mononuclear cytotrophoblasts into the layer. The syncytiotrophoblast secretes enzymes that facilitate the further invasion of the newly forming placenta into the uterine decidua. As the trophoblast layer expands, it forms projections into the decidua which are referred to as trabeculae with gaps in the maternal tissue between the trabeculae being referred to as lacunae. This state is thought to persist only until about day 12 post-fertilization at which point the trabeculae are invaded by mononuclear cytotrophoblasts which form a layer on the embryonic side of the syncytiotrophoblast, giving rise to structures called primary villi. From this point on the trabeculae are referred to as villi and the lacunae between them as the intervillous space. During the next stage of villous development, cells of the extra-embryonic mesenchyme invade the primary villi to form a loose stromal core. These villi are now referred to as secondary villi. Then by approximately days 19–20 post-conception, vascular structures arise in the villi which are then termed tertiary villi. By the end of the third week after conception, a true arterio-capillary-venous circulation has developed and the fetal heart has commenced activity. New villous branches arise as the placenta expands, but for the remainder of the pregnancy the majority of villi are tertiary villi. Thus during the first trimester, most villi are characterized by an outer syncytiotrophoblast, underlain by an obvious villous cytotrophoblast layer and a minimally cellular stromal core containing a few

---

*Early Pregnancy*, ed. Roy G. Farquharson and Mary D. Stephenson. Published by Cambridge University Press.

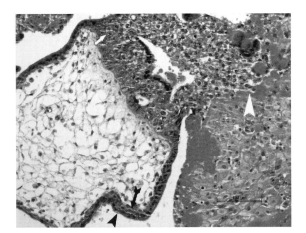

**Figure 21.1** An example of an anchoring villous from a first trimester placenta. The anchoring villous is on the left of the image with a column of extravillous cytotrophoblasts invading out of the villous (white arrows) and migrating toward the uterine decidua (white arrow head). The double layer of villous trophoblasts can be clearly seen with the syncytiotrophoblast facing the intervillous space (black arrowhead) and the villous cytotrophoblast on the fetal side (tailed black arrow). Hematoxylin and eosin stained.

fetal capillaries (Figure 21.1). At the same time as the villi are forming vasculogenesis begins in the extraembryonic mesoderm of the yolk sac, the connecting stalk and the chorion [1]. The early embryonic circulation has been visualized by Doppler ultrasound using transvaginal scanning [3]. These studies have shown detectable yolk sac circulation (blood flow velocities) by 5+ gestational weeks which declined to being undetectable again after 10 gestational weeks. During this period the umbilico-placental circulation was established with blood flow velocities increasing from a mean of 7.2 cm/s at 8 weeks to 13 cm/s at 10 weeks consistent with the placenta replacing the yolk sac as the major source of blood/nutrient supply to the embryo-fetus.

## Trophoblast invasion of the decidua

Throughout pregnancy the villi are covered by an essentially continuous layer of syncytiotrophoblast. However early in gestation, in structures known as anchoring villi (Figure 21.1), villous cytotrophoblasts breach the syncytiotrophoblast layer and form columns of migratory extravillous trophoblast which move away from the placenta spreading laterally around the implantation site to form the cytotrophoblastic shell which eventually completely encompasses the implantation site. More importantly from a functional point of view, these

extravillous trophoblasts invade both the maternal decidual stroma, and the decidual spiral arteries. Extravillous trophoblasts that invade the decidual stroma would appear to function to attach the placenta to the uterine wall but also assist in the transformation of the spiral arteries. These stromal (or interstitial) trophoblasts appear to migrate preferentially towards the spiral arteries and to be involved in the remodeling of the spiral artery walls [4]. It seems intuitively likely that the initial route of entry of the trophoblasts to the spiral artery lumens is via the decidual stroma. Endovascular trophoblasts occupy the lumen of the maternal spiral arteries and migrate deeper into the uterus as gestation progresses such that, in a normal pregnancy, by about 20 weeks' gestation the endovascular trophoblasts have migrated as far as one-third of the distance through the myometrium from the decidua/myometrial boundary [5]. The invasive trophoblasts that are associated with the spiral arteries perform two crucial tasks. Firstly, between them the endovascular and perivascular trophoblasts transform the spiral arteries from narrow-bore muscular vasoactive vessels that are capable of responding to maternal vasoconstrictive stimuli into larger flaccid vessels that are not responsive to maternal vasoconstricting signals [5]. This transformation of the spiral arteries is referred to as the "physiological changes of pregnancy" [5]. Transformation of the spiral arteries is achieved by digestion of the muscular wall of the vessels and digestion of the elastic lamina while endovascular trophoblasts replace the endothelial cells that line the spiral arteries. It appears that the invading extravillous trophoblasts are able to induce the death, by apoptosis (i.e. physiological cell death), of both the vascular endothelial cells and smooth muscle cells of the spiral arteries [6–9]. Using in vitro models, it has been shown that the invading trophoblasts induce vascular cell death by a combination of systems that induce apoptotic cell death including the Fas/Fas-ligand pathway, although other systems may also be involved [6,8]. In the same experimental model, invasive trophoblasts were shown to upregulate the expression of metalloproteinases which aid the digestion of the protein components of the spiral artery walls [7]. This transformation of the spiral arteries is essential to allow the massively increased blood supply that will be required by the fetus for growth during the second and third trimesters. Initially these observations of spiral artery transformation were determined following the examination of whole or biopsied implantation sites [1,5]. More recently, alterations in the uteroplacental blood flow, measured by Doppler ultrasound examinations, have confirmed these findings. By 11 post-menstrual weeks, uterine arterial Doppler signals may be reliably recorded and standards have been developed [10]. Gomez et al. [10] using transvaginal scanning between 11 and 14 weeks found that the greatest changes in pulsatility indices (fetal – umbilical and maternal – uterine) occurred at 13–14 weeks. This may be a biophysical correlate to the establishment of the early definitive placental circulation and increase in perfusion of the intervillous space. To date, uterine arterial Doppler velocimetry has not been shown to have sufficient predictive power to be a screen for later conditions of utero-placental vascular impairment, in the general population. Recent work combining 11–13 week and 20–24 week velocimetry has shown high detection rates for pre-eclampsia in a study group. Of interest the changes in pulsatility indices between 11–13[6] and 20–24[6] were also independently predictive of pre-eclampsia [11]. In that study [11] and in a prospective study of nulliparous women only [12], uterine artery Doppler velocimetry had higher predictive values for fetal growth restriction than pre-eclampsia, suggesting that in the latter condition an abnormal maternal response to the pregnancy occurs in addition to inadequate trophoblast invasion and decidual vascularization.

A second crucial function of endovascular trophoblasts is their formation of plugs in the spiral arteries. These trophoblast plugs prevent maternal red blood cells accessing the intervillous space in early pregnancy and dissipate between 10 and 12 gestational weeks [13,14]. These trophoblast plugs may act as pressure reducing valves isolating the delicate placenta from the full force of maternal arterial blood pressure although protection from high oxygen concentrations too early in placental development may be an equally, or more, important role of the trophoblast plugs since, prior to the dissipation of the trophoblast plugs, the placenta is not well equipped with the antioxidant systems that are required to protect the tissues from the oxidative damage that would be induced by the levels of oxygen present in arterial blood [15]. The presence of the trophoblast plugs means that during the first trimester the placenta develops normally in a physiologically low-oxygen environment. Despite the inability of maternal red cells to reach the placental surface during the 10–12 weeks of pregnancy, in their classic work, Boyd and Hamilton [1] demonstrated that the trophoblast plugs are loosely cohesive and allow the passage of maternal plasma through the spiral arteries (which they tracked by injection of Indian Ink into pregnant hysterectomy specimens). Thus, it seems likely that soluble material and subcellular particulate material could reach the placenta from the maternal circulation, albeit at a low rate, during the first trimester and further that due to the inflow of maternal plasma there is the clear possibility for this flow to facilitate the transport of material away from the placental site into the maternal circulation during early pregnancy. Outflow of material from the placenta/intervillous space into the maternal circulation may well be important for the development of maternal disease, particularly pre-eclampsia. Morphological studies indicating lack of maternal blood flow in the intervillous space during the first trimester have been confirmed by direct measurement of the oxygen content of the decidua and placentae of pregnancies about to undergo elective termination. These studies confirmed that oxygen levels rise from less than 20 mm Hg at 8 weeks to greater than 50 mm Hg at 12 weeks' gestation and that these changes in oxygenation of the placenta are accompanied by increases in expression of placental antioxidant systems that would protect the placental tissue from normal arterial blood oxygen levels [15].

# The consequences of failed transformation of the spiral arteries

Failure of the extravillous trophoblasts to invade adequately along the spiral arteries is associated with both pre-eclampsia [16–18] and intrauterine growth restriction [16], as well as later gestation pregnancy loss [19] but not early gestation sporadic miscarriage [20]. In early pregnancy, failure to transform the spiral arteries is associated with recurrent miscarriages in the presence of antiphospholipid antibodies [21] but evidence for this in women without these antibodies is less clear.

It is a widely held theory that failure of the spiral arteries to undergo the physiological changes of pregnancy is an underlying cause of pre-eclampsia. In essence the theory suggests that if the spiral arteries are not transformed then the placenta will become hypoxic and this hypoxic insult will, in due course, lead the placenta to produce an as-yet unknown factor which causes widespread activation of maternal vascular endothelial cells resulting in the symptoms of pre-eclampsia, especially hypertension. However, this theory is based largely on evidence from biopsies of the placental bed which is the region where the uterus is invaded by the trophoblasts containing the transformed spiral arteries. Since biopsies may not be truly representative of the entire placental bed they may give a misleading picture of the development, or lack of development, of the physiological changes in pre-eclampsia. Since the advent of ultrasound and in particular of Doppler ultrasound it has become increasingly apparent that there are many cases of preeclampsia in which there appears to be relatively normal uterine blood flow. This is especially the case where pre-eclampsia occurs late in pregnancy after 32 weeks' gestation and in addition to the low prevalence of pre-eclampsia in the general pregnant population this may explain the low predictive value of uterine arterial Doppler studies [22]. It has been proposed recently that an inherent defect in the trophoblast and trophoblast turnover may be responsible for the placental trigger for pre-eclampsia rather than a failure of the transformation of the spiral arteries in early and mid gestation [23]. The failure of transformation of the spiral arteries in pre-eclampsia is often presented overly simplistically as an all-or-none event in which either the depth of trophoblast invasion or the number of spiral arteries transformed is drastically reduced in pre-eclampsia compared with normal pregnancy. However, biology seldom works in such a black and white fashion and one group has shown that even in severe early-onset pre-eclampsia a spectrum of deficiencies in the extent of transformation of the spiral arteries occurs [24]. These authors also point to the problematic nature of studying biopsies of the placental bed since there was considerable variation in the extent of trophoblast invasion even within biopsies [24].

Thus while it is clear that inadequate transformation of the spiral arteries is associated with IUGR, it is now less certain that inadequate trophoblast invasion of these vessels contributes significantly to the pathogenesis of pre-eclampsia.

## The consequences of premature exposure of the placenta to maternal blood

Recent evidence suggests that premature exposure of the placenta to maternal blood is likely to result in miscarriage [25]. These workers, using Doppler ultrasound, demonstrated an increased flow of maternal blood to the placenta in missed miscarriage at 8–9 weeks' gestation compared with normal controls [25]. Further, this increased premature maternal blood flow to the placenta was distributed centrally and across the placenta whereas, in normal pregnancies, the maternal blood flow was more likely to be observed at the periphery of the placenta only [25,26].

## What allows/promotes trophoblast invasion?

As can be seen from the preceding discussion, appropriate invasion of the spiral arteries by trophoblasts is crucial to the establishment of normal pregnancy. Given this, one might expect that the factors controlling trophoblast invasion should be well established, yet we have, at best, a very poor understanding of these control mechanisms. This is in large part because human placentation, especially with regard to the extent/depth of trophoblast invasion of the spiral arteries is unique, with even closely related primates differing on these points. Therefore, much of what we do know about the controls of trophoblast invasion is derived from placental bed biopsies or in vitro examination of factors affecting primary placental cell and explant cultures, or from trophoblast-like cells including choriocarcinoma cell lines. It has long been debated which of these is the best model since many studies produce conflicting results on, for example, whether a particular growth factor does or does not promote trophoblast invasion. In a recent study [27] in which micro-arrays were used to determine similarities and differences between several widely used cell lines including the trophoblast cell lines SGHPL-5, HTR8/SVneo, ACH3P, the trophoblast-derived choriocarcinoma cell lines Jeg-3 and BeWo, and cultured primary cytotrophoblasts, it was clear that substantial differences existed in the expressed mRNAs between each of these cell types. The differences identified in this study clearly displayed the limitations imposed by our existing models. Bearing these limitations in mind numerous studies have examined the role of growth factors such as TGF-$\beta$ [28], activin [29] CSF-1 [30] and insulin-like growth factors [31] in regulating trophoblast proliferation and invasion (trophoblasts are usually considered to be able to either invade or proliferate but not both). However, often there are conflicting reports in the literature as to how these growth factors affect trophoblasts and frequently the inconsistencies in experimental results can be traced at least in part to the use of different experimental model systems.

Knock-out mouse models have also been used to try to elucidate the role of growth factors in controlling trophoblast behavior [32] but the dissimilarity of murine and human placentae means these studies, while very interesting, can not be extrapolated directly to the human situation [32].

While the mechanism of the control of the depth of invasion of trophoblasts into the human decidua remains unclear, abnormally deep implantation appears to be associated with thin or poorly formed decidua basalis which may occur where there has been previous uterine surgery such as curettage or cesarean section. Clinically, this results in a placenta that is abnormally adherent to the uterus where anchoring villi attach to the myometrium, instead of being confined to the decidua, and this condition is termed placenta accreta.

## Trophoblast deportation

Trophoblast deportation was first described by the German pathologist Schmorl in 1893 [33]. Schmorl found multinucleated fragments of syncytiotrophoblast, which are now referred to as syncytial knots, trapped in the pulmonary capillaries of women who had died of eclampsia. After Schmorl's initial report [33] it rapidly became apparent that syncytial knots were also deported in normal pregnancy, with the definitive study by Attwood and Park indicating that trophoblast deportation is readily detectable in most pregnancies but is exacerbated in pre-eclampsia/eclampsia [34]. It is now apparent that syncytial knots are derived from aged or damaged regions of the syncytiotrophoblasts which are extruded into the maternal blood. This is thought to be part of the normal life cycle of the trophoblast layer and is analogous to the shedding of skin or gut epithelia. Syncytial knots may vary in size up to several hundred micrometers and contain hundreds of nuclei (Figure 21.2) [35]. Syncytial knots are deported from the uteroplacental site via the draining veins. Since the majority of syncytial knots are too large to traverse through capillaries they become lodged in the first capillary bed they encounter, that is, in the maternal lungs. However, a few syncytial knots can pass through the lungs to enter the peripheral circulation and several groups have been able to harvest syncytial knots from maternal peripheral blood [36–39]. In addition to syncytial knots, mononuclear cytotrophoblasts are also shed from the placenta and can be harvested from the maternal blood. Since these smaller cells pass more

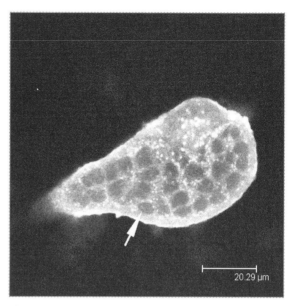

**Figure 21.2** A photomicrograph of a syncytial knot shed from a first trimester placenta. Multiple dark stained nuclei can be seen within the syncytial knot (one nucleus is indicated by the white arrow). The syncytial knot has been immunofluorescently stained with an antibody to cytokeratin, demonstrating trophoblastic nature of the knot (white staining). Image kindly provided by Dr Q Chen, University of Auckland.

readily through the maternal pulmonary capillaries they appear to be more abundant numerically in the maternal circulation [38,39]. Although one study reported the deported cytotrophoblasts to be villous rather than extravillous cytotrophoblasts, it would seem likely that at least some circulating mononuclear trophoblast might be derived from extravillous trophoblasts during the period in which the trophoblast plugs in the spiral arteries dissipate. Subcellular trophoblast micro and/or nano particles are also found in the maternal blood in both normal and pre-eclamptic pregnancies with possibly increased quantities in pre-eclampsia [40]. Trophoblast subcellular debris, micro and nanoparticles, are thought to be derived from the microvillous surface of the syncytiotrophoblast and importantly unlike larger deported trophoblast cells these subcellular remnants can pass freely through the maternal lungs to enter the peripheral circulation where they could affect many maternal physiological functions. Since the harvesting of trophoblasts from the peripheral blood is extremely challenging technically, we do not understand fully when trophoblast shedding and deportation commences. However, at least one study has shown trophoblasts in the peripheral blood of pregnant women as early as

6 weeks' gestation [36] and syncytial knots are certainly present in maternal blood late in the first and early second trimesters [37]. In a small unpublished study, we were able to isolate both syncytial knots and mononuclear trophoblasts from maternal blood at 12–14 weeks' gestation. Most studies of deported trophoblasts are aimed at harvesting these cells for diagnosis of fetal genetic abnormalities. However, deported trophoblasts have huge potential for diagnostic purposes not only of fetal genetic abnormalities, but also potentially for the prediction of placental pathologies since they may provide a "window" to assess, by virtue of their number or nature, the state of the placenta.

The physiological role of deported trophoblasts may not be limited to simply being a disposal system for aged and damaged trophoblasts. Deported trophoblasts may play a key role in the success of pregnancy via their effects on the maternal immune system. The fetus is genetically derived from two unrelated individuals, mother and father, and therefore those components that are encoded by paternal genes should, if they are different from the maternal gene products, be identified by the maternal immune system as immunologically foreign and rejected. Thus, the placenta is essentially a semiallogenic tissue graft and in the case of a donor embryo or donor oocyte pregnancy the fetus and placenta are true allografts, similar in many respects to any other tissue graft. A question which has intrigued reproductive immunologists for nearly a century is: "Why is the fetal allograft not rejected by the maternal immune system?" Deported trophoblasts may be part of the answer to this question. It is now well established that apoptotic cells (that is, cells that have died via programmed cell death) when phagocytosed induce an anti-inflammatory or immunosuppressive type of immune response, regardless of whether the cells are derived from the host organism or are allogeneic (foreign) [41]. Thus, phagocytosis of apoptotic deported trophoblasts may lead to tolerization of the maternal immune system to paternally derived proteins from placenta. In support of this hypothesis, we have recently shown, that when macrophages phagocytose apoptotic trophoblasts shed from placental explants in vitro, the macrophages increased their secretion of anti-inflammatory IL-10 and decreased secretion of proinflammatory IL-1β [42]. The macrophages also increased their production of the tryptophan metabolizing enzyme, indoleamine 2–3 dioxygenase, which would also be likely to have an antigen-specific tolerizing effect on maternal T cells [42]. In stark contrast, when necrotic trophoblasts are phagocytosed, endothelial cells become activated [43]. Thus deported trophoblasts, dying physiologically, in a normal pregnancy are hypothesized to tolerize the maternal immune system to paternally derived antigens, but deported trophoblasts dying by necrosis, following a placental insult, may lead to pathological activation of the maternal endothelium, as is seen in pre-eclampsia.

## Effects of trisomies and other genetic abnormalities on trophoblasts

The long history of maternal serum screening for aneuploidy illustrates that trophoblastic cellular function is affected by aneuploidy and potentially by genetic abnormalities.

The majority of very early miscarriages are associated with aneuploidy although this is not always the case in recurrent miscarriage [44]; non-aneuploid losses are unlikely to be due to defective trophoblast invasion or spiral arterial transformation as no differences between aneuploid or euploid conceptions were found in a study of the pathology of early embryonic demise [20].

In addition to abnormal first-trimester marker levels predicting outcome in threatened miscarriage [45], abnormal levels of pregnancy associated placental protein A (PAPP-A) in euploid conceptions are associated with subsequent poor obstetric outcomes such as pregnancy loss, pre-term birth or fetal growth restriction [46] but such markers have insufficient predictive power to be individually useful as screening tests for these conditions.

Confined placental mosaicism (CPM) is a complex situation where aneuploidy exists in the trophoblast (cytotrophoblast – CPM type I, villous stroma – CPM type II or both cytotrophoblast and villous stroma – type III) and depending on the chromosomes involved may be associated with normal or abnormal fetal outcomes. Confined placental mosaicism may occur in around 2% of villous samples obtained at chorionic villus sampling in the first trimester [47]. The outcomes in CPM may be chromosome specific but CPM of meiotic origin involving chromosomes 2, 7 or 16 is associated with poor outcomes including pregnancy loss, fetal growth restriction or intrauterine death.

# Heparin and aspirin in in vitro models

Antiphospholipid antibodies (aPL) are the single largest identifiable, non-genetic cause of recurrent pregnancy losses, accounting for approximately 20% of cases of recurrent miscarriage. These antibodies are associated with thrombotic disease of the systemic circulation and were originally thought to induce recurrent miscarriage by causing thrombosis of the spiral arteries with subsequent infarction of the regions of the placenta supplied by the affected vessels. Based on this hypothetical mechanism of action, heparin and aspirin therapy was introduced for women with recurrent miscarriage and aPL. While not all trials confirm the utility of heparin and/or aspirin [48–50] other trials do suggest the clinical efficacy of this treatment [51]. However, it has become apparent that aPL do not induce recurrent miscarriage by a thrombotic mechanism and several in vitro studies have shown that these antibodies can disrupt a variety of normal functions carried out by trophoblasts during implantation and early pregnancy including proliferation, invasion and hormone secretion (reviewed in [52] and [53]). Likewise, several studies have shown that heparin (which is now known to have multiple functions unrelated to its effects on coagulation such as activating or sequestering growth factors/regulators), and/or aspirin, can reverse these adverse effects of aPL on trophoblasts in vitro [54–56]. However, it must be noted that in the absence of aPL, heparin may have adverse effects on trophoblast invasion in vitro [57].

# Conclusions

Trophoblasts, and particularly their invasion of the uterus, are key to developing a healthy placenta and therefore, fetus. Our understanding of the very early stages of implantation, as well as of the factors that control trophoblast invasion remain limited despite intensive investigations. Much work remains to be done before we understand the processes involved in establishment of the placenta in normal pregnancy and how these processes are disrupted in diseased pregnancies. Only with a fuller understanding of these processes will we be able to develop better diagnostics and therapies for conditions such as recurrent miscarriage and intrauterine growth restriction, the pathogenesis of which are routed, at least in part, in abnormal trophoblast behavior.

# References

1. Boyd JD, Hamilton WJ. *The Human Placenta*. Cambridge, MA: W Heffer and Sons, 1970.

2. Wulff C, Weigand M, Kreienberg R, Fraser HM. Angiogenesis during primate placentation in health and disease. *Reproduction* 2003; **126**: 569–77.

3. Makikallio K, Tekay A, Jouppila P. Yolk sac and umbilicoplacental hemodynamics during early human embryonic development. *Ultrasound Obstet Gynecol* 1999; **14**: 175–9.

4. Frank HG, Kaufmann P. Nonvillous parts and trophoblast invasion. In K Benirschke, P Kaufmann, R Baergen (eds.), *Pathology of the Human Placenta*. 5th edition.. New York: Springer, 2006, pp. 191–312.

5. Brosens I, Robertson WB, Dixon HG. The physiological response of the vessels of the placental bed to normal pregnancy. *J Pathol Bacteriol* 1967; **93**: 569–79.

6. Harris LK, Keogh RJ, Wareing M *et al.* Invasive trophoblasts stimulate vascular smooth muscle cell apoptosis by a fas ligand-dependent mechanism. *Am J Pathol* 2006; **169**: 1863–74.

7. Harris LK, Keogh RJ, Wareing M *et al.* BeWo cells stimulate smooth muscle cell apoptosis and elastin breakdown in a model of spiral artery transformation. *Hum Reprod* 2007; **22**: 2834–41.

8. Keogh RJ, Harris LK, Freeman A *et al.* Fetal-derived trophoblast use the apoptotic cytokine tumor necrosis factor-alpha-related apoptosis-inducing ligand to induce smooth muscle cell death. *Circ Res* 2007; **100**: 834–41.

9. Chen Q, Stone PR, McCowan LM, Chamley LW. Interaction of Jar choriocarcinoma cells with endothelial cell monolayers. *Placenta* 2005; **26**: 617–25.

10. Gomez O, Figueras F, Martinez JM *et al.* Sequential changes in uterine artery blood flow pattern between the first and second trimesters of gestation in relation to pregnancy outcome. *Ultrasound Obstet Gynecol* 2006; **28**: 802–8.

11. Plasencia W, Maiz N, Poon L, Yu C, Nicolaides KH. Uterine artery Doppler at 11 + 0 to 13 + 6 weeks and 21 + 0 to 24 + 6 weeks in the prediction of pre-eclampsia. *Ultrasound Obstet Gynecol* 2008; **32**: 138–46.

12. Groom KM, North RA, Stone PR *et al.* Patterns of change in uterine artery Doppler studies between 20 and 24 weeks of gestation and pregnancy outcomes. *Obstet Gynecol* 2009; **113**: 332–8.

13. Foidart JM, Hustin J, Dubois M, Schaaps JP. The human placenta becomes haemochorial at the 13th week of pregnancy. *Int J Dev Biol* 1992; **36**: 451–3.

14. Jauniaux E, Watson A, Burton G. Evaluation of respiratory gases and acid-base gradients in human fetal fluids and uteroplacental tissue between 7 and 16 weeks' gestation. *Am J Obstet Gynecol* 2001; **184**: 998–1003.

15. Jauniaux E, Watson AL, Hempstock J et al. Onset of maternal arterial blood flow and placental oxidative stress. A possible factor in human early pregnancy failure. *Am J Pathol* 2000; **157**: 2111–22.

16. Khong TY, De Wolf F, Robertson WB, Brosens I. Inadequate maternal vascular response to placentation in pregnancies complicated by pre-eclampsia and by small-for-gestational age infants. *Br J Obstet Gynaecol* 1986; **93**: 1049–59.

17. Robertson WB, Brosens I, Dixon HG. The pathological response of the vessels of the placental bed to hypertensive pregnancy. *J Pathol Bacteriol* 1967; **93**: 581–92.

18. Naicker T, Khedun SM, Moodley J, Pijnenborg R. Quantitative analysis of trophoblast invasion in preeclampsia. *Acta Obstet Gynecol Scand* 2003; **82**: 722–9.

19. Ball E, Bulmer JN, Ayis S, Lyall F, Robson SC. Late sporadic miscarriage is associated with abnormalities in spiral artery transformation and trophoblast invasion. *J Pathol* 2006; **208**: 535–42.

20. Ball E, Robson SC, Ayis S, Lyall F, Bulmer JN. Early embryonic demise: no evidence of abnormal spiral artery transformation or trophoblast invasion. *J Pathol* 2006; **208**: 528–34.

21. Sebire NJ, Fox H, Backos M et al. Defective endovascular trophoblast invasion in primary antiphospholipid antibody syndrome-associated early pregnancy failure. *Hum Reprod* 2002; **17**: 1067–71.

22. Chien PF, Arnott N, Gordon A, Owen P, Khan KS. How useful is uterine artery Doppler flow velocimetry in the prediction of pre-eclampsia, intrauterine growth retardation and perinatal death? An overview. *BJOG* 2000; **107**: 196–208.

23. Huppertz B. Placental origins of preeclampsia: challenging the current hypothesis. *Hypertension* 2008; **51**: 970–5.

24. Meekins JW, Pijnenborg R, Hanssens M, McFadyen IR, van Asshe A. A study of placental bed spiral arteries and trophoblast invasion in normal and severe pre-eclamptic pregnancies. *Br J Obstet Gynaecol* 1994; **101**: 669–74.

25. Jauniaux E, Hempstock J, Greenwold N, Burton GJ. Trophoblastic oxidative stress in relation to temporal and regional differences in maternal placental blood flow in normal and abnormal early pregnancies. *Am J Pathol* 2003; **162**: 115–25.

26. Jauniaux E, Greenwold N, Hempstock J, Burton GJ. Comparison of ultrasonographic and Doppler mapping of the intervillous circulation in normal and abnormal early pregnancies. *Fertil Steril* 2003; **79**: 100–6.

27. Lash GE, Ansari T, Bischof P et al. IFPA meeting 2008 workshops report. *Placenta* 2009; 30: S4–S14.

28. Caniggia I, Grisaru-Gravnosky S, Kuliszewsky M, Post M, Lye SJ. Inhibition of TGF-beta 3 restores the invasive capability of extravillous trophoblasts in preeclamptic pregnancies. *J Clin Invest* 1999; **103**: 1641–50.

29. Caniggia I, Lye SJ, Cross JC. Activin is a local regulator of human cytotrophoblast cell differentiation. *Endocrinology* 1997; **138**: 3976–86.

30. Hamilton GS, Lysiak JJ, Watson AJ, Lala PK. Effects of colony stimulating factor-1 on human extravillous trophoblast growth and invasion. *J Endocrinol* 1998; **159**: 69–77.

31. Hamilton GS, Lysiak JJ, Han VK, Lala PK. Autocrine-paracrine regulation of human trophoblast invasiveness by insulin-like growth factor (IGF)-II and IGF-binding protein (IGFBP)-1. *Exp Cell Res* 1998; **244**: 147–56.

32. Constancia M, Hemberger M, Hughes J et al. Placental-specific IGF-II is a major modulator of placental and fetal growth. *Nature* 2002; **417**: 945–8.

33. Schmorl G. *Pathologisch-Anatomische Untersuchungen Uber Puerperal-Eklampsie.* Verlag von FC Vogel: Leipzig, 1893.

34. Attwood HD, Park WW. Embolism to the lungs by trophoblast. *J Obstet Gynaecol Br Commonw* 1961; **68**: 611–17.

35. Abumaree MH, Stone PR, Chamley LW. An in vitro model of human placental trophoblast deportation/shedding. *Mol Hum Reprod* 2006; **12**: 687–94.

36. Covone AE, Mutton D, Johnson PM, Adinolfi M. Trophoblast cells in peripheral blood from pregnant women. *Lancet* 1984; **2**: 841–3.

37. Hawes CS, Suskin HA, Petropoulos A, Latham SE, Mueller UW. A morphologic study of trophoblast isolated from peripheral blood of pregnant women. *Am J Obstet Gynecol* 1994; **170**: 1297–300.

38. Johansen M, Redman CW, Wilkins T, Sargent IL. Trophoblast deportation in human pregnancy – its relevance for pre-eclampsia. *Placenta* 1999; **20**: 531–9.

39. Chua S, Wilkins T, Sargent I, Redman C. Trophoblast deportation in pre-eclamptic pregnancy. *Br J Obstet Gynaecol* 1991; **98**: 973–9.

40. Knight M, Redman CW, Linton EA, Sargent IL. Shedding of syncytiotrophoblast microvilli into the maternal circulation in pre-eclamptic pregnancies. *Br J Obstet Gynaecol* 1998; **105**: 632–40.

41. Bittencourt MC, Perruche S, Contassot E et al. Intravenous injection of apoptotic leukocytes enhances bone marrow engraftment across major histocompatibility barriers. *Blood* 2001; **98**: 224–30.

42. Abumaree MH, Stone PR, Chamley LW. The effects of apoptotic, deported human placental trophoblast on macrophages: possible consequences for pregnancy. *J Reprod Immunol* 2006; **72**: 33–45.

43. Chen Q, Stone PR, McCowan LM, Chamley LW. Phagocytosis of necrotic but not apoptotic trophoblasts

induces endothelial cell activation. *Hypertension* 2006; **47**: 116–21.

44. Sullivan AE, Silver RM, LaCoursiere DY, Porter TF, Branch DW. Recurrent fetal aneuploidy and recurrent miscarriage. *Obstet Gynecol* 2004; **104**: 784–8.

45. Johns J, Muttukrishna S, Lygnos M, Groome N, Jauniaux E. Maternal serum hormone concentrations for prediction of adverse outcome in threatened miscarriage. *Reprod Biomed Online* 2007; **15**: 413–21.

46. Barrett SL, Bower C, Hadlow NC. Use of the combined first-trimester screen result and low PAPP-A to predict risk of adverse fetal outcomes. *Prenat Diagn* 2008; **28**: 28–35.

47. Robinson WP, Barrett IJ, Bernard L *et al.* Meiotic origin of trisomy in confined placental mosaicism is correlated with presence of fetal uniparental disomy, high levels of trisomy in trophoblast, and increased risk of fetal intrauterine growth restriction. *Am J Hum Genet* 1997; **60**: 917–27.

48. Farquharson RG, Quenby S, Greaves M. Antiphospholipid syndrome in pregnancy: a randomized, controlled trial of treatment. *Obstet Gynecol* 2002; **100**: 408–13.

49. Pattison NS, Chamley LW, Birdsall M *et al.* Does aspirin have a role in improving pregnancy outcome for women with the antiphospholipid syndrome? A randomized controlled trial. *Am J Obstet Gynecol* 2000; **183**: 1008–12.

50. Laskin CA, Spitzer KA, Clark CA *et al.* Low molecular weight heparin and aspirin for recurrent pregnancy loss: results from the randomized, controlled HepASA trial. *J Rheumatol* 2009; **36**: 279–87.

51. Rai R, Cohen H, Dave M, Regan L. Randomised controlled trial of aspirin and aspirin plus heparin in pregnant women with recurrent miscarriage associated with phospholipid antibodies (or antiphospholipid antibodies). *Br Med J* 1997; **314**: 253–7.

52. Chamley LW. Antiphospholipid antibodies: biological basis and prospects for treatment. *J Reprod Immunol* 2002; **57**: 185–202.

53. Di Simone N, Luigi MP, Marco D *et al.* Pregnancies complicated with antiphospholipid syndrome: the pathogenic mechanism of antiphospholipid antibodies: a review of the literature. *Ann N Y Acad Sci* 2007; **1108**: 505–14.

54. Bose P, Black S, Kadyrov M *et al.* Adverse effects of lupus anticoagulant positive blood sera on placental viability can be prevented by heparin in vitro. *Am J Obstet Gynecol* 2004; **191**: 2125–31.

55. Bose P, Black S, Kadyrov M *et al.* Heparin and aspirin attenuate placental apoptosis in vitro: implications for early pregnancy failure. *Am J Obstet Gynecol* 2005; **192**: 23–30.

56. Di Simone N, Caliandro D, Castellani R *et al.* Low-molecular weight heparin restores in-vitro trophoblast invasiveness and differentiation in presence of immunoglobulin G fractions obtained from patients with antiphospholipid syndrome. *Hum Reprod* 1999; **14**: 489–95.

57. Ganapathy R, Whitley GS, Cartwright JE, Dash PR, Thilaganathan B. Effect of heparin and fractionated heparin on trophoblast invasion. *Hum Reprod* 2007; **22**: 2523–7.

235

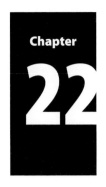

# Implantation failure: an embryologist's view

Dominique Royère and Etienne Van den Abbeel

## Introduction

Failed implantation is one of the most difficult challenges for clinicians and embryologists involved in assisted reproductive technologies (ART). Besides some irrational attitudes which might lead a clinician to consider such failure as the embryologist's failure or vice versa, or both to consider failed implantation as a definitely unsolved question, the "embryologist's view" might focus on which factors might impair implantation at the level of the embryo and its close environment, while factors involved in the implantation process itself (dialog between embryo and endometrium) are considered elsewhere in this book. In this chapter we consider how far genetic abnormalities or morphological characteristics may impair or favor implantation, then review the main strategies usually proposed to counteract implantation failure, while new approaches for non-invasive embryo quality assessment will be presented as perspectives, since they need clinical validation. Alternatives for recurrent implantation failure will finally be briefly discussed.

## Genetic abnormalities

Following the extensive use of preimplantation genetic aneuploidy screening, the possible link between recurrent implantation failure and an increased aneuploidy rate was thoroughly assessed and confirmed by many studies [1]. However almost no studies confirmed that aneuploidy screening was able to improve the chances of implantation in recurrent implantation failure [2] while most studies lacked an adequate control group. So far only one randomized controlled trial has been reported but with a very low size sample and no benefit on clinical outcome [3]. The impact of larger-scale analysis using comparative genomic hybridization, the higher frequency of post-zygotic errors in recurrent

implantation failure as compared with recurrent miscarriage or advanced maternal age and its possible link with some intrinsic mechanism to the embryo rather to any abnormality in parental meiosis remain to be further studied [4,5]. Interestingly one of the two randomized controlled trials concerning the assessment of pre-implantation genetic diagnosis (PIGD) for advanced maternal age mentioned an increased proportion (65%) of euploid embryos able to reach the blastocyst stage, while combined abnormalities were mainly excluded by such a development [6].

## Morphological characteristics

Despite their limited contribution to predict both further development and implantation of the embryo, the morphological and kinetic assessment of early and later embryo development as well as oocyte assessment before fertilization remain most widely used in clinical embryology (Figure 22.1).

## Early embryo development

### Embryo morphology at days 2/3

Early embryo development has been the focus of attention from the beginning of ART for several reasons, including the efficacy of transfer of embryos at days 2 or 3, and the increase in multifollicular stimulations that are imposed to select the embryo(s) for transfer with the best accuracy. Based on unique or homogeneous transfers or on various scores, many studies have confirmed how both number and size of the blastomeres and the proportion of exudates might influence the implantation rate [7,8]; 4–5-cell embryos at day 2 (Figure 22.1B) and 6–8-cell embryos at day 3 with a low rate or absence of fragmentation, and without any multinucleated blastomere, have the highest chances of implantation.

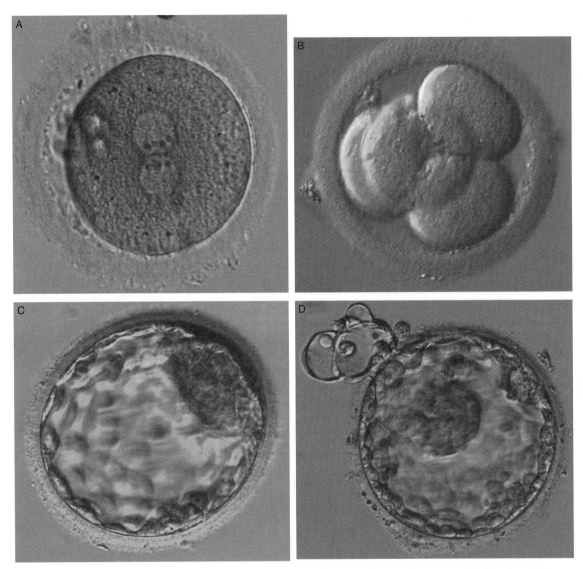

**Figure 22.1** Morphological aspects of pre-implantation embryo: A. "Typical" pattern of zygote adjacent pronuclei aligned nucleolar precursor bodies. B. Day 2 embryo with four equal-sized cells, each with a unique interphase nucleus, without cytoplasmic exudate. C. Expanded day 5 blastocyst, with a dense and continue monolayer of trophectoderm cells, a compact and cohesive inner cell mass. D. Day 5 hatching blastocyst.

Later videomicrographic studies have addressed the importance of kinetics in embryo development particularly concerning the presence of cytoplasmic exudates [9].

## Zygote and early cleavage assessment

Pronuclei observation is available using non-invasive simple optical microscopy (Figure 22.1A). Assembling, growth and fusion between nucleolar precursor bodies (NPB) are stages of early nucleogenesis following a chronology described for human zygotes [10]. A day-1 score integrating the location of pronuclei, both position and number of NPB, cytoplasmic halo and early cleavage was correlated with the rate of implantation for transferred embryos and later simplified for routine use [11,12]. A different method of zygote scoring, assessing NPB number and polarization, pronuclei size and respective position was related to developmental ability of the issued embryos with a particular emphasis on pronuclei synchrony [13]. Using a simplified approach derived from this last classification, an individual follow-up of more than 4000 embryos allowed us to relate the typical pattern of zygotes with the highest probability for an embryo to reach the blastocyst stage as opposed to non-typical zygote patterns [14]. Other classifications were later proposed, which brought similar results. Cytoplasmic halo [15] and early cleavage [16–18] were proposed as additional criteria, while this last criterion is less debated [14]. The link between early cleavage and embryo developmental ability has to be elucidated; better nucleocytoplasmic synchronization with lower risk for critical level of maternal RNA before genomic activation [19] as well as paternal contribution for first cell cycle and some key events in metabolism [20] have been hypothesized which might at least partly explain this link.

### Oocyte characteristics before fertilization

Legal constraints may in some way stimulate the research concerning additional criteria, when embryo freezing is forbidden (for example in Germany and Switzerland) as opposed to zygote freezing, but also when the number of oocytes is strictly limited (Italy). Assessment of the second metaphase spindle based on its spontaneous fluorescence under polarized light was reported as a valuable tool to select oocyte for fertilization and further development, while anisotropy of the zona pellucida was also proposed as an additional tool for oocyte selection [21–24].

## Late embryo development

### Extended culture to the blastocyst stage

While transferring human embryos at the blastocyst stage appeared the best strategy, its use did not really expand before cocultures, then sequential media, were proposed to sustain it. Beside the natural arrival and implantation of the blastocyst into the uterus, another reason to promote such a strategy was based on the timing of embryo genomic activation in our species, which lasts between 4- and 8-cell stages [25]. Morphological criteria (Figure 22.1C, D) including the size of the blastocoelic cavity, density and continuity of trophectodermal cells, density and cohesiveness of the inner cell mass were clearly related with higher implantation potential [14,26]. Whether blastocyst transfer should be preferred to day 2/3 embryo transfer remains a matter of debate [27,28], even though about half of the day 2/3 embryos will be unable to reach the blastocyst stage. Such embryo leakage was partly explained by chromosomal abnormalities, unadapted genome expression,

suboptimal culture conditions or inadequate oocyte maturation [29].

### Reaching the blastocyst stage: an additional criteria?

While the debate about blastocysts is still open, several observations may argue for its impact on further development and implantation of the embryo. Firstly, the increase in euploidy rate for embryos reaching the blastocyst stage as compared with those arresting their development was already underlined [6], even if mosaics, some mono or trisomies were not concerned by this development arrest. Then hierarchical analysis brought a limited value to morphological parameters of early embryo development (area under the curve 0.688) to predict the ability to reach the blastocyst stage. However, once the blastocyst stage is achieved, implantation rates remain similar whatever the initial criteria of early development [14], since none of these criteria could discriminate between implanting and non-implanting blastocysts.

## Strategies aimed at overcoming implantation failure

We will consider successively blastocyst transfer, assisted hatching, transfer media, co-cultures, cytoplasmic transfer and zygote intra-fallopian transfer.

## Blastocyst transfer

Few studies have reported on this topic. A prospective randomized study reported on a higher pregnancy rate following blastocyst transfer after at least three previous failed day 2/3 embryo transfers, but the number of patients was too small to be statistically significant [30]. Another prospective non-randomized study that included larger groups (147 for day 2 versus 129 for day 5/6 respectively) reported on both higher clinical pregnancy and implantation rates following blastocyst transfer in failed implantations [31].

## Assisted hatching

Artificial disruption of the zona pellucida has been proposed as a method to overcome hatching difficulties as a possible explanation for implantation failure. One meta-analysis including 23 RCTs did not draw any difference with controls among the six RCTs assessing the live-birth rate as the endpoint (OR 1.33, 95% CI 0.81–1.73), whereas clinical pregnancy rate was increased (OR 1.33, 95% CI 1.12–1.57) among the 23 RCTs [32]. Therefore the conclusion was that there is insufficient evidence to recommend assisted hatching.

## Transfer medium

The impact of adding recombinant hyaluronan and albumin (HA) was assessed in an RCT including 103 patients with repeated implantation failures [33]. An increase in implantation rate was reported (16.3% vs 4.8%) which argued for a beneficial effect of adding HA to the transfer medium. Such a result has to be confirmed before any conclusion might be made.

## Coculture

Attempts to circumvent the suboptimal culture conditions as factors associated with poor success rates in human IVF were done in the early 1990s using co-cultures of embryos with epithelial cell lines. However safety constraints led to the discarding of any non-human cell lines for coculture, while new media were developed to sustain embryo development beyond day 2/3. Later trials using human autologous cells (mainly endometrial cells but also granulosa or cumulus cells) claimed for a beneficial effect of such a coculture to improve implantation rates. However RCTs involving autologous cells are lacking to allow any definite conclusion, whereas the recently published meta-analysis combined both heterologous and autologous support of coculture to draw its conclusion [34].

## Cytoplasmic transfer

The possibility to alleviate the 2-cell block by transfer of cytoplasm was performed in mice during the early 1980s. The first human pregnancy following the transfer of cytoplasm from donor oocytes into the oocytes of a patient with a history of poor embryo development and recurrent implantation failure was reported in 1997. Since then more births have been reported following cytoplasmic transfer in human in the early 2000s, however potential risks of mitochondrial heteroplasmy, mitochondrial disease, nuclear–mitochondrial interaction and epigenetic changes have been stressed [35,36] therefore restraining this technique to an experimental procedure.

## Zygote intra-fallopian transfer

The literature remains controversial about the benefit, if any, of zygote intra-fallopian transfer (ZIFT). Following some optimistic reports several RCTs have failed to demonstrate any advantage for ZIFT in recurrent implantation failure [37].

# Perspectives: functional approaches of developmental competence of the oocyte/embryo

As in many fields of human pathology, "omics" techniques have been applied in recent years in the field of implantation and embryo development. Beside direct investigations on oocyte or embryo, which belong to an experimental approach due to their invasiveness, other non-invasive approaches based on oocyte: embryo environment might have a clinical input on our practice.

## Direct "omics" approaches on oocyte or embryo

### Transcriptional analysis of embryos

First experimental large-scale transcriptional analysis was reported in cattle [38], with several genes identified with an expression level related with implantation failure (e.g. TNFα), ongoing gestation (e.g. CDX2), or both implantation and ongoing gestation (TXN thioredoxin). Similar strategies were applied to human blastocysts with trophectoderm biopsies [39]. Genes involved in adhesion or cellular communication were identified as their expression was related with implantation.

### Proteomic analysis

This technique was applied at the level of the embryo itself [40] as well as its own environmental medium [41,42], in the two latter studies with perspectives to relate a protein profile in the medium with embryo viability in a non-invasive manner.

## Metabolomic analysis

While embryo metabolism was experimentally studied for a long time to define its metabolic requirements, more recent studies have focused on embryo respirometry [43,44] to better define embryo quality. Despite their value in terms of knowledge, their use in clinical embryology remains questionable. Recent approaches based on various techniques of spectroscopy (Raman, Near InfraRed) were applied to culture media with promising results through viability scores deduced from such metabolomic profiles [45].

# Indirect approaches on oocyte or embryo environment

## Cytokines or hormones in the follicular fluid

Various components in the follicular fluid were studied as a function of oocyte follow-up. In this way anti-Mullerian hormone (AMH) levels in the dominant follicle were related with both implantation and ongoing pregnancy rates [46]. Recently the follicular level of the granulocyte colony stimulating factor (G-CSF) was related with the developmental potential of the oocyte issued from that follicle [47]. Such interesting results need to be confirmed in a prospective study.

## Transcriptomic analysis of cumulus cells

This non-invasive indirect approach is based on the oocyte–cumulus dialog as a key event of oocyte maturation. Such dialog not only involves metabolic synergy between both compartments [48] but also gene expression at the level of granulosa/cumulus cells [49]. The possibility to integrate some granulosa/cumulus cell genetic markers in oocyte/embryo selection needs further clinical validation.

# Concluding remarks

It is difficult at the present time to say which parameters among all the criteria presented in this review will be robust enough (simple, non-invasive, reproducible, with a reasonable cost) to be used in a clinical embryology routine. Such evaluations will progress in parallel with knowledge on the implantation process on the endometrium side, keeping in mind that the best embryo does not fulfill all the superlatives (most rapid, most energy consuming …) but rather some precise and stressless pattern of genomic, proteic and metabolic activity in a "quiet embryo" hypothesis [50]. Alternatives to recurrent implantation failure like oocyte or sperm donation may be proposed to patients, keeping in mind that with the exception of identified genetic abnormalities, developmental or implantation failure may involve the male or female partner as well, while discriminative studies on that subject are presently lacking.

# References

1. Donoso P, Staessen C, Fauser BCJ et al. Current value of preimplantation genetic aneuploidy screening in IVF. Hum Reprod Update 2007; 13: 15–25.

2. Caglar GS, Asimakopoulos B, Nikolettos N et al. Preimplantation genetic diagnosis for aneuploidy screening in repeated implantation failure. Reprod Biomed Online 2005; 10: 381–8.

3. Werlin L, Rodi I, DeCherney A et al. Preimplantation genetic diagnosis as both a therapeutic and diagnostic tool in assisted reproductive technology. Fertil Steril 2003; 80: 467–8.

4. Wilton L. Preimplantation genetic diagnosis and chromosome analysis of blastomeres using comparative genomic hybridization. Hum Reprod 2005; 11: 22–41.

5. Mantzouratou A, Mania A, Fragouli E et al. Variable aneuploidy mechanisms in embryos from couples with poor reproductive histories undergoing preimplantation genetic screening. Hum Reprod 2007; 22: 1844–53.

6. Staessen C, Platteau P, Van Assche E et al. Comparison of blastocyst transfer with or without preimplantation genetic diagnosis for aneuploidy screening in couples with advanced maternal age: a propective randomized controlled trial. Hum Reprod 2004; 19: 2849–58.

7. Ebner T, Moser M, Sommergruber M, Tews G. Selection based on morphological assessment of oocytes and embryos at different stages of preimplantation development: a review. Hum Reprod Update 2003; 9: 252–62.

8. Scott L. The biological basis of non-invasive strategies for selection of human oocytes and embryos. Hum Reprod Update 2003; 9: 237–49.

9. Lemmen JG, Agerholm I, Ziebe S. Kinetic markers of human embryo quality using time-lapse recordings of IVF/ICSI-fertilized oocytes. Reprod Biomed Online 2008; 17: 385–91. Hum Reprod 2004; 19: 288–93.

10. Tesarik J, Kopecny V. Development of human male pronucleus: ultrastructure and timing. Gamete Res 1989; 24: 135–49.

11. Scott LA, Smith S. The successful use of pronuclear embryo transfers the day following oocyte retrieval. Hum Reprod 1998; 13: 1003–13.

12. Scott LA, Alvero R, Leondires M, Miller B. The morphology of human pronuclear embryos is positively related to blastocyst development and implantation. Hum Reprod 2000; 15: 2394–403.

13. Tesarik J, Greco E. The probability of abnormal preimplantation development can be predicted by a single static observation on pronuclear stage morphology. Hum Reprod 1999; 14: 1318–23.

14. Guerif F, Le Gouge A, Giraudeau B et al. Limited value of morphological assessment at days 1 and 2 to predict blastocyst development potential: a prospective study based on 4042 embryos. Hum Reprod 2007; 22: 1973–81.

15. Ebner T, Moser M, Sommergruber M *et al.* Presence, but not type or degree of extension, of a cytoplasmic halo has a significant influence on preimplantation development and implantation behaviour. *Hum Reprod* 2003; **18**: 2406–12.

16. Shoukir Y, Campana A, Farley T, Sakkas D. Early cleavage of in vitro fertilized human embryos to the 2-cell stage: a novel indicator of embryo quality and viability. *Hum Reprod* 1997; **12**: 1531–6.

17. Lundin K, Bergh C, Hadarson T. Early embryo cleavage is a strong indicator of embryo quality in human IVF. *Hum Reprod* 2001; **16**: 2652–7.

18. Van Montfoort APA, Dumoulin JCM, Kester ADM, Evers JLH. Early cleavage is a valuable addition to existing embryo selection parameters: a study using single embryo transfers. *Hum Reprod* 2004; **19**: 2103–8.

19. Bachvarova R, de Leon V. Polyadenylated RNA of mouse ova and loss of maternal RNA in early development. *Dev Biol* 1980; **74**: 1–8.

20. Comizzoli P, Urner F, Sakkas D, Renard JP. Up-regulation of glucose metabolism during male pronucleus formation determines the early onset of the S Phase in bovine zygotes. *Biol Reprod* 2003; **68**: 1934–40.

21. Wang WH, Mang L, Hackett RJ, Keefe DL. Developmental ability of human oocytes with or without birefringent spindles imaged by Polscope before insemination. *Hum Reprod* 2001; **16**: 1464–8.

22. Rienzi L, Ubaldi F, Martinez F *et al.* Relationship between meiotic spindle location with regard to the polar body position and oocyte developmental potential after ICSI. *Hum Reprod* 2003; **18**: 1289–93.

23. Rama Raju GA, Prakash GJ, Krishna KM, Madan K. Meiotic spindle and zona pellucida characteristics as predictors of embryonic development: a preliminary study using Polscope imaging. *Reprod BioMed Online* 2007; **14**: 166–74.

24. Shen Y, Stalf T, Mehnert C, Eichenlaub-Ritter U, Tinneberg HR. High magnitude light retardation by the zona pellucida is associated with conception cycles. *Hum Reprod* 2005; **20**: 1596–606.

25. Braude P, Bolton V, Moore S. Human gene expression first occurs between the four-and eight-cell stages of preimplantation development. *Nature* 1988; **332**: 459–61.

26. Gardner DK, Lane JD, Stevens J, Schlenker T, Schoolcraft WB. Blastocyst score affects implantation and pregnancy outcome: towards a single blastocyst transfer. *Fertil Steril* 2000; **73**: 1155–8.

27. Blake D, Proctor M, Johnson N, Olive D. Cleavage stage versus blastocyst stage embryo transfer in assisted conception. *Cochrane Database Syst Rev* 2002; **2**: CD002118 [update in *Cochrane Database Syst Rev* 2005; **4**: CD002118].

28. Papanikolaou EG, Kolibianakis EM, Tournaye H *et al.* Live birth rates after transfer of equal number of blastocysts or cleavage-stage embryos in IVF. A systematic review and meta-analysis. *Hum Reprod* 2008; **23**: 91–9.

29. Hardy K, Spanos S, Becker D *et al.* From cell death to embryo arrest: mathematical models of human preimplantation embryo development. *Proc Natl Acad Sci USA* 2001; **98**: 1655–60.

30. Levitas E, Lunenfeld Z, Har-Vardu I *et al.* Blastocyst-stage embryo transfer in patients who failed to conceive in three or more day 2–3 embryo transfer cycles: a prospective, randomized study. *Fertil Steril* 2004; **81**: 567–71.

31. Guerif F, Bidault R, Gasnier O *et al.* Efficacy of blastocyst transfer after implantation failure. *Reprod BioMedicine Online* 2004; **9**: 630–6.

32. Seif M, Edi-Osagie E, Farquhar C *et al.* Assisted hatching on assisted conception (IVF & ICSI). *Cochrane Database Syst Rev* 2005; **4**: CD001894.

33. Friedler S, Schachter M, Strassburger *et al.* A randomized clinical trial comparing recombinant hyaluronan/recombinant albumin versus human tubal fluid for cleavage stage embryo transfer in patients with multiple IVF-embryo transfer failure. *Hum Reprod* 2007; **22**: 2444–8.

34. Kattal N, Cohen J, Barmat LI. Role of coculture in human in vitro fertilization: a meta-analysis. *Fertil Steril* 2008; **90**: 1069–76.

35. Levy R, Elder K, Menezo Y. Cytoplasmic transfer in oocytes: biochemical aspects. *Hum Reprod Update* 2004; **10**: 241–50.

36. Spiking EC, Alderson J, St. John JC. Transmission of mitochondrial DNA following assisted reproduction and nuclear transfer. *Hum Reprod Update* 2006; **12**: 401–15.

37. Aslan D, Elizur SE, Levran J *et al.* Comparison of zygote intrafallopian tube transfer and transcervical uterine embryo transfer in patients with repeated implantation failure. *Eur J Obstet Gynecol Reprod Biol* 2005; **122**: 191–4.

38. El-Sayed A, Hoelker M, Rings F *et al.* Large-scale transcriptional analysis of bovine biopsies in relation to pregnancy success after transfer to recipients. *Physiol Genomics* 2006; **28**: 84–96.

39. Jones GM, Cram DS, Song B *et al.* Novel strategy with potential to identify developmentally competent IVF blastocysts. *Hum Reprod* 2008; **23**: 1748–59.

40. Katz-Jaffe MG, Gardner DK, Schoolcraft WB. Proteomic analysis of individual embryos to identify novel biomarkers of development and viability. *Fertil Steril* 2006; **85**: 101–7.

41. Katz-Jaffe MG, Schoolcraft WB, Gardner DK. Analysis of protein expression (secretome) by human and mouse preimplantation embryos. *Fertil Steril* 2006; **86**: 678–85.

42. Dominguez F, Gadea B, Esteban FJ *et al.* Comparative protein-profile analysis of implanted versus non-implanted human blastocysts. *Hum Reprod* 2008; **23**: 1993–2000.

43. Lopes A, Greve T, Callesen H. Quantification of embryo quality by respirometry. *Theriogenology* 2007; **67**: 21–31.

44. Scott L, Berntsen J, Davies D *et al.* Human oocyte respiration-rate measurement – potential to improve oocyte and embryo selection? *Reprod Biomed Online* 2008; **17**: 461–9.

45. Botros L, Sakkas D, Seli E. Metabolomics and its application for non-invasive embryo assessment in IVF. *Mol Hum Reprod* 2008; **14**: 679–90.

46. Fanchin R, Mendez Lozano DH, Frydman N *et al.* Anti-Mullerian hormone concentrations in the follicular fluid of the preovulatory follicle are predictive of the implantation potential of the ensuing embryo obtained by in vitro fertilization. *J Clin Endocrinol Metab* 2007; **92**: 1796–802.

47. Ledee N, Lombroso R, Lombardelli L *et al.* Cytokines and chemokines in follicular fluids and potential of the corresponding embryo: the role of granulocyte colony-stimulating factor. *Hum Reprod* 2008; **23**: 2001–9.

48. Su YQ, Sugiura K, Wigglesworth K *et al.* Oocyte regulation of metabolic cooperativity between mouse cumulus cells and oocytes: BMP15 and GDF9 control cholesterol biosynthesis in cumulus cells. *Development* 2008; **135**: 111–21.

49. Li Q, McKenzie LJ, Matzuk MM. Revisiting oocyte-somatic cell interactions: in search of novel intrafollicular predictors and regulators of oocyte developmental competence. *Mol Hum Reprod* 2008; **14**: 673–8.

50. Leese HJ. Quiet please, do not disturb: a hypothesis of embryo metabolism and viability. *BioEssays* 2002; **24**: 845–9.

# Chapter 23

# Embryo reduction in multiple pregnancies

Eduard Gratacos and Fatima Crispi

## Introduction

Embryo reduction (ER) may be indicated in a number of situations in fetal medicine. The most common and well-known by general ob/gyn specialists is the reduction of triplets, or higher-order multiple pregnancies, to twins. The number of high-order multiple pregnancies has increased several-fold after the introduction of assisted reproductive techniques (ART), and the classical figure of one twin pair in 90 pregnancies is now over 2% or more in developed countries [1]. Over the last two decades the rate of higher-order pregnancies has incremented by more than 10-fold, although there is evidence that the sustained rise in the number of triplet deliveries seems to have come to a plateau over recent years [2]. About 20 years ago, the classically poor outcome associated with high-order multiple pregnancies prompted a small number of groups in Europe and the USA [3] to start offering reduction of the number of embryos, in an attempt to improve the chances of survival and quality of life of the remaining fetuses. Embryo reduction has demonstrated to result in roughly similar outcomes for the remaining twins as if the pregnancy had started with twins, and today is offered to couples carrying triplets worldwide. As a trade off, the procedure is associated with an increased risk of miscarriage of the whole pregnancy. This stresses the need to provide parents with comprehensive information on the benefits and risks of the procedure. Although no randomized clinical trial (RCT) on ER has been conducted [4], a number of recent large collaborative studies and systematic reviews now allow reasonable estimates of the perinatal outcome that parents can expect after ER in comparison with expectant management.

Selective ER may also be contemplated in twin pregnancies, normally for fetal or maternal reasons. In contrast with ER in triplets, which is normally performed in the first trimester, selective reduction in twins is in most instances carried out from the second trimester onwards.

In this chapter we will summarize the available evidence on ER and we will discuss the impact of several factors which might influence results. In addition, we will briefly summarize currently used techniques and available data on the perinatal outcome after ER in multiple pregnancies.

## Indications and justification of elective embryo reduction

### Triplets and higher-order pregnancies

Embryo reduction in triplet or higher-order pregnancies is in most cases an elective procedure, performed with the intention to improve the poor outcome associated with high-order multiplets. In spite of advances in perinatal medicine, the perinatal outcome of triplets has not improved over the last 30 years [5]. A compilation of the available data in the English literature compared two different periods, reporting a mean gestational age at delivery of 33.6 weeks in 1979–1989, and 33.3 weeks in 1991–1999. The rates of delivery before 32 and 28 weeks were 24% and 8% respectively in the first time interval, and 25% and 9% respectively in the second. Aside from prematurity, the incidence of fetal growth restriction is also significantly increased. After a given gestational age, 32 weeks in twins and 29 weeks in triplets, the mean birth weights become progressively lower than those in singletons [6]. This does not reflect a different growth curve, but the increased incidence of fetal growth restriction, which affects up to 10% of twins and 25% of triplets [6]. Since prematurity and fetal growth restriction are the most important factors for adverse neonatal outcome [7], not surprisingly the

*Early Pregnancy*, ed. Roy G. Farquharson and Mary D. Stephenson. Published by Cambridge University Press.
© Cambridge University Press 2010.

245

exceedingly high rates of prematurity in high-order multiplets result in an increased risk for neonatal mortality and long-term neurological morbidity. A large population-based study in Australia reported the prevalence of cerebral palsy to be 28 per 1000 in triplets, in comparison with 7.3 in twins and 1.6 in singletons [8]. A similar study in the UK [9] calculated the cerebral palsy rates per 1000 survivors at 44.8 per 1000 in triplets, in comparison with 12.6 in twins and 1.5 in singletons. As expected, the perinatal outcome for pregnancies of higher order than triplets is progressively worse. The rate of delivery before 28 weeks of gestation may be as high as 25% for quadruplets and quintuplets, and the rate of intra-uterine growth restriction (IUGR) 62% [10]. The mean gestational age at delivery for quadruplets is 30 weeks, with 44% delivering between 24 and 30 weeks [11], and the mean birth weight has been reported to be 1414 g [12].

A second indication for ER in triplets is the presence of a discordant malformation in one or more embryos [13]. In a substantial number of cases the anomaly is found on the 20-week scan, and consequently most of these procedures are carried out in the second trimester. Most of the results discussed over the following sections correspond to elective ER procedures.

## Twin pregnancies

Selective ER in twins may be indicated for elective reasons, because of the parents' desires to reduce the number of embryos and/or improve pregnancy outcome [3], the presence of an increased fetal or maternal risk, or the presence of a discordant anomaly [13,14]. The prevalence of malformations in dichorionic twins does not differ from that in singletons, which implies that about 2–3% of all twins will present with a discordant anomaly in one fetus. Selective reduction may also be indicated for maternal safety reasons, in patients with previous severe pre-term births, or in twin pregnancies with an early (<24 weeks) premature rupture of membranes [3].

## Technical and practical aspects of embryo reduction

### Gestational age

Elective ER is normally performed as early as possible in pregnancy. Data on large collaborative series suggest that reduction after the first trimester does not increase

pregnancy loss or early pre-term birth rates [13]. However, the psychological impact of ER in parents is important, and earlier procedures are likely to minimize this impact [15]. At present the gestational age for the procedure is conditioned by the need to perform an evaluation for structural defects and ultrasound markers of chromosomal abnormalities at 11–14 weeks. Thus, most ERs in fetal medicine units are today performed around 12 weeks' gestation [16].

## Chorionicity

As stated above, detailed ultrasound assessment is mandatory before performing an ER. The first step is diagnosis of chorionicity (Figures 23.1 and 23.2). The existence of vascular anastomoses in the common placenta of monochorionic twins is the basis for the development of severe complications and the complexity of invasive procedures. Thus, reduction of one monochorionic twin by injection of potassium chloride is not possible due to the high risks that this method involves for the co-twin [17].

Therefore selective ER must be managed differently in dichorionic and monochorionic twins. Fetal reduction in monochorionic twins is always a complex procedure, thus, techniques for selective fetocide must include a method for completely and permanently arresting flow in the cord of the target fetus, such as cord coagulation or ligation [18]. These techniques are mainly applied in the second trimester of pregnancy and therefore not being discussed in this chapter. In the next sections, we will discuss the techniques and outcomes of selective ER in dichorionic twin pregnancies.

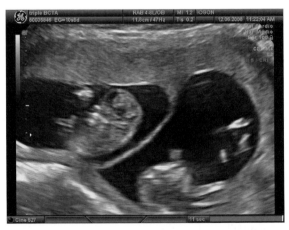

**Figure 23.1.** Diagnosis of chorionicity in dichorionic pregnancies: lambda sign.

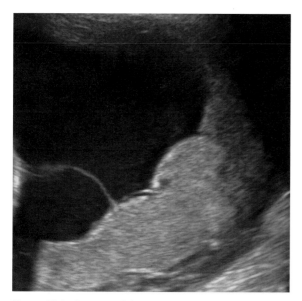

**Figure 23.2.** Diagnosis of chorionicity in monochorionic pregnancies: "T" sign.

In triplets and higher-order multiple pregnancies chorionicity has major implications in the decision of which embryo to reduce. Triplets with one monochorionic pair have a six to ten-fold risk of poor perinatal outcome as compared with trichorionic triplets, due to the development of complications of monochorionic pregnancy such as twin – twin transfusion [19]. Consequently most parents will choose to reduce the monochorionic twin pair instead of reducing the "singleton" embryo. Failing to identify chorionicity might substantially worsen the overall pregnancy outcome after ER.

## Assessment for embryo malformations prior to reduction

The second essential step in the ultrasound evaluation prior to ER is evaluation of embryo anatomy. In expert hands, high-definition ultrasound at 11–14 weeks' gestation may rule out about 70% of major malformations occurring during pregnancy [20]. Additionally, at that time embryos can be screened for ultrasound markers for chromosomal abnormalities. A nuchal translucency thickness over the 95th percentile has 75% sensitivity for the detection of Down's syndrome [21]. The presence of any embryo abnormality or ultrasound marker will determine the embryo to reduce. On the contrary, a normal ultrasound will substantially reduce the risk of a later diagnosis of malformation in one of the remaining fetuses.

A recent study suggested that cervical length measurements could be of help in predicting the risk of pre-term delivery in 25 triplets undergoing ER [22]. The authors reported an increased risk of delivering earlier than 33 weeks in patients with a cervical length below 35 mm. Cervical length is strongly associated with the risk of pre-term delivery regardless of the number of fetuses [23], but it is normally evaluated in the second trimester. It seems unlikely that at 12 weeks' gestation cervical length provides meaningful information concerning the chances for pregnancy loss after ER, but in any case the answer to this question requires a larger sample size. In a small series of 35 twins reduced in the first trimester and 83 non-reduced triplets, ER did not result in cervical length differences at 15–19 weeks [24].

## Technical aspects and influence of experience

Embryo reduction can be performed transvaginally or transabdominally. The transvaginal approach may be used from very early in gestation [25] and it is a technically simpler procedure. Transabdominal reduction must be performed later and requires a substantially higher level of expertise [26]. The transvaginal approach has been associated with a higher risk of miscarriage [25]. Today, most experienced groups perform the procedure transabdominally [16]. The typical transabdominal procedure consists of an ultrasound-guided cardiac or thoracic embryo puncture with a 20–22 Ga needle and injection of a small amount of potassium chloride, normally 1–5 ml, as required to observe complete cardiac arrest. In the transvaginal route, most reports have used injection of potassium chloride [25], although alternative techniques have been described, including aspiration of the embryo [27] or simple puncture until observing cardiac arrest [28].

In the presence of a sign suggesting an increased risk of embryo anomaly, reduction is performed on the affected embryo. In the absence of any embryo defect, it is common practice to avoid reducing the presenting embryo [16]. In a series of selective reduction in twins or triplets with discordant malformations, Eddleman et al. [14] reported that reduction of the presenting embryo was associated with a modest but significant decrease in gestational age at delivery (37 vs 38 weeks), and a significant increase in the rate of pre-term delivery before <32 weeks (22.5% vs 6.1%).

Embryo reduction may occasionally be a technically demanding procedure. The uterus and embryo are very small, the maternal abdominal wall may be thick and access to the target embryo is not always straightforward. In their fourth report on the international collaborative experience with ER, Evans *et al.* reported the impact of the learning curve over a period of 12 years in 3513 procedures. The rate of pregnancy loss decreased from an initial 13% to a 6% for losses before 24 weeks, and from 4.5% to 0.2% for losses beyond 24 weeks [29]. The improvement in pregnancy outcome is thought to be largely due to increased experience, possibly in combination with improvements in the quality of ultrasound equipments. As with any invasive procedure in fetal medicine, the duration and the degree of manipulation, and the number of attempts, must substantially affect the rate of procedure-related complications. Consequently, ER should be performed by fetal medicine specialists highly experienced in ultrasound guided intrauterine procedures.

## Combining prenatal diagnosis with embryo reduction

Non-invasive assessment of the risk for chromosomal anomalies in triplets is limited to the use of ultrasound markers, since biochemical markers are not useful for pregnancies of a higher order than twins [30]. On the other hand, the rate of chromosomal defects is higher in patients conceiving by ART [31]. Consequently, the number of patients with triplets or higher-order pregnancies considering prenatal diagnosis is expected to be high. One possible option is to undergo a second-trimester amniocentesis 3–4 weeks after ER. In a study comparing the impact of amniocentesis in twin pregnancies resulting from a previous ER, the rate of pregnancy loss was 3.1% in 127 patients who had an amniocentesis, compared with 7.2% in 167 patients who did not, the difference being non-significant [32]. One of the main drawbacks of amniocentesis is that if a chromosomal abnormality is found, patients are then faced for the second time with the decision of performing a selective fetal reduction, a procedure which will in turn increase further the risks of losing the full pregnancy.

The second, and most accepted option today, is to perform a chorionic villous sampling (CVS) in all embryos before the procedure. The existence of aneuploidy in the chromosomes 13, 18, 21, X and Y can be ruled out within 24–48 hours by QF-PCR or fluorescent in-situ hybridization (FISH). With this approach the full karyotype is not available until 2 weeks later, and therefore there is a residual risk for chromosomal anomalies. However, the combination of rapid diagnosis techniques with a detailed ultrasound assessment

reduces considerably the chances of leaving a non-reduced fetus with a severe anomaly [16]. Most parents would feel reasonably reassured with this approach, and thus the combination of CVS followed by ER is routinely offered in an increasing number of reference centers [33]. Recently, Brambati *et al.* [34] reported their extended experience with 424 consecutive multiple pregnancies reduced to twins or singletons at 8–13 weeks' gestation after transabdominal CVS with a successful CVS in 100% of cases, and an accuracy of karyotyping of 99%. The overall pregnancy loss rate after reduction (3.3%) was similar to other studies [29]. The overall rate of chromosomal abnormalities in the study series was higher (relative risk = 2) than in a singleton control series. The study further confirms a higher pregnancy rate of chromosomal abnormalities in multiple pregnancies, and provides strong evidence that CVS prior to ER is a safe procedure.

## Ethical and psychological issues concerning embryo reduction and selective reduction in multiple pregnancies

Intrauterine reduction of an embryo, either electively or in the presence of a malformation, is by definition a controversial issue. When considered in the context of a purely ethical discussion, thus devoid of any other connotation, the most widely accepted consideration is that the procedure follows the principle of treating to achieve the most good for the least harm [16]. A detailed discussion on the ethical issues is beyond the objectives of this chapter. For very good texts on this matter we refer the reader to several reviews over the last decade [16,35].

Embryo reduction is normally a stressful experience for most parents [15]. In one study, 14 of 44 women described the procedure as "horrible," although in the year following the procedure no apparent increased risk of depression was noted [36]. In our experience, first-trimester procedures are normally well tolerated, while later procedures, mainly those performed after 16–18 weeks, are associated with intense feelings of grief, normally persisting after delivery of the unaffected fetus, and we normally recommend and offer psychological support during and after pregnancy to these patients.

## Outcomes after embryo reduction

A Cochrane review in 2002 [4] confirmed the absence of randomized controlled trials evaluating the outcome of ER. It seems unlikely that such a trial will be carried out, considering on the one hand the numbers required for such study and on the other hand that most parents have already strong preferences against or for reduction before counseling [37]. There is a huge body of data on pregnancy outcome in reduced and non-reduced multiple pregnancies. The available data further demonstrate that the outcome is different according to the starting or finishing number of fetuses. Thus, over the following sections we will analyze separately the available evidence on pregnancy outcome in four possible types of ER: triplets to twins, triplets to singletons, and higher-order pregnancies in general, and finally selective reduction in dichorionic twins.

The two most important adverse outcomes in multiple pregnancies are the rate of early pre-term delivery, normally defined as less than 32 weeks' gestation, and the rate of pregnancy loss, defined as that occurring before 24 weeks. The first complication is precisely the one that ER is supposed to improve, while the second is the complication that the procedure may increase. To compare pregnancy loss rates in published studies has a major problem, since for any pregnancy the chance for having a loss rate decreases with gestational age. Thus, one question is the rate of pregnancy loss for the whole pregnancy, and the other, and most relevant for clinical comparisons and counseling, is what the chances are of losing a viable pregnancy at a certain moment. Most pregnancy losses

occur over the first weeks of gestation. For instance, the likelihoods of delivering liveborn fetuses change from early to late first trimester from 63% to 90% in twins, and 45% to 90% in triplets [38]. Furthermore, after the diagnosis of a viable pregnancy at 14 weeks' gestation, the rate of miscarriage is substantially reduced; less than 1% in singletons [39], 1.8% in dichorionic twins [40] and 4% in triplets [37]. If we apply this to comparisons between reduced and non-reduced multiple pregnancies, comparing groups with different gestational age at inclusion might lead to substantially biased conclusions. We have kept this concept in mind in the presentation of available data over the next sections, and have therefore purposely omitted any reference to background loss rates where the gestational age of the population at enrolment was not stated.

## Reduction of triplets to twins

The best available evidence on reduction of triplets to twins (Table 23.1) comes from a large study by Papageorghiou et al. [37], in which the authors combined their own results with a systematic review of previously published data, including a total of 482 pregnancies with ER and 411 managed expectantly. Embryo reduction was performed at a range of 7–14 weeks' gestation. In the group treated with ER the rate of pregnancy loss was higher at 8.1%, compared with 4.4% in the expectantly managed group (relative

**Table 23.1** Embryo reduction in triplet pregnancies: rough estimates of the pregnancy outcomes in comparison with the expected outcome in triplet, twin and singleton pregnancies with live fetuses at 11–14 weeks' gestation. Numbers are based on published studies on selective reduction and/or national birth statistics from Europe and the USA, and are given in round figures in order to facilitate comparison of the expected outcomes with either management. The baby take-home rate, where not reported in published studies, has been estimated on the basis of pregnancy loss rate and expected mortality rates in very pre-term births.

| | Pregnancy loss (>24 weeks) | Early pre-term delivery (<32 weeks) | Gestational age at delivery (weeks) | Baby take-home rate |
|---|---|---|---|---|
| Background outcomes | | | | |
| Triplets | 4% | 25% | 33.5 | 93% |
| Dichorionic twins | 2% | 10% | 36 | 96% |
| Singleton | <1% | <1% | 40 | 98% |
| Reduced triplets | | | | |
| 3 to 2 | 6% | 10% | 36 | 90% |
| 3 to 1 | 8% | 2% | 38 | 90% |

risk = 1.83). The rate of pregnancy loss is somewhat higher than the 4.8% reported by Evans *et al.* [29] in 1318 triplets reduced to twins. The spontaneous pregnancy loss for non-reduced triplets in other series may appear too "benign" if one considers previous studies reporting background loss rates for triplets. However, as stated above, it is essential to consider the chances of pregnancy loss adjusted for gestational age.

In the systematic review by Papageorghiou *et al.* [37], the rate of early pre-term delivery was lower in the ER group (10.4 vs 26.7%, relative risk 0.37). The figures are remarkably similar to the 10% reported by Evans *et al.* [29] in their large collaborative series including 1749 reduced triplets, although their series included a small proportion of reductions of three to one fetuses.

The mean gestational age at delivery in triplets reduced to twins has consistently been reported to be significantly higher by about 2.5 weeks than in non-reduced triplets. Papageorghiou *et al.* [37] reported a mean gestational age at delivery was 33.8 weeks in cases managed expectantly, and 36.1 weeks in cases reduced to twins. The results are similar to those reported by Evans *et al.* [29] in their large collaborative study (35.8 weeks in triplets reduced to twins).

The number of pregnancies with at least one survivor can not be calculated in most published studies. In the study by Papageorghiou *et al.* [37], including 180 non-reduced and 185 reduced triplets, the proportions were 93.5% for the expectant management groups and 91.1% for the reduced group. Aside from the interest that these numbers may have for parents, it is important to make these comparisons in order to realize that the final differences in survival are not as important as the differences in the miscarriage rate may suggest. The rate of deliveries between 24–28 weeks is two- to four-fold higher in non-reduced as compared with reduced triplets [37], and this carries a substantially higher risk of neonatal mortality. Therefore, the differences in miscarriage in favor of non-reduced triplets are later compensated by a higher rate of neonatal morbidity due to the increment in very early pre-term delivery.

## Reduction of triplets to singletons

Reduction of triplets to singletons (Table 23.1) may be the option of choice on certain occasions. Although there is an increase in the number of patients electively requesting this option [33], the general recommendation is still to reduce to twins, since the outcomes of twins are acceptable and the chances of achieving a

new pregnancy in the future may be uncertain. Thus, for the moment the most common reason for reducing to a singleton remains the presence of a triplet pregnancy with a monochorionic twin pair, also named dichorionic triplet. As stated above, dichorionic triplets have a six- to ten-fold risk of poor perinatal outcome as compared with trichorionic triplets [19]. For instance, twin – twin transfusion syndrome may develop in 15–25% of cases and fetal weight discordance may complicate a similar proportion [19]. Therefore, provided that the 'singleton' embryo appears to be normal on first-trimester ultrasound evaluation, most parents would probably choose for reduction of the monochorionic pair. In a recent review, Evans and Britt [41] estimate that the pregnancy loss rate in triplets reduced to singletons is 7%, the gestational age at delivery is around 39 weeks, and the proportion of pregnancies with a birth weight <1500 g would be <2% (compared with about 7% in triplets reduced to twins). Data on the number of pregnancies with at least one survivor in pregnancies reduced from three to one can not be obtained from published studies.

In summary, the available information suggests that reducing triplets to singletons could result in similar rates of pregnancy loss, with a higher gestational age at delivery and a substantial reduction in neonatal morbidity as compared with triplets reduced to twins.

## Reduction of higher-order (four or more) pregnancies

Unfortunately there are no case – control studies comparing the outcome of reduced and non-reduced higher-order pregnancies in the same centers, and therefore results must be compared with historical series from other studies. In order to make comparisons as meaningful as possible we will mostly refer to the large collaborative study by Evans *et al.* [29], reporting the outcome of ER in higher-order pregnancies in 1610 pregnancies. More than 80% of quadruplets are reduced to twins [29]. In general, the rate of pregnancy loss in reduced quadruplets seems to be very similar to that of twins. Evans *et al.* [29] reported an initial 13% rate in quadruplets reduced to twins for procedures performed before 1994, which decreased to 6.6% from 1995 to 1998. The rate of early pre-term delivery was 14.2%, a small but significant increase with respect to reduced triplets (10.1%). Mean gestational age at delivery was 35.1 weeks, but it is not possible to estimate the number of pregnancies with at least one survivor. In summary, reduction of quadruplet pregnancies results in a slight increase in the rates of pregnancy loss and early pre-term delivery with respect to reduced triplets, but mean gestational age at delivery is similar. However, it must be noted that these conclusions should only be applied to quadruplets reduced to twins. The loss rate in quadruplets reduced to other numbers was 20%. Therefore, in the light of current available literature, it is likely that the outcome for quadruplets reduced to singletons or triplets is not as good as for triplets reduced to twins, and patients should be counseled accordingly (Table 23.2).

The best evidence on the outcome for quintuplets or higher-order pregnancies comes also from the collaborative review by Evans et al. [29]. Reduced quintuplets had a pregnancy loss rate of 15.1%, and an early pre-term delivery rate of 15.7%. Reduced sextuplets of higher-order pregnancies showed a pregnancy loss rate of 21.6%, and a rate of early pre-term delivery of 16.9%. The mean gestational age for the combined set of pregnancies with quintuplets or more was 34.8 weeks. Therefore, although the results become poorer with increasing starting numbers, in the hands of an experienced operator, reduction of very high-order pregnancies is associated with acceptable outcomes.

## Selective reduction in dichorionic twin pregnancies

Pregnancy loss rates in reduced twins (Table 23.3) due to selective fetal malformations range between 3–7% [13,26]. Evans et al. [13] reported a loss rate of 5.4% in procedures performed between 9–12 weeks, and of 8.7% in those performed at 13–18 weeks. The rate of early pre-term delivery was 12.4%. Eddleman et al. [14] reported a loss rate of 2.4%, early delivery rate of 13.2% and a mean gestational age at delivery of 38 weeks. When dealing with the issue of reduction in twins, it is also important to consider the rate of severe

prematurity (delivery before 28 weeks). For instance, the cumulative rate of delivery before and after 28 weeks was 12% in the collaborative series reported by Evans et al. [13]. To avoid this complication, several groups have proposed to delay the moment of termination beyond 24 weeks, even at 28–32 weeks [42]. Such "late" selective termination procedures have been reported to be associated with survival rates of the unaffected twin of 97–100% [42,43]. Consequently, this possibility could be offered to parents in countries where the law permits late pregnancy termination.

Available data suggest that the outcomes of *elective* reduction of twins to singletons are similar to reductions performed for medical reasons during the first trimester, although the rate of delivery before 28 weeks might be lower. In the large collaborative series reported by Evans et al. [29], the pregnancy loss rate was 5.8% and early pre-term birth was 7.1%. In a later study, Evans et al. [3] reported their own experience with a pregnancy loss rate of 1.9%, early pre-term birth of 7.5%, mean gestational age at delivery of 37.5 weeks, and a baby take-home rate of 96%.

In summary, the outcome of dichorionic twins electively reduced to singletons in the first trimester is clearly worse than in singleton pregnancies; they deliver earlier (roughly 37.5–38 weeks) and have an increased rate of early pre-term delivery (2.5–7.5%). However, the perinatal outcome seems to modestly improve on the outcome of non-reduced twins (36.0 weeks at delivery and 10% early pre-term birth). Whether this is a sufficient argument in favor of elective reduction or not remains a complex question and it is not the purpose of this review to enter into such debate.

### Impact of embryo reduction on long-term neurological outcome

The balance between the pregnancy loss and early pre-term delivery are the most commonly used figures for

**Table 23.2** Embryo reduction in quadruplet or higher-order pregnancies: rough estimates of the pregnancy outcomes in comparison with the expected outcomes in higher-order non-reduced pregnancies. Numbers are based on published studies on selective reduction and/or national birth statistics from Europe and the USA, and are given in round figures in order to facilitate comparison of the expected outcomes with either management.

| | Pregnancy loss (>24 weeks) | Early pre-term delivery (<32 weeks) | Gestational age at delivery (weeks) |
|---|---|---|---|
| Background outcomes | 10% | ≥50% | ≥30 |
| Embryo reduction | 10% | 15% | 35 |

**Table 23.3** Embryo reduction in dichorionic twin pregnancies: rough estimates of the pregnancy outcomes in comparison with the expected outcome in twin and singleton pregnancies with live fetuses at 11–14 weeks' gestation. Numbers are based on published studies on selective reduction and/or national birth statistics from Europe and the USA, and are given in round figures in order to facilitate comparison of the expected outcomes with either management. The baby take-home rate, where not reported in published studies, has been estimated on the basis of pregnancy loss rate and expected mortality rates in very pre-term births.

| | Pregnancy loss (>24 weeks) | Early pre-term delivery (<32 weeks) | Gestational age at delivery (weeks) | Baby take-home rate |
|---|---|---|---|---|
| Background outcomes | | | | |
| Dichorionic twins | 2% | 10% | 36 | 96% |
| Singleton | <1% | <1% | 40 | 98% |
| Reduced twins | | | | |
| >15 weeks | 4% | 6% | 38 | >95% |
| 15–24 weeks | 6% | 12.5% | 38 | 90% |

evaluating the risks and benefits of embryo reduction. However, at the time of counseling, the issue of long-term neurological morbidity usually comes into the discussion as the most feared by parents. The relevance of neurological outcome is normally better understood than that of prematurity, a more diffuse concept for most parents.

There are no direct estimates on the rate of cerebral palsy after ER. Geva et al. [44], in a small retrospective study on 14 neonates, reported that the rate of periventricular leukomalacia, the strongest neonatal predictor of cerebral palsy, was overrepresented in survivors after ER and suggested this could be a direct effect of the procedure. In contrast, none of the prospective studies recording the neonatal outcome after reduction from triplets to twins has reported an increased prevalence of leukomalacia [43,45–47]. In addition, Dimitriou et al. [48] assessed 72 children from trichorionic triplet pregnancies reduced to twins by selective reduction and found a prevalence of cerebral palsy of 13 per 1000, which does not differ from previously reported rates of cerebral palsy in spontaneous twin pregnancies [8–9]. Therefore, in the light of current evidence, it is unlikely that ER increases per se the rate of adverse neurological outcome, and that the prevalence of long-term neurological injury in survivors from reduced and non-reduced triplets should be mainly dependent on gestational age and birth weight. Papageorghiou et al. [37] estimated that severe handicap decreases from 28% at 24 weeks to less than 5% at 32 weeks, and calculated that ER from triplets to twins would reduce

the handicap rate from 1.5% to 0.6%. Another way to approach the same issue would be to anticipate that, since the rate of cerebral palsy in triplets has been consistently reported to be four-fold that of twins, 28–44/1000 versus 7–12/1000 [8–9], ER is likely to reduce by the same proportion the risk of cerebral palsy in survivors. In the absence of prospective studies assessing the long-term follow-up in survivors from ER, the above estimations may be helpful for parents with high-order pregnancies to understand the risks and benefits of expectant management versus ER.

# References

1. Blondel B, Macfarlane A, Gissler M, Breart G, Zeitlin J; PERISTAT Study Group. Preterm birth and multiple pregnancy in European countries participating in the PERISTAT project. *Br J Obstet Gynecol* 2006; **113**: 528–35.

2. Martin JA, Hamilton BE, Sutton PD et al. Births: Final Data for 2003. *National Vital Statistics Reports* 2005; **54**(2).

3. Evans MI, Kaufman MI, Urban AJ et al. Fetal reduction from twins to a singleton: a reasonable consideration. *Obstet Gynecol* 2004; **104**: 102–9.

4. Dodd JM, Crowther CA. Reduction of the number of fetuses for women with triplet and higher order multiple pregnancies. *Cochrane Database Syst Rev* 2003; **2**: CD003932.

5. Stone J, Eddleman K. Multifetal pregnancy reduction. *Curr Opin Obstet Gynecol* 2000; **12**: 491–6.

6. Garite TJ, Clark RH, Elliott JP, Thorp JA. Twins and triplets: the effect of plurality and growth on neonatal

outcome compared with singleton infants. *Am J Obstet Gynecol* 2004; **191**: 700–7.

7. Larroque B, Ancel PY, Marret S *et al.* Neurodevelopmental disabilities and special care of 5-year-old children born before 33 weeks of gestation (the EPIPAGE study): a longitudinal cohort study. *Lancet* 2008; **371**: 813–20.

8. Petterson B, Nelson KB, Watson L, Stanely F. Twins, triplets, and cerebral palsy in births in Western Australia in the 1980s. *Br Med J* 1993; **307**: 1239–43.

9. Pharoah PO, Cooke T. Cerebral palsy and multiple births. *Archives Dis Child Fetal Neonatal Ed* 1996; **75**: F174–9.

10. Skrablin S, Kuvacic I, Pavicic D, Kalafatic D, Goluza T. Maternal neonatal outcome in quadruplet and quintuplet versus triplet gestations. *Eur J Obstet Gynecol Reprod Biol* 2000; **88**: 147–52.

11. Angel JL, Kalter CS, Morales WJ, Rasmussen C, Caron L. Aggressive perinatal care for high-order multiple gestations: does good perinatal outcome justify aggressive assisted reproductive techniques? *Am J Obstet Gynecol* 1999; **181**: 253–9.

12. Seoud MA, Toner JP, Kruithoff C, Muasher SJ. Outcome of twin, triplet and quadruplet in vitro fertilization pregnancies: the Norfolk experience. *Fertil Steril* 1992, **57**: 825–34.

13. Evans MI, Goldberg JD, Horenstein J *et al.* Selective termination for structural, chromosomal, and mendelian anomalies: international experience. *Am J Obstet Gynecol* 1999; **181**: 893–7.

14. Eddleman K, Stone J, Lynch L, Berkowitz R. Selective termination of anomalous fetuses in multifetal pregnancies: 200 cases at a single center. *Am J Obst Gynecol* 2002; **185**: S79.

15. Britt DW, Risinger ST, Mans M, Evans MI. Anxiety among women who have undergone fertility therapy and who are considering multifetal pregnancy reduction: trends and implications. *J Matern Fetal Neonatal Med* 2004; **13**: 271–8.

16. Evans MI, Ciorica D, Britt DW, Fletcher JC. Update on selective reduction. *Prenat Diagn* 2005; **25**: 807–13.

17. Olivennes F, Doumerc S, Senat MV, Audibert F, Fanchin R, Frydman R. Evidence of early placental vascular anastomosis during selective embryo reduction in monozygotic twins. *Fertil Steril* 2002; **77**: 183–4.

18. Lewi L, Van Schoubroeck D, Gratacos E *et al.* Monochorionic diamniotic twins: complications and management options. *Curr Opin Obstet Gynecol* 2003; **15**: 177–94.

19. Bajoria R, Ward SB, Adegbite AL. Comparative study of perinatal outcome of dichorionic and trichorionic iatrogenic triplets. *Am J Obstet Gynecol* 2006; **194**: 415–24.

20. Souka AP, Pilalis A, Kavalakis Y *et al.* Assessment of fetal anatomy at the 11–14 weeks ultrasound examination. *Ultrasound Obstet Gynecol* 2004; **24**: 730–4.

21. Nicolaides KH. Nuchal translucency and other first-trimester sonographic markers of chromosomal abnormalities. *Am J Obstet Gynecol* 2004; **191**: 45–67.

22. Fait G, Har-Toov J, Gull I *et al.* Cervical length, multifetal pregnancy reduction, and prediction of preterm birth. *J Clin Ultrasound* 2005; **33**: 329–32.

23. To MS, Fonseca EB, Molina F, Cacho AM, Nicolaides KH. Maternal characteristics and cervical length in the prediction of spontaneous early preterm delivery in twins. *Am J Obstet Gynecol* 2006; **194**: 1360–5.

24. Rebarber A, Carreno CA, Lipkind H *et al.* Cervical length after multifetal pregnancy reduction in remaining twin gestations. *Am J Obstet Gynecol* 2001; **185**: 1113–17.

25. Timor-Tritsch IE, Peisner DB, Monteagudo A, Lerner JP, Sharma S. Multifetal pregnancy reduction by transvaginal puncture: evaluation of the technique used in 134 cases. *Am J Obstet Gynecol* 1993; **168**: 799–804.

26. Berkowitz RL, Stone JL, Eddleman KA. One hundred consecutive cases of selective termination of an abnormal fetus in a multifetal gestation. *Obstet Gynecol* 1997; **90**: 606–10.

27. Mansour RT, Aboulghar MA, Serour GI *et al.* Multifetal pregnancy reduction: modification of the technique and analysis of the outcome. *Fertil Steril* 1999; **71**: 380–4.

28. Ibérico G, Navarro J, Blasco L *et al.* Embryo reduction of multifetal pregnancies following assisted reproduction treatment: a modification of the transvaginal ultrasound-guided technique. *Hum Reprod* 2000; **15**: 2228–33.

29. Evans MI, Berkowitz R, Wapner R *et al.* Multifetal pregnancy reduction (MFPR): improved outcomes with increased experience. *Am J Obstet Gynecol* 2001; **184**: 97–103.

30. Cleary-Goldman J, Berkowitz RL. First trimester screening for Down syndrome in multiple pregnancy. *Semin Perinatol* 2005; **29**: 395–400.

31. Pinborg A, Loft A, Schmidt L, Andersen AN. Morbidity in a Danish national cohort of 472 IVF/ICSI twins, 1132 non-IVF/ICSI twins and 634 IVF/ICSI singletons: health related and social implications for the children and their families. *Hum Reprod* 2003; **18**: 1234–43.

32. Selam B, Torok O, Lembet A *et al.* Genetic amniocentesis after multifetal pregnancy reduction. *Am J Obstet Gynecol* 1999; **180**: 226–30.

33. Stone J, Belogolovkin V, Matho A *et al.* Evolving trends in 2000 cases of multifetal pregnancy reduction: a single center experience. *Am J Obstet Gynecol* 2007; **197**: 394.e1–4.

34. Brambati B, Tului L, Camurri L, Guercilena S. First-trimester fetal reduction to a singleton infant or twins: outcome in relation to the final number and karyotyping before reduction by transabdominal chorionic villus sampling. *Am J Obstet Gynecol* 2004; **191**: 2035–40.

35. Chervenak FA, McCullough LB, Wapner R. Three ethically justified indications for selective termination in multifetal pregnancy: a practical and comprehensive management strategy. *J Assist Reprod Genet* 1995; **12**: 531–6.

36. McKinney MK, Tuber SB, Downey JI. Multifetal pregnancy reduction: psychodynamic implications. *Psychiatry* 1996; **59**: 393–407.

37. Papageorghiou AT, Avgidou K, Bakoulas V, Sebire NJ, Nicolaides KH. Risks of miscarriage and early preterm birth in trichorionic triplet pregnancies with embryo reduction versus expectant management: new data and systematic review. *Hum Reprod* 2006; **21**: 1912–17.

38. Dickey RP, Olar TT, Curole DN *et al*. The probability of multiple births when multiple gestational sacs or viable embryos are diagnosed at first trimester ultrasound. *Hum Reprod* 1990; **5**: 880–2.

39. Tabor A, Philip J, Madsen M *et al*. Randomised controlled trial of genetic amniocentesis in 4606 low-risk women. *Lancet* 1986; **7**: 1287–93.

40. Sebire NJ, Snijders RJ, Hughes K, Sepulveda W, Nicolaides KH. The hidden mortality of monochorionic twin pregnancies. *Br J Obstet Gynaecol* 1997; **104**: 1203–7.

41. Evans MI, Britt DW. Fetal reduction. *Semin Perinatol* 2005; **29**: 321–9.

42. Shalev J, Meizner I, Rabinerson D *et al*. Improving pregnancy outcome in twin gestations with one malformed fetus by postponing selective feticide in the third trimester. *Fertil Steril* 1999; **72**: 257–60.

43. Lipitz S, Shalev E, Meizner I *et al*. Late selective termination of fetal abnormalities in twin pregnancies: a multicentre report. *Br J Obstet Gynecol* 1996; **103**: 1212–16.

44. Geva E, Lerner-Geva L, Stavorovsky Z *et al*. Multifetal pregnancy reduction: a possible risk factor for periventricular leukomalacia in premature newborns. *Fertil Steril* 1998; **69**: 845–50.

45. Selam B, Lembet A, Stone J, Lapinski R, Berkowitz RL. Pregnancy complications and neonatal outcomes in multifetal pregnancies reduced to twins compared with nonreduced twin pregnancies. *Am J Perinatol* 1999; **16**: 65–71.

46. Dietterich C, Check JH, Lurie D. Comparison of pregnancy outcome of natural twin pregnancies versus multifetal pregnancies selectively reduced to twins. *Clin Exp Obstet Gynecol* 1997; **24**: 17–18.

47. Nevo O, Avisar E, Tamir A *et al*. Neonatal course and outcome of twins from reduced multifetal pregnancy versus non-reduced twins. *Isr Med Assoc J* 2003; **5**: 245–8.

48. Dimitriou G, Pharoah PO, Nicolaides KH, Greenough A. Cerebral palsy in triplet pregnancies with and without iatrogenic reduction. *Eur J Pediatr* 2004; **163**: 449–51.

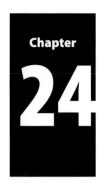

# Miscarriage after in-vitro fertilization

Ruth Bunker Lathi and Mary D. Stephenson

Case #1: A 39-year-old woman with tubal factor infertility conceives with IVF. Ultrasound evaluation at 6 weeks' gestation reveals an empty gestational sac. Cytogenetic analysis reveals trisomy 15, specifically, 47, XX, +15.

Case #2: A 30-year-old woman with unexplained infertility conceives for the first time after IVF. Ultrasound evaluation at 8 weeks' gestation reveals an embryonic pole of 10 mm, without cardiac motion. Cytogenetic analysis reveals a diploid male result, 46, XY.

## How should these patients be managed?

Miscarriage after IVF can heighten the emotional roller coaster of infertility treatments. Patients often equate "miscarriage" with "IVF failure," rather than concluding that miscarriage is a common occurrence, even with assisted reproductive technology (ART). It is important to discuss the frequency of miscarriage with patients, prior to initiating IVF. The risk of miscarriage increases with advancing maternal age, primarily due to the increasing frequency of maternally derived trisomy [1]. Unfortunately, the risk of infertility also increases with advancing maternal age. Women over 35 years of age commonly consider IVF in their desire to start a family. As shown in Figure 24.1, when autologous oocytes are used, the likelihood of an ART cycle ending in miscarriage increases with advancing maternal age.

Numeric chromosome errors, specifically, trisomy, monosomy and polyploidy, are the most common cause of first-trimester miscarriage, in both spontaneous and IVF conceptions [1]. It is important to consider factors associated with the couple's history of infertility, as well as medications and techniques required for IVF, in your assessment of miscarriage

risk. This information needs to be discussed with the couple so an informed decision can be made, in regard to whether to proceed with IVF.

The objectives of this chapter are two-fold:

(1) To review factors associated with miscarriage following IVF.
(2) To outline an evidence-based approach to counseling such couples.

Infertility is a common problem among couples of reproductive age. It is estimated that over 6 million women in the USA have difficulty conceiving and approximately 1.2 million seek treatment every year in the USA [2]. There are many non-IVF therapies, which are less invasive and complicated, for infertility but because IVF has the highest success rate per cycle, many couples choose IVF initially or after failing other treatments.

In the year 2004, 127 977 IVF cycles were reported to the Centers for Disease Control and Prevention (CDC), mostly from the USA and Canada, and 367 066 were reported to the European Society of Human Reproduction and Embryology (ESHRE), mostly from European countries [3,4]. The clinical miscarriage rate after IVF increases from 10% at 25 years of age to 50% at 43 years of age [2].

Sending the miscarriage tissue for cytogenetic analysis is the crucial first step to understanding why miscarriage occurred. If there is a numeric chromosome error, termed non-euploidy, such as trisomy, monosomy or polyploidy, or an unbalanced structural chromosome rearrangement, then the miscarriage is "explained." If the result is euploid, specifically diploid female or male, or a balanced structural chromosome rearrangement, the cause of the miscarriage is unknown, or "unexplained." If a structural chromosome rearrangement is found, such as a reciprocal or Robertsonian translocation, the parents should be

*Early Pregnancy*, ed. Roy G. Farquharson and Mary D. Stephenson. Published by Cambridge University Press.
© Cambridge University Press 2010.

**Table 24.1** Frequency of chromosome errors in clinical miscarriage following IVF.

| Author | Mean maternal age at miscarriage (years) | Clinical miscarriages (n) | Chromosome errors |
| --- | --- | --- | --- |
| Causio et al. [7] | 32 | 64 | 45% |
| Plachot [8] | 35 | 21 | 62% |
| Ma et al. [9] | 36 | 80 | 64% |
| Bettio et al. [5] | 37 | 119 | 61% |
| Spandorfer et al. [10] | 37 | 71 | 71% |
| Lathi et al. [11] | 37 | 152 | 62% |

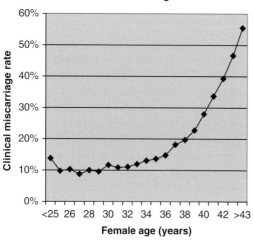

**Percentage of IVF pregnancies that end in clinical miscarriage**

**Figure 24.1** National summary of fresh non-donor egg ART cycles in US from the Centers for Disease Control and Prevention, US department of Heath and Human Services [2].

screened. If one of the parents has the rearrangement, genetic counseling is recommended. If neither is affected, then the structural chromosome rearrangement occurred *de novo* and the couple has a low risk of recurrence. .

## Numeric chromosome errors in miscarriages following IVF

The risk of miscarriage dramatically increased with advancing maternal age, primarily due to trisomy [1]. Several researchers have examined the frequency of chromosome abnormalities in miscarriages following IVF, as shown in Table 24.1. Although few direct comparisons have been published, the frequency of

numeric chromosome errors in miscarriages following IVF are comparable to those following spontaneous conception[5,6]. The differences seen, between these studies, are likely due to differences in the mean maternal ages [7–11].

Ovarian stimulation protocols have been evolving since the first successful human IVF procedure was performed in 1978 [12]. In a natural cycle, typically only one mature follicle is produced. Since not every follicle produces a viable oocyte and not every oocyte becomes fertilized in the laboratory, ovarian stimulation is performed to increase oocyte yield and embryo number. By increasing the numbers of embryos available for transfer, pregnancy rates per cycle have increased [13,14]. With an aggressive stimulation protocol, which typically consists of a GnRH agonist or antagonist, and high doses of FSH with or without LH, 10–20 oocytes can be obtained, whereas with a more mild stimulation, 5–10 oocytes are typically obtained. The effects of ovarian stimulation on the developing oocyte are poorly understood.

Studies on preimplantation embryos show a high rate of numeric chromosome errors in embryos produced through IVF [15,16]. Such findings have led researchers to study the impact of ovarian stimulation on oocyte and embryo development. Baart and colleagues compared the impact of a standard ovarian stimulation to a milder ovarian stimulation in a randomized controlled trial (RCT) [17]. The standard ovarian stimulation protocol consisted of 225 IU of recombinant FSH following 2 weeks of pre-treatment with a GnRH agonist. The mild ovarian stimulation protocol consisted of 150 IU of recombinant FSH starting 5 days after onset of menses for ovarian stimulation followed by a GnRH antagonist to prevent ovulation. There were 44 and 67 patients in standard and mild stimulation groups, respectively. Pre-implantation genetic analysis was performed by 10 chromosome FISH, of 1–2 blastomeres per cleavage stage embryo. The results showed that the subjects in the standard ovarian stimulation group had a higher percentage of embryos with numeric chromosome errors compared with the mild ovarian stimulation group, 63% vs 45% ($P = 0.016$). Despite this difference, because there were a higher number of eggs and embryos in the standard ovarian stimulation group, there was no difference in the absolute number of euploid embryos available for transfer per cycle between the two groups. Baart et al. concluded that a more aggressive stimulation results in more aneuploid embryos without an increase in viable embryos for transfer. The increased frequency of chromosome errors could be due to the increased dose of FSH in the standard ovarian stimulation group but other factors, such as pre-treatment with a GnRH agonist or the use of a GnRH antagonist, could have also influenced the results. It is interesting to note that the 45% chromosome error rate in the mild ovarian stimulation group is comparable to the 36% seen in natural cycle PGD [18]. This study certainly illustrates how stimulation protocols may impact the frequency of numeric chromosome errors in oocytes, and thus embryos, in IVF cycles.

In the case of the 39-year-old woman who conceived through IVF, but, unfortunately, had a miscarriage associated with trisomy 15, the question of whether pre-implantation genetic screening (PGS) could improve her subsequent likelihood of success has been raised by many IVF clinicians and scientists. In theory, PGS would allow selection of euploid embryos, which would be advantageous, especially in woman of advanced maternal age [19]. Unfortunately, morphological assessment of embryos prior to transfer is not effective in identifying embryos with chromosome errors; 60% of aneuploid embryos have good embryo scores at the cleavage stage and 30–50% progress to the blastocyst stage [20].

Initial retrospective PGS reports showed lower miscarriage rates in women over 35 years of age [21,22]. However, several subsequent RCTs found no clear benefit of PGS, with respect to live birth or miscarriage rates [23–27]; see Table 24.2.

In 2007, Mastenbroek and colleagues reported a large multicentered RCT comparing standard IVF with or without PGS[23]. Four hundred and two subjects between 35 and 41 years of age were randomized to standard IVF or IVF with PGS. They underwent

up to three cycles of their assigned treatments. This study showed a statistically significant reduction in the ongoing pregnancy rate in the IVF/PGS group compared with the control group. In addition, the miscarriage rate in the IVF/PGS group was not decreased [23]. Later, a subgroup analysis of this data set showed no differences in miscarriage rates even in patients with a history of one or more prior miscarriages [28]. Several smaller RCTs showed similar results, therefore, there appears to be no benefit of IVF/PGS to improve the live birth rate in women of advanced maternal age [24–27,29].

- All studies included one cycle per patient except in Mastenbroek et al. [23], where up to three cycles were performed per patient.
- Clinical miscarriage rate was calculated per clinical pregnancy rate.

As the effectiveness of the technique is called into question, accuracy and safety appear to be among the limitations of PGS. The required biopsy is performed using a laser to remove a portion of the zona pellucida, followed by gentle suction to aspirate a single blastomere. The blastomere is then fixed and analyzed using fluorescent in-situ hybridization (FISH) probes to a chromosome-specific loci. If no nucleus is seen, a second cell is removed and tested [30,31]. Since all chromosomes cannot be screened with FISH, specific chromosome probes are chosen; typically 3–12 probes are used. With a lower number of probes, fewer errors are detected but many errors could be missed. However, with a higher number of chromosome probes, the false positive rate increases, leading to fewer embryos to transfer. Critics of PGS have stated that the results of a single cell do not accurately represent the embryo because of mosaicism among blastomeres [32–36]. As new embryo screening options become available, we may be able to screen for more chromosomes and have fewer errors, but concerns about embryo mosaicism and embryo biopsy techniques will remain.

To date, all prospective RCTs demonstrate no advantage of IVF/PGS over conventional IVF in terms of live birth rate or miscarriage rate, in either young or older IVF patients (see Table 24.2). Despite the knowledge that women over the age of 35 years have a higher proportion of non-euploid embryos, all IVF/PGS RCTs for this cohort show poorer outcomes with IVF/PGS. Even in younger women desiring a single embryo transfer, there was no benefit of

**Table 24.2** Randomized controlled trials of in-vitro fertilization with pre-implantation genetic screening (IVF/PGS) versus IVF alone.

| | Number of patients (n) | Female age criteria (years) | Age (mean) | Chromosomes screened | Live birth rate/ patient | Clinical miscarriage rate |
|---|---|---|---|---|---|---|
| Mastenbroek, et al. IVF/PGS [23] | 206 | 35–41 | 38 | X, Y, 1, 13, 16, 17, 18, 21 | 24% | 18% |
| IVF controls (without PGS) | 202 | 35–41 | 37.9 | | 35% | 18% |
| Hardarson et al. IVF/PGS [24] | 56 | >38 | 40.5 | X, Y, 13, 16, 18, 21, 22 | 5% | 70% |
| IVF controls | 53 | >38 | 40.6 | | 19% | 37% |
| Staessen et al. IVF/PGS [25] | 148 | >37 | 40.1 | X, Y, 13, 16, 18, 21, 22 | 15% | 24% |
| IVF controls | 141 | >37 | 39.9 | | 21% | 25% |
| Schoolcraft et al. IVF/PGS [26] | 32 | >35 | 38.2 | X, Y, 13, 15, 16, 17, 18, 21, 22 | 50% | 26% |
| IVF controls [26] | 30 | >35 | 38.3 | | 52% | 32% |
| Meyer et al. IVF/PGS [27] | 21 | <39 | 31.6 | X, Y, 13, 16, 17, 18, 21, 22 | 29% | 46% |
| IVF controls | 22 | <39 | 31.1 | | 68% | 6% |
| Hardarson et al. IVF/PGS [24] | 56 | ≥38 | 40.5 | X, Y, 13, 16, 18, 21, 22 | 5.4% | 70% |
| IVF controls | 53 | ≥38 | 40.6 | | 19% | 38% |
| Staessen et al. IVF/PGS [29] | 107 | <36 | 30.0 | X, Y, 13, 16, 18, 21, 22 | 31% | 21% |
| IVF controls | 107 | <36 | 29.7 | | 31% | 28% |

IVF/PGS [29]. Staessen *et al.* showed that embryos selected for transfer by visual inspection were just as likely to result in a live birth or miscarriage as those selected for transfer based on IVF/PGS with 7-probe FISH.

In summary, chromosome errors are commonly found in miscarriages, whether the pregnancy was achieved spontaneously or through IVF. Clinicians should have a clear understanding of the common chromosome errors [37] and their frequencies, so that they can counsel their patients appropriately. At least 90% of pregnancies with chromosome errors end in demise prior to 10 weeks' gestation. It appears that the overwhelming majority of miscarriages with chromosome errors are not associated with an increased risk of miscarriage in the next pregnancies, as it appears to be a random event. Hence, sending miscarriage tissue for chromosome testing can be informative for the patient and clinician. If the

miscarriage is found to be non-euploid, no further evaluation is needed and IVF/PGS should not be recommended based on currently available data from the RCTs described above. A milder stimulation protocol without pretreatment with a GnRH agonist could be considered, based on the RCT by Baart *et al.* [17]. However, further studies are needed in this area.

# Approach to patients with euploid miscarriages after IVF

With a euploid miscarriage, a careful review of the patient's obstetric and medical history is warranted. For example, if this is her second or third miscarriage, a thorough evaluation for recurrent pregnancy loss would be indicated, as described in Chapter 7. In Case #2, this was the patient's first miscarriage, which occurred prior to 10 weeks' gestation. Since the cytogenetics result was diploid male, 46, XY, miscarriage risk factors should be carefully evaluated.

Counseling women after miscarriages with euploid chromosome results is challenging because the etiology is often unknown. If the result is diploid female, 46, XX, discussion with the cytogenetics laboratory is required, to determine whether further studies could be performed to assess for maternal cell contamination, due to culturing of the maternal decidua, rather than the miscarriage tissue.

Despite euploid results, developmental defects often occur. In fact, embryoscopy studies of the miscarriage prior to uterine evacuation reveal that major embryonic developmental abnormalities are often seen in euploid miscarriages. Philipp *et al.* found that 71% of euploid miscarriages had major morphological abnormalities, including neural tube defects, microcephaly, as well as face and limb defects. Only 7% of the miscarriages examined were both chromosomally and morphologically normal [38]. In a subsequent publication, Philipp *et al.* reported embryoscopy and cytogenetic results of 23 IVF pregnancies ending in miscarriage [39]. They found that 15 of the 23 miscarriages had numeric chromosome errors and that six out of eight of the embryos with euploid results had grossly abnormal developmental defects. Although embryoscopy is not widely available, these results can be used for counseling. Despite normal chromosome results, an embryo may have had a major developmental defect, which was incompatible with life.

## Lifestyle modification

Lifestyle factors should be carefully evaluated and modified, when possible, following a euploid miscarriage and, ideally, for all women who are considering starting a family. Sometimes, having a miscarriage can motivate prospective mothers to improve their prepregnancy health. Such factors include obesity and substance use, such as tobacco and caffeine. Maternal obesity has been associated with an increased risk of miscarriage and poor pregnancy outcomes in several studies of spontaneous [40–43] and IVF conceptions [44,45]. Although studies on the effect of weight loss on miscarriage are often small and retrospective, they do show a reduction in miscarriage rates [43,46].

The link between caffeine consumption and the risk of miscarriage has been debated for years. The largest prospective study in the literature suggests a link between increased caffeine consumption and

early pregnancy loss [47]. In addition, a study by Cnattingius *et al.* demonstrated that the increased miscarriage rate was due to demise of euploid pregnancies [48].

Cigarette smoking is another modifiable risk factor for infertility and history of miscarriage [49,50]. A meta-analysis of 17 studies examining the outcome of assisted reproduction found that women who smoked had an increased odds of miscarriage compared with non-smokers, OR 2.65 (95% CI 1.33–5.30) [51]. In addition, smoking was associated with higher ectopic pregnancy rates and lower implantation rates. Despite such risks, some women continue to smoke throughout pregnancy [49]. Counseling patients to stop smoking prior to IVF is likely to improve the live birth rate and decrease the risk of miscarriage.

In summary, caffeine, tobacco and secondhand smoke exposure have been associated with a modest increase in early miscarriage [48,52,53]. It should be recommended that patients minimize or avoid caffeine ingestion and exposure to tobacco smoke prior to and during pregnancy to reduce the risk of adverse pregnancy outcomes [54].

The optimal amount of physical exercise during pregnancy is unknown. Patients with a history of miscarriage will often ask if bedrest is necessary to prevent miscarriage. These patients should be reassured that typical or routine non-vigorous activity does not appear to be a risk factor for miscarriage. Secondly, several studies have shown that bedrest does not appear to reduce the risk of miscarriage [55]. However, there are data that suggest that intense and long duration of physical exertion may be associated with a higher risk of miscarriage [56,57]. Therefore, it may be reasonable to recommend that women consider reducing the intensity and duration of their exercise in pregnancy, especially if there is a history of miscarriage.

## Tubal disease

Several studies have shown that hydrosalpinx is associated with an increased miscarriage rate in IVF, compared with control patients with other infertility factors or proximal tubal occusion [58–62]. The mechanism of this detrimental effect is thought to be due to a direct effect of the hydrosalpinx fluid on embryo development or endometrial receptivity [63,64]. The biochemical markers of implantation, such as ß3 integrins, *Hoxa* genes, LIF and IL-1 appear to be altered in the setting of hydrosalpinges

[54,64–67]. Treatment of hydrosalpinx either by proximal tubal ligation or salpingectomy, has been shown to improve the success of IVF by reducing the miscarriage rate [68–71]. Typically, a hydrosalpinx is diagnosed during the initial infertility evaluation by hysterosalpingogram (HSG). However, HSG may not be uniformly performed, for example, in cases of severe male factor infertility. If a hydrosalpinx is suspected, based on ultrasound findings or history, an HSG should be performed. If present, ligation or salpingectomy should be considered before another IVF cycle.

## Endocrine evaluation

Several endocrine factors, most notably thyroid disease, are also linked to an increased miscarriage risk after IVF. The most common etiology of clinical and subclinical hypothyroidism in developed countries is autoimmune disease. Several studies have shown an increased incidence of autoimmune thyroid disease in the infertile population, particularly associated with endometriosis and ovarian failure [72–74]. In 1990, Stagnaro-Green et al. published the first study showing an association between antithryoid antibodies and miscarriage. Since then, this association has been confirmed by others and appears to be independent of demographics, age and obstetric history [75–81]. A meta-analysis of these studies reported an OR of 2.73 (95% CI 2.20–3.40) for miscarriage in antibody-positive euthyroid women, compared with controls [82]. The cause of this association is unknown, but preliminary data suggest that the risk of miscarriage may be reduced with thyroid supplementation [83,84].

For women with known thyroid disease, the Endocrine Society guidelines recommend that thyroid supplementation be adjusted so that the TSH level is below 2.5 prior to conception. Thyroid requirements are known to increase during pregnancy and an increase in thyroid supplementation by 30–50% during early pregnancy should be anticipated [85]. A sensitive TSH assay should be performed after a euploid miscarriage. Recent evidence suggests that 2.5 mIU/ml should be considered the upper limit of normal in women contemplating pregnancy and that higher levels are considered to be subclinical or overt thyroid disease [86].

Fertility treatments can also stress the secretory capacity of the thyroid, therefore, women with subclinical thyroid disease may develop overt hypothyroidism with the initiation of IVF. In a pilot study, Baker et al. found that TSH levels between 2.5 and 4 mIU/mL prior to an IVF cycle were associated with an increased miscarriage rate [87]. Therefore, thyroid supplementation should be considered in the IVF population when the pre-pregnancy TSH level is greater than 2.5 mIU/mL, with dosing adjusted to maintain the TSH below this cut-off prior to attempting conception and throughout pregnancy.

In-vitro fertilization patients with a euploid miscarriage should be re-evaluated for prolactin disorders. Hyperprolactinemia typically presents with oligomenorrhea or galactorrhea, however, otherwise asymptomatic patients with hyperprolactinemia may suffer from altered steroid hormone production [88,89]. Treatment of asymptomatic recurrent miscarriage patients with bromocriptine was shown to decrease miscarriage risk in an RCT [90]. Although this study was limited by size and did not address IVF patients with a euploid miscarriage, it seems reasonable to treat hyperprolactinemia in this setting.

Although uncontrolled diabetes is rare in the reproductive age population, it is an important factor associated with first-trimester miscarriage. Since women with polycystic ovary syndrome (PCOS) are at increased risk for both insulin resistance and overt diabetes, it is recommended that PCOS patients be screened for diabetes [91]. Diagnosing and treating diabetes is essential for women attempting pregnancy, both to reduce the miscarriage rate [92], but also to reduce the risk of congenital malformations [93,94]. Strict blood-sugar control during preconception and in early pregnancy is necessary to reduce the miscarriage risk [95,96]. While ideally glycosylated hemoglobin levels should be kept below 6.1%, any reduction in HgA1c can be associated with improved pregnancy outcomes [97,98].

## Endometrial factors

Successful implantation and pregnancy depends on a complex interaction between the developing endometrium and the embryo. Aberrations in markers of endometrial receptivity, such as LIF and IL-11 [99,100], have been seen in both infertile and recurrent miscarriage patients [101–104]. Studies examining endometrial dating have shown accelerated endometrial maturation and dysregulation of endometrial transcripts in the luteal phase of gonadotropin-stimulated cycles [105–108]. Studies have revealed these changes are more pronounced with a more aggressive ovarian stimulation protocol and higher estradiol levels[109,110]. The impact of these changes on the miscarriage rate is poorly understood. In a retrospective review of IVF cycles, Santoro *et al.* found a trend toward increasing miscarriage rate with increasing dose of gonatropins, however, due to confounders, such as age and decreased ovarian reserve, this trend did not reach statistical significance [111]. Well-powered studies are needed to evaluate the impact of ovarian stimulation protocols on endometrial function and miscarriage risk.

## Uterine factors

Congenital and acquired anomalies of the uterus are found in patients with infertility and recurrent miscarriage. If not performed prior to an IVF cycle, a uterine evaluation should be performed after a euploid miscarriage to assess for congenital and acquired uterine anomalies. A uterine septum, either partial or complete, is the most frequent of the müllerian fusion anomalies. If a septum is found, counseling about treatment options, specifically, a hysteroscopy metroplasty, should be discussed to reduce the risk of miscarriage in the IVF population [112].

Uterine fibroids are common among women of reproductive age; submucosal and intramural fibroids have been associated with an increased miscarriage rate [113–115]. Although no RCT has been performed, retrospective studies suggest that removal of fibroids reduces miscarriage rates in women with a history of miscarriage [116,117]. Therefore, surgery could be considered for an IVF patient with a euploid miscarriage, if clinically significant fibroids are present.

Intrauterine synechiae may form after any type of endometrial trauma, most commonly infection or surgery. Synechiae are found in 5–25% of patients with infertility and/or recurrent miscarriage [118]. In order to optimize future pregnancy outcomes, consideration should be given to hysteroscopic adhesiolysis.

Fortunately, müllerian fusion anomalies, such as the unicornuate uterus, bicornuate uterus and uterine didelphys, all of which cannot be surgically repaired, have a good prognosis for a subsequent live birth [119,120].

## Conclusions

Miscarriages after an IVF cycle are frustrating for the patient and physician. Performing cytogenetic analysis on the miscarriage tissue is useful for counseling the patient and for determining whether further evaluation is warranted. Based on several RCTs, IVF/PGS does not appear to reduce the risk of miscarriage in IVF. After a euploid miscarriage, underlying medical and obstetric factors should be carefully evaluated. Hydrosalpinx, subclinical and overt hypothyroidism, obesity and diabetes should be treated. Lifestyle factors can also contribute to excess miscarriage, so those should also be modified to create the optimal environment for early pregnancy.

If a factor is not identified, patients should be encouraged to try again. Presently, IVF live birth rates are no different for women with a history of miscarriage compared with those without, or with no prior pregnancy [2]. There is a paucity of randomized controlled data on ovarian stimulation protocols and their impact on euploid or non-euploid miscarriages. Further studies are urgently needed so that optimal care can be provided to reduce the risk of miscarriage following an IVF cycle.

## References

1. Hassold T, Chiu D. Maternal age-specific rates of numerical chromosome abnormalities with special reference to trisomy. *Hum Genet* 1985; **70**(1): 11–17.

2. Centers for Disease Control and Prevention; ASfRM, Society for Assisted Reproductive Technology. 2006 Assisted Reproductive Technology Success Rates: National Summary and Fertility Clinic Reports. US Department of Health and Human Services CfDcaP, 2008.

3. Andersen AN, Goossens V, Ferraretti AP *et al.* Assisted reproductive technology in Europe, 2004: results generated from European registers by ESHRE. *Hum Reprod* 2008; **23**(4): 756–71.

4. Martinez GM, Chandra A, Abma JC, Jones J, Mosher WD. Fertility, contraception, and fatherhood: data on men and women from cycle 6 (2002) of the 2002 National Survey of Family Growth. *Vital Health Stat* 2006 **23**: 1–142.

5. Bettio D, Venci A, Levi Setti PE. Chromosomal abnormalities in miscarriages after different assisted reproduction procedures. *Placenta* 2008; **29** (Suppl. B): 126–8.

6. Schieve LA, Tatham L, Peterson HB, Toner J, Jeng G. Spontaneous abortion among pregnancies conceived using assisted reproductive technology in the United States. *Obstet Gynecol* 2003; **101**(5 Pt 1): 959–67.

7. Causio F, Fischetto R, Sarcina E, Geusa S, Tartagni M. Chromosome analysis of spontaneous abortions after in vitro fertilization (IVF) and intracytoplasmic sperm injection (ICSI). *Eur J Obstet Gynecol Reprod Biol* 2002; **105**(1): 44–8.

8. Plachot M. Chromosome analysis of spontaneous abortions after IVF. A European survey. *Hum Reprod* 1989; **4**(4): 425–9.

9. Ma S, Philipp T, Zhao Y *et al.* Frequency of chromosomal abnormalities in spontaneous abortions derived from intracytoplasmic sperm injection compared with those from in vitro fertilization. *Fertil Steril* 2006; **85**(1): 236–9.

10. Spandorfer SD, Davis OK, Barmat LI, Chung PH, Rosenwaks Z. Relationship between maternal age and aneuploidy in in vitro fertilization pregnancy loss. *Fertil Steril* 2004; **81**(5): 1265–9.

11. Lathi RB, Westphal LM, Milki AA. Aneuploidy in the miscarriages of infertile women and the potential benefit of preimplanation genetic diagnosis. *Fertil Steril* 2008; **89**(2): 353–7.

12. Steptoe PC, Edwards RG. Birth after the reimplantation of a human embryo. *Lancet* 1978; **2**(8085): 366.

13. Phillips SJ, Kadoch IJ, Lapensee L *et al.* Controlled natural cycle IVF: experience in a world of stimulation. *Reprod Biomed Online* 2007; **14**(3): 356–9.

14. Fishel SB, Edwards RG, Purdy JM *et al.* Implantation, abortion, and birth after in vitro fertilization using the natural menstrual cycle or follicular stimulation with clomiphene citrate and human menopausal gonadotropin. *J In Vitro Fert Embryo Transf* 1985; **2**(3): 123–31.

15. Simon C, Rubio C, Vidal F *et al.* Increased chromosome abnormalities in human preimplantation embryos after in-vitro fertilization in patients with recurrent miscarriage. *Reprod Fertil Dev* 1998; **10**(1): 87–92.

16. Rubio C, Pehlivan T, Rodrigo L *et al.* Embryo aneuploidy screening for unexplained recurrent miscarriage: a minireview. *Am J Reprod Immunol* 2005; **53**(4): 159–65.

17. Baart EB, Martini E, Eijkemans MJ *et al.* Milder ovarian stimulation for in-vitro fertilization reduces aneuploidy in the human preimplantation embryo: a randomized controlled trial. *Hum Reprod* 2007; **22**(4): 980–8.

18. Verpoest W, Fauser BC, Papanikolaou E *et al.* Chromosomal aneuploidy in embryos conceived with unstimulated cycle IVF. *Hum Reprod* 2008; **23**(10): 2369–71.

19. Baruch S, Kaufman D, Hudson KL. Genetic testing of embryos: practices and perspectives of US in vitro fertilization clinics. *Fertil Steril* 2008; **89**(5): 1053–8.

20. Rubio C, Rodrigo L, Mercader A *et al.* Impact of chromosomal abnormalities on preimplantation embryo development. *Prenat Diagn* 2007; **27**(8): 748–56.

21. Munne S, Chen S, Fischer J *et al.* Preimplantation genetic diagnosis reduces pregnancy loss in women aged 35 years and older with a history of recurrent miscarriages. *Fertil Steril* 2005; **84**(2): 331–5.

22. Munne S, Sandalinas M, Escudero T *et al.* Improved implantation after preimplantation genetic diagnosis of aneuploidy. *Reprod Biomed Online* 2003; **7**(1): 91–7.

23. Mastenbroek S, Twisk M, van Echten-Arends J *et al.* In vitro fertilization with preimplantation genetic screening. *New Engl J Med* 2007; **357**(1): 9–17.

24. Hardarson T, Hanson C, Lundin K *et al.* Preimplantation genetic screening in women of advanced maternal age caused a decrease in clinical pregnancy rate: a randomized controlled trial. *Hum Reprod* 2008; **23**(12): 2806–12.

25. Staessen C, Platteau P, Van Assche E *et al.* Comparison of blastocyst transfer with or without preimplantation genetic diagnosis for aneuploidy screening in couples with advanced maternal age: a prospective randomized controlled trial. *Hum Reprod* 2004; **19**(12): 2849–58.

26. Schoolcraft WB, Katz-Jaffe MG, Stevens J, Rawlins M, Munne S. Preimplantation aneuploidy testing for infertile patients of advanced maternal age: a randomized prospective trial. *Fertil Steril* 2009; **92**: 157–62.

27. Meyer LR, Klipstein S, Hazlett WD, Nasta T, Mangan P, Karande VC. A prospective randomized controlled trial of preimplantation genetic screening in the "good prognosis" patient. *Fertil Steril* 2009; **91**: 1731.

28. Twisk M, Mastenbroek S, van Wely M *et al.* Preimplantation genetic screening for abnormal number of chromosomes (aneuploidies) in in vitro fertilisation or intracytoplasmic sperm injection. *Cochrane Database Syst Rev* 2006; **1**: CD005291.

29. Staessen C, Verpoest W, Donoso P *et al.* Preimplantation genetic screening does not improve delivery rate in women under the age of 36 following single-embryo transfer. *Hum Reprod* 2008; **23**(12): 2818–25.

30. Cohen J, Wells D, Munne S. Removal of 2 cells from cleavage stage embryos is likely to reduce the efficacy of chromosomal tests that are used to enhance implantation rates. *Fertil Steril* 2007; **87**(3): 496–503.

31. Goossens V, De Rycke M, De Vos A *et al.* Diagnostic efficiency, embryonic development and clinical outcome after the biopsy of one or two blastomeres for preimplantation genetic diagnosis. *Hum Reprod* 2008; **23**(3): 481–92.

32. Gonzalez-Merino E, Emiliani S, Vassart G *et al.* Incidence of chromosomal mosaicism in human embryos at different developmental stages analyzed by fluorescence in situ hybridization. *Genet Test* 2003; **7**(2): 85–95.

33. Munne S, Sandalinas M, Escudero T, Marquez C, Cohen J. Chromosome mosaicism in cleavage-stage human embryos: evidence of a maternal age effect. *Reprod Biomed Online* 2002; **4**(3): 223–32.

34. Bielanska M, Tan SL, Ao A. Chromosomal mosaicism throughout human preimplantation development in vitro: incidence, type, and relevance to embryo outcome. *Hum Reprod* 2002; **17**(2): 413–19.

35. Munne S, Weier HU, Grifo J, Cohen J. Chromosome mosaicism in human embryos. *Biol Reprod* 1994; **51**(3): 373–9.

36. Harper JC, Coonen E, Handyside AH *et al*. Mosaicism of autosomes and sex chromosomes in morphologically normal, monospermic preimplantation human embryos. *Prenat Diagn* 1995; **15**(1): 41–9.

37. Morton NE, Jacobs PA, Hassold T, Wu D. Maternal age in trisomy. *Ann Hum Genet* 1988; **52**(Pt 3): 227–35.

38. Philipp T, Philipp K, Reiner A, Beer F, Kalousek DK. Embryoscopic and cytogenetic analysis of 233 missed abortions: factors involved in the pathogenesis of developmental defects of early failed pregnancies. *Hum Reprod* 2003; **18**(8): 1724–32.

39. Philipp T, Feichtinger W, Van Allen MI *et al*. Abnormal embryonic development diagnosed embryoscopically in early intrauterine deaths after in vitro fertilization: a preliminary report of 23 cases. *Fertil Steril* 2004; **82**(5): 1337–42.

40. Metwally M, Li TC, Ledger WL. The impact of obesity on female reproductive function. *Obes Rev* 2007; **8**(6): 515–23.

41. Satpathy HK, Fleming A, Frey D *et al*. Maternal obesity and pregnancy. *Postgrad Med* 2008; **120**(3): E01–9.

42. Metwally M, Ledger WL, Li TC. Reproductive endocrinology and clinical aspects of obesity in women. *Ann N Y Acad Sci* 2008; **1127**: 140–6.

43. Bilenka B, Ben-Shlomo I, Cozacov C, Gold CH, Zohar S. Fertility, miscarriage and pregnancy after vertical banded gastroplasty operation for morbid obesity. *Acta Obstet Gynecol Scand* 1995; **74**(1): 42–4.

44. Fedorcsak P, Storeng R, Dale PO, Tanbo T, Abyholm T. Obesity is a risk factor for early pregnancy loss after IVF or ICSI. *Acta Obstet Gynecol Scand* 2000; **79**(1): 43–8.

45. Bellver J, Busso C, Pellicer A, Remohi J, Simon C. Obesity and assisted reproductive technology outcomes. *Reprod Biomed Online* 2006; **12**(5): 562–8.

46. Clark AM, Thornley B, Tomlinson L, Galletley C, Norman RJ. Weight loss in obese infertile women results in improvement in reproductive outcome for all forms of fertility treatment. *Hum Reprod* 1998; **13**(6): 1502–5.

47. Weng X, Odouli R, Li DK. Maternal caffeine consumption during pregnancy and the risk of miscarriage: a prospective cohort study. *Am J Obstet Gynecol* 2008; **198**(3): 279 e1–8.

48. Cnattingius S, Signorello LB, Anneren G *et al*. Caffeine intake and the risk of first-trimester spontaneous abortion. *New Engl J Med* 2000; **343**(25): 1839–45.

49. Einarson A, Riordan S. Smoking in pregnancy and lactation: a review of risks and cessation strategies. *Eur J Clin Pharmacol* 2009; **65**(4): 325–30.

50. Castles A, Adams EK, Melvin CL, Kelsch C, Boulton ML. Effects of smoking during pregnancy. Five meta-analyses. *Am J Prev Med* 1999; **16**(3): 208–15.

51. Waylen AL, Metwally M, Jones GL, Wilkinson AJ, Ledger WL. Effects of cigarette smoking upon clinical outcomes of assisted reproduction: a meta-analysis. *Hum Reprod Update* 2009; **15**(1): 31–44.

52. George L, Granath F, Johansson AL, Anneren G, Cnattingius S. Environmental tobacco smoke and risk of spontaneous abortion. *Epidemiology* 2006; **17**(5): 500–5.

53. Windham GC, Von Behren J, Waller K, Fenster L. Exposure to environmental and mainstream tobacco smoke and risk of spontaneous abortion. *Am J Epidemiol* 1999; **149**(3): 243–7.

54. Meyer WR, Castelbaum AJ, Somkuti S, *et al*. Hydrosalpinges adversely affect markers of endometrial receptivity. *Hum Reprod* 1997; **12**(7): 1393–8.

55. Aleman A, Althabe F, Belizan J, Bergel E. Bed rest during pregnancy for preventing miscarriage. *Cochrane Database Syst Rev* 2005; **2**: CD003576.

56. Madsen M, Jorgensen T, Jensen ML *et al*. Leisure time physical exercise during pregnancy and the risk of miscarriage: a study within the Danish National Birth Cohort. *BJOG* 2007; **114**(11): 1419–26.

57. Morris SN, Missmer SA, Cramer DW *et al*. Effects of lifetime exercise on the outcome of in vitro fertilization. *Obstet Gynecol* 2006; **108**(4): 938–45.

58. Camus E, Poncelet C, Goffinet F *et al*. Pregnancy rates after in-vitro fertilization in cases of tubal infertility with and without hydrosalpinx: a meta-analysis of published comparative studies. *Hum Reprod* 1999; **14**(5): 1243–9.

59. Ozmen B, Diedrich K, Al-Hasani S. Hydrosalpinx and IVF: assessment of treatments implemented prior to IVF. *Reprod Biomed Online* 2007; **14**(2): 235–41.

60. Strandell A, Waldenstrom U, Nilsson L, Hamberger L. Hydrosalpinx reduces in-vitro fertilization/embryo transfer pregnancy rates. *Hum Reprod* 1994; **9**(5): 861–3.

61. Fleming C, Hull MG. Impaired implantation after in vitro fertilisation treatment associated with hydrosalpinx. *Br J Obstet Gynaecol* 1996; **103**(3): 268–72.

62. Zeyneloglu HB, Arici A, Olive DL. Adverse effects of hydrosalpinx on pregnancy rates after in vitro fertilization-embryo transfer. *Fertil Steril* 1998; **70**(3): 492–9.

63. Strandell A, Lindhard A. Why does hydrosalpinx reduce fertility? The importance of hydrosalpinx fluid. *Hum Reprod* 2002; **17**(5): 1141–5.

64. Daftary GS, Kayisli U, Seli E *et al.* Salpingectomy increases peri-implantation endometrial HOXA10 expression in women with hydrosalpinx. *Fertil Steril* 2007; **87**(2): 367–72.

65. Bildirici I, Bukulmez O, Ensari A, Yarali H, Gurgan T. A prospective evaluation of the effect of salpingectomy on endometrial receptivity in cases of women with communicating hydrosalpinges. *Hum Reprod* 2001; **16**(11): 2422–6.

66. Copperman AB, Wells V, Luna M *et al.* Presence of hydrosalpinx correlated to endometrial inflammatory response in vivo. *Fertil Steril* 2006; **86**(4): 972–6.

67. Savaris RF, Pedrini JL, Flores R, Fabris G, Zettler CG. Expression of alpha 1 and beta 3 integrins subunits in the endometrium of patients with tubal phimosis or hydrosalpinx. *Fertil Steril* 2006; **85**(1): 188–92.

68. Johnson NP, Mak W, Sowter MC. Laparoscopic salpingectomy for women with hydrosalpinges enhances the success of IVF: a Cochrane review. *Hum Reprod* 2002; **17**(3): 543–8.

69. Kontoravdis A, Makrakis E, Pantos K *et al.* Proximal tubal occlusion and salpingectomy result in similar improvement in in vitro fertilization outcome in patients with hydrosalpinx. *Fertil Steril* 2006; **86**(6):1642–9.

70. Strandell A, Lindhard A, Waldenstrom U *et al.* Hydrosalpinx and IVF outcome: a prospective, randomized multicentre trial in Scandinavia on salpingectomy prior to IVF. *Hum Reprod* 1999; **14**(11): 2762–9.

71. Bontis JN, Theodoridis TD. Laparoscopic management of hydrosalpinx. *Ann N Y Acad Sci* 2006; **1092**: 199–210.

72. Poppe K, Velkeniers B, Glinoer D. The role of thyroid autoimmunity in fertility and pregnancy. *Nat Clin Pract Endocrinol Metab* 2008; **4**(7): 394–405.

73. Poppe K, Glinoer D. Thyroid autoimmunity and hypothyroidism before and during pregnancy. *Hum Reprod Update* 2003; **9**(2): 149–61.

74. Karabinas CD, Tolis GJ. Thyroid disorders and pregnancy. *J Obstet Gynaecol* 1998; **18**(6): 509–15.

75. Stagnaro-Green A, Glinoer D. Thyroid autoimmunity and the risk of miscarriage. *Best Pract Res Clin Endocrinol Metab* 2004; **18**(2): 167–81.

76. Muller AF, Berghout A. Consequences of autoimmune thyroiditis before, during and after pregnancy. *Minerva Endocrinol* 2003; **28**(3): 247–54.

77. Kutteh WH, Yetman DL, Carr AC, Beck LA, Scott RT, Jr. Increased prevalence of antithyroid antibodies identified in women with recurrent pregnancy loss but not in women undergoing assisted reproduction. *Fertil Steril* 1999; **71**(5): 843–8.

78. Glinoer D. Miscarriage in women with positive anti-TPO antibodies: is thyroxine the answer? *J Clin Endocrinol Metab* 2006; **91**(7): 2500–2.

79. Trokoudes KM, Skordis N, Picolos MK. Infertility and thyroid disorders. *Curr Opin Obstet Gynecol* 2006; **18**(4): 446–51.

80. Poppe K, Glinoer D, Tournaye H *et al.* Assisted reproduction and thyroid autoimmunity: an unfortunate combination? *J Clin Endocrinol Metab* 2003; **88**(9): 4149–52.

81. Glinoer D. Thyroid autoimmunity and spontaneous abortion. *Fertil Steril* 1999; **72**(2): 373–4.

82. Prummel MF, Wiersinga WM. Thyroid autoimmunity and miscarriage. *Eur J Endocrinol* 2004; **150**(6): 751–5.

83. Negro R, Formoso G, Coppola L, *et al.* Euthyroid women with autoimmune disease undergoing assisted reproduction technologies: the role of autoimmunity and thyroid function. *J Endocrinol Invest* 2007; **30**(1): 30–8.

84. Vaquero E, Lazzarin N, De Carolis C *et al.* Mild thyroid abnormalities and recurrent spontaneous abortion: diagnostic and therapeutical approach. *Am J Reprod Immunol* 2000; **43**(4): 204–8.

85. Abalovich M, Amino N, Barbour LA *et al.* Management of thyroid dysfunction during pregnancy and postpartum: an Endocrine Society Clinical Practice Guideline. *J Clin Endocrinol Metab* 2007; **92**(8 Suppl.): S1–47.

86. Wartofsky L, Dickey RA. The evidence for a narrower thyrotropin reference range is compelling. *J Clin Endocrinol Metab* 2005; **90**(9): 5483–8.

87. Baker VL, Rone HM, Pasta DJ *et al.* Correlation of thyroid stimulating hormone (TSH) level with pregnancy outcome in women undergoing in vitro fertilization. *Am J Obstet Gynecol* 2006; **194**(6): 1668–74; discussion 74–5.

88. Katz E, Adashi EY. Hyperprolactinemic disorders. *Clin Obstet Gynecol* 1990; **33**(3): 622–39.

89. Ranta T, Lehtovirta P, Stenman UH, Seppala M. Serum prolactin and progesterone concentrations in ovulatory infertility. *J Endocrinol Invest* 1979; **2**(1): 71–3.

90. Hirahara F, Andoh N, Sawai K, Hirabuki T, Uemura T, Minaguchi H. Hyperprolactinemic recurrent miscarriage and results of randomized bromocriptine treatment trials. *Fertil Steril* 1998; **70**(2): 246–52.

91. Peppard HR, Marfori J, Iuorno MJ, Nestler JE. Prevalence of polycystic ovary syndrome among premenopausal women with type 2 diabetes. *Diabetes Care* 2001; **24**(6): 1050–2.

92. Miodovnik M, Mimouni F, Siddiqi TA, Khoury J, Berk MA. Spontaneous abortions in repeat diabetic pregnancies: a relationship with glycemic control. *Obstet Gynecol* 1990; **75**(1): 75–8.

93. Nielsen GL, Sorensen HT, Nielsen PH, Sabroe S, Olsen J. Glycosylated hemoglobin as predictor of adverse fetal outcome in type 1 diabetic pregnancies. *Acta Diabetol* 1997; **34**(3): 217–22.

94. Temple R, Aldridge V, Greenwood R *et al.* Association between outcome of pregnancy and glycaemic control in early pregnancy in type 1 diabetes: population based study. *BR Med J* 2002; **325**(7375): 1275–6.

95. Pearson DW, Kernaghan D, Lee R, Penney GC. The relationship between pre-pregnancy care and early pregnancy loss, major congenital anomaly or perinatal death in type I diabetes mellitus. *BJOG* 2007; **114**(1): 104–7.

96. Langer O, Conway DL. Level of glycemia and perinatal outcome in pregestational diabetes. *J Matern Fetal Med* 2000; **9**(1): 35–41.

97. Management of diabetes from preconception to the postnatal period: summary of NICE guidance. *Br Med J* 2008; **336**(7646): 714–7.

98. Hanson U, Persson B, Thunell S. Relationship between haemoglobin A1C in early type 1 (insulin-dependent) diabetic pregnancy and the occurrence of spontaneous abortion and fetal malformation in Sweden. *Diabetologia* 1990; **33**(2): 100–4.

99. Laird SM, Tuckerman EM, Li TC. Cytokine expression in the endometrium of women with implantation failure and recurrent miscarriage. *Reprod Biomed Online* 2006; **13**(1): 13–23.

100. Haddad-Filho J, Cedenho AP, Katz SG. Endometrial expression of IL-1RtI in patients undergoing miscarriage or unsuccessful IVF cycles. *Reprod Biomed Online* 2007; **14**(1): 117–24.

101. Kralickova M, Ulcova-Gallova Z, Sima R *et al.* Association of the leukemia inhibitory factor gene mutation and the antiphospholipid antibodies in the peripheral blood of infertile women. *Folia Microbiol (Praha)* 2007; **52**(5): 543–8.

102. Mikolajczyk M, Wirstlein P, Skrzypczak J. The impact of leukemia inhibitory factor in uterine flushing on the reproductive potential of infertile women – a prospective study. *Am J Reprod Immunol* 2007; **58**(1): 65–74.

103. Skrzypczak J, Wirstlein P, Mikolajczyk M. Could the defects in the endometrial extracellular matrix during the implantation be a cause for impaired fertility? *Am J Reprod Immunol* 2007; **57**(1): 40–8.

104. Lass A, Weiser W, Munafo A, Loumaye E. Leukemia inhibitory factor in human reproduction. *Fertil Steril* 2001; **76**(6): 1091–6.

105. Thomas K, Thomson AJ, Sephton V *et al.* The effect of gonadotrophic stimulation on integrin expression in the endometrium. *Hum Reprod* 2002; **17**(1): 63–8.

106. Bourgain C, Devroey P. The endometrium in stimulated cycles for IVF. *Hum Reprod Update* 2003; **9**(6): 515–22.

107. Papanikolaou EG, Bourgain C, Kolibianakis E, Tournaye H, Devroey P. Steroid receptor expression in late follicular phase endometrium in GnRH antagonist IVF cycles is already altered, indicating initiation of early luteal phase transformation in the absence of secretory changes. *Hum Reprod* 2005; **20**(6): 1541–7.

108. Macklon NS, van der Gaast MH, Hamilton A, Fauser BC, Giudice LC. The impact of ovarian stimulation with recombinant FSH in combination with GnRH antagonist on the endometrial transcriptome in the window of implantation. *Reprod Sci* 2008; **15**(4): 357–65.

109. Liu Y, Lee KF, Ng EH, Yeung WS, Ho PC. Gene expression profiling of human peri-implantation endometria between natural and stimulated cycles. *Fertil Steril* 2008; **90**(6): 2152–64.

110. Makkar G, Ng EH, Yeung WS, Ho PC. Reduced expression of interleukin-11 and interleukin-6 in the periimplantation endometrium of excessive ovarian responders during in vitro fertilization treatment. *J Clin Endocrinol Metab* 2006; **91**(8): 3181–8.

111. Pal L, Jindal S, Witt BR, Santoro N. Less is more: increased gonadotropin use for ovarian stimulation adversely influences clinical pregnancy and live birth after in vitro fertilization. *Fertil Steril* 2008; **89**(6): 1694–701.

112. Ban-Frangez H, Tomazevic T, Virant-Klun I *et al.* The outcome of singleton pregnancies after IVF/ICSI in women before and after hysteroscopic resection of a uterine septum compared to normal controls. *Eur J Obstet Gynecol Reprod Biol* 2009; **146**: 184–7.

113. Kolankaya A, Arici A. Myomas and assisted reproductive technologies: when and how to act? *Obstet Gynecol Clin North Am* 2006; **33**(1): 145–52.

114. Gianaroli L, Gordts S, D'Angelo A *et al.* Effect of inner myometrium fibroid on reproductive outcome after IVF. *Reprod Biomed Online* 2005; **10**(4): 473–7.

115. Klatsky PC, Tran ND, Caughey AB, Fujimoto VY. Fibroids and reproductive outcomes: a systematic literature review from conception to delivery. *Am J Obstet Gynecol* 2008; **198**(4): 357–66.

116. Bajekal N, Li TC. Fibroids, infertility and pregnancy wastage. *Hum Reprod Update* 2000; **6**(6): 614–20.

117. Khaund A, Lumsden MA. Impact of fibroids on reproductive function. *Best Pract Res Clin Obstet Gynaecol* 2008; **22**(4): 749–60.

118. Yu D, Wong YM, Cheong Y, Xia E, Li TC. Asherman syndrome – one century later. *Fertil Steril* 2008; **89**(4): 759–79.

119. Raga F, Bauset C, Remohi J *et al.* Reproductive impact of congenital Müllerian anomalies. *Hum Reprod* 1997; **12**(10): 2277–81.

120. Simon C, Martinez L, Pardo F, Tortajada M, Pellicer A. Müllerian defects in women with normal reproductive outcome. *Fertil Steril* 1991; **56**(6): 1192–3.

# Chapter 25

# Vanishing twin syndrome and long-term outcome

Anja Pinborg

## Introduction

Three decades ago the existence of "vanishing twins" was only hypothesized and the term encumbered with mystical overtones. As ultrasonography is a prerequisite for the diagnosis, the vanishing twin phenomenon – described as embryonic loss of one twin and survival of its co-twin – was first documented in the early days of this technique [1]. As neither the number of vanished twins nor the total number of twin gestations can be determined when first-trimester ultrasonography is not universally performed, the true prevalence of the syndrome is unknown. Further, the use of strict diagnostic criteria is very important for the definition to avoid the confusion between a vanishing gestational (but empty) sac and a disappearing embryo, and between a prominent yolk sac and a gestational sac [2].

Thirty years have passed and more than 2 million assisted reproductive technologies (ART) children have been born worldwide since the first in-vitro fertilization (IVF) baby was delivered in 1978. The incidence of multiple pregnancies has simultaneously increased dramatically owing to the expanded use of infertility therapies and higher childbearing age. Advocated in the late 1990s, the move from triple- to double-embryo transfer almost eliminated higher-order births, but hardly affected the incidence of twin pregnancies. It is well known that twin pregnancies are associated with considerable risks for the mother and offspring and strategies to reduce the frequency of ART twin pregnancies are developing. Arising evidence has proven that compared with their spontaneously conceived counterparts even ART singletons carry higher risks of adverse short- and long-term outcomes [3–9]. The explanation for this is multifactorial and includes (1) higher maternal age, (2) higher frequency of first-time mothers in ART and (3) infertility per se or the

unfavorable parental characteristics of the infertile couples [10–15]. Vanishing twin pregnancies are also a considerable contributor. Whether the IVF/intracytoplasmic sperm injection (ICSI) methods themselves including the ovarian stimulation plays a role in the poorer outcome is currently being discussed.

Although the concept of the vanishing twin was developed in the 1970s, the term has gained new focus as the dual-embryo transfer policy in ART has contributed not only to the rise in twin pregnancies but also to an increasing number of vanishing twin pregnancies. The routine of early ultrasonography in ART pregnancies has provided new information of the true frequency.

This chapter addresses the prevalence of vanishing twins with considerations of the early implantation process including possible pathological mechanisms of the vanishing twin and the vanishing embryo syndrome. The main part is focusing on obstetric and long-term outcome for the surviving fetus in both spontaneously conceived (SC) and ART pregnancies. Finally, vanishing twin syndrome in a broader perspective of elective single-embryo transfer in ART is discussed.

## Pathology

In 1945, long before the advent of ultrasound, the vanishing twin phenomenon was commented on by Stoeckel, who suggested: "It thus appears that twins are more often conceived than born; not only in addition to the evidence of feti papyracei, it may be that twin material is reabsorbed due to early death, without leaving any trace" [16]. Ultrasound has decades later confirmed the events described by Stoeckel, characterized as the vanishing twin phenomenon and also designated as spontaneous reduction. In 1979 Finberg and Birnholz were the first to postulate that a collection of blood seen during pregnancy termination represented an earlier sonographic finding of a second sac that had been adjacent to a 6-week viable gestation and had the statement pathologically confirmed afterwards [17]. The routine use of ultrasonography has later confirmed that spontaneous reduction is a relatively frequent event and histological findings from the fetal surface of placenta have been documented such as well-defined cysts or sacs, degenerated chorion villi, fibrin deposition or fibrinoid degeneration, placental nodules or plaques, embryonic remnants and macerated or stunted fetuses [2].

The precise pathophysiological mechanism of the vanishing twin is still unknown, but early pregnancy disappearance seems to involve resorption and/or formation of a blighted ovum or fetus papyraceus and several explanations are offered: inferior implantation, insufficient placental function, chromosomal abnormalities, malformations and iso-immunization. Chromosomal abnormalities including trisomy 9 and 16, triploidy, tetraploidy and sex chromosomal abnormalities in one of the twins are a documented cause of a resorbed co-twin. Trisomy 16 arising from residual villi belonged to a trisomic twin that never developed, which was supported by a cytogenic analysis of a placental nodule identified at the time of delivery of a healthy infant [18]. Theoretically, iso-immunization developing during pregnancy in a previously unsensitized rhesus-negative mother, in which a rhesus-positive fetus disappears and a rhesus-negative twin continues could be responsible for disappearance of the co-twin [19].

Landy and Keith defined the vanishing twin as the disappearance of one of two gestational sacs or embryos after documented fetal activity [1]. The "lower" gestational age limit involves ultrasound documentation of an embryo or gestation, but an "upper" gestational age limit is not implemented in the definition. Therefore this "upper" limit varies in different studies with both first, second and third trimester disappearances, which is important when comparing outcome of the surviving co-twin.

## The vanishing embryo syndrome

Commonly two or more embryos are transferred in ART pregnancies with a potential risk of losing co-embryos in early pregnancy. Very early, unrecognized twin gestations or "incipient twins" are impossible to quantify, as this entity cannot be verified by ultrasound. A quantitative estimate of the "incipient twin" is the difference between the number of embryos transferred and the number of implanted embryos measured as the number of gestational sacs. The number of implanted embryos is less likely to be reported and therefore some authors have looked at the "vanishing embryo syndrome" as the outcome in pregnancies, where the number of embryos transferred is greater than the number of children born.

Hypothetical mechanisms for the poorer pregnancy outcome in singleton births with an incipient twin are first-trimester "crowding" of the developing gestations or lack of appropriate sites for placental implantation. These factors may determine placental expansion and ultimate fetal nourishment and growth. A hypothetical but unspecific indicator of the incipient twin is first-trimester bleeding, which is present in one-third of all ART pregnancies and is associated with a higher rate of spontaneous abortions [20–21]. Disappearance of a fetus or a gestational sac is associated with vaginal bleeding or spotting, and the clinical presentation of bleeding seems to coincide with the vanishing process [19]. In spontaneously conceived (SC) pregnancies first-trimester vaginal bleeding is associated with higher obstetric risks, which in a population-based study were directly proportional to the amount of bleeding [22–23]. A similar association between first-trimester bleeding and pregnancy outcome including a three-fold increased risk of extreme pre-term birth (OR 3.0, 95% CI 1.1–8.3) was shown in 1432 ART singleton pregnancies [24]. The authors found a correlation between the incidence of first-trimester bleeding and the number of embryos transferred, and first-trimester bleeding was more prevalent in ART than in SC pregnancies, which could point to differences in the implantation process after ART. Moreover there were significantly more vanishing twin pregnancies with first-trimester bleeding (8.7%) than in singleton controls (4.0%).

Early vanishing twins including incipient twins following the transfer of two or more embryos may increase the incidence of first-trimester bleeding in ART pregnancies. Another indicator of the incipient twin in the study by De Sutter was the linear correlation between the incidence of first-trimester bleeding and the number of embryos transferred, which is very suggestive of the early vanishing twin effect. The authors conclude that significantly more embryos were transferred in the first-trimester bleeding group than in controls, which may point to the fact that in some of the patients this bleeding is associated with both recognized and unrecognized vanishing twins [24].

Schieve et al. found that infants conceived with ART were more likely to be of low birth weight in pregnancies with vanishing embryos [25]. In accord with this, Dickey et al. showed that the length of gestation in ART pregnancies was inversely related to the initial numbers of gestational sacs in singletons and twins [26]. A Danish national population-based cohort study has looked at the association between vanishing co-embryos and the risk of cerebral palsy in 9444 IVF/ICSI children [27]. In a Cox regression analysis adjusted for all the relevant covariates the hazard rate ratio of cerebral palsy was 2.3 (95% CI 0.99–5.32) in pregnancies where the number of children at delivery was smaller than the number of embryos transferred compared with pregnancies where the number of embryos was equal to the number of children born.

# The vanishing twin

## Diagnosis and frequency

The true incidence of vanishing twin pregnancies remains unknown and precise assessment is very difficult, as it requires (1) strict definition, (2) routine ultrasonography of both ART and SC pregnancies and (3) clearly defined ultrasound criteria. There is uncertainty whether the term refers to two gestational sacs or two live fetuses and some authors have included the disappearance of a gestational sac (where inevitably there is a possibility that one might be a pseudo-sac) while others include the demise of a fetus with fetal heart beat. Regarding the upper limits both first-, second- and third-trimester discarded fetuses have been included. As no routine ultrasonography up to now has been performed in early SC pregnancies, the true incidence of SC vanishing twin pregnancies has not been verified. On the other hand ART pregnancies with the obligatory early viability scans have provided valuable new information on vanishing twins, though the incidence in ART pregnancies is probably higher than in SC pregnancies due to the dual-embryo transfer policy. Sonographic findings such as normal early embryonic structures including amniotic cavity, chorionic sac, yolk sac, extraembryonic coelom and also subchorionic hemorrhage or hydropic changes in chorion villi can be misinterpreted as additional gestational sacs [2]. Hence the skills of the sonographer and the quality of the equipment used mean an inherent possibility of both exaggeration and underestimation of the true incidence.

Landy and Keith included all relevant publications since 1990 to determine the frequency of resorption in the first trimester in ART and SC pregnancies after early sonography had demonstrated either two gestational sacs or fetuses [2]. The frequencies of vanishing twins in this review together with more recent publications are presented in Table 25.1. The review, with a total of 317 ART pregnancies with initially two sacs, showed very similar pregnancy outcomes to a later thoroughly designed prospective study by Dickey with 866 ART pregnancies with initially two sacs; 9% with miscarriage, 27% singleton delivery and 64% twin delivery [2,26]. In these studies 27% had a vanishing twin pregnancy after the diagnosis of initially two gestational sacs.

The pregnancy outcome of the studies classified with two viable fetuses including a total of 871 ART pregnancies is less consistent as frequencies of miscarriage, singleton and twin pregnancy vary from 5–12%, 12–38% and 57–83%, respectively [2,28,29]. In a Danish multicenter study of delivery outcome in 2137 ART pregnancies after the diagnosis of two viable fetuses in early pregnancy, 4% had a miscarriage, 9% a singleton delivery and 88% a twin delivery (Table 25.1) [30]. These divergences are attributable to the controversy in the definition of spontaneous reduction, inter-study variability in gestational age at early ultrasound and various study populations. Not surprisingly studies with very early ultrasonography had a higher vanishing twin and miscarriage rate.

Dickey et al., in a debate with additional analyses on their primary cohort [31], presented the vice versa frequency as the authors stated that 15% of singleton births following IVF began as a higher-order gestation [31]. This finding was consistent with Tummers, who in 397 early ART twin pregnancies found a vanishing twin rate of 12% in singleton births [28] and with a Danish multicenter cohort study on 8542 clinical IVF pregnancies with a 10% vanishing twin rate in the singleton births [30]. A lower rate of only 6% vanishing twins was found in the Australian and New Zealand national register of assisted conception after two gestational sacs were present at the early ultrasonography. This diminished rate could be a consequence of less optimal recording in the registers and with diverging gestational ages at early ultrasound [32]. However, a similarly low rate was recently found in an Austrian case–control study with 5.8% of ART singletons originating from a twin gestation [33].

With no solid data available the true incidence of vanishing twins in SC pregnancies is widely unknown.

**Table 25.1** Pregnancy/delivery outcome in assisted reproductive technology (ART) and non-ART conceptions after two fetuses or two sacs were observed by ultrasonography in the first trimester.

| Reference | Type of study | Type of conception | Study period | UL GA week | Pregnancies N | Twins % | Singleton % | Miscarriage % |
|---|---|---|---|---|---|---|---|---|
| | | | | | | Pregnancy/delivery outcome | | |
| Two gestational sacs | | | | | | | | |
| [26]* | Retrospective | ART | 1976–2000 | 6–7 | 549 | 63.9% | 26.8% | 9.3% |
| [2]* | Review (n = 3) | ART | 1976–92 | early | 317 | 64.0% | 27.1% | 8.8% |
| [2]* | Review (n = 1) | Non-ART | 1976–92 | early | 37 | 40.5% | 40.5% | 19.0% |
| Two fetuses | | | | | | | | |
| [30]** | Registry | ART | 1995–2001 | 6–7 | 2137 | 87.7% | 8.8% | 3.5% |
| [28]* | Retrospective | ART | 1993–2000 | 6–7 | 397 | 82.8% | 12.1% | 5.1% |
| [29]* | Retrospective | ART | 1992–2002 | 4–5 | 261 | 64.8% | 23.7% | 11.5% |
| [2]* | Review (n = 7) | ART | 1976–1992 | early | 213 | 57.3% | 38.0% | 4.7% |
| [2]* | Review (n = 4) | Non-ART | 1976–1992 | early | 41 | 82.9% | 7.3% | 9.8% |

* Outcome of pregnancy in second trimester;
** Outcome of pregnancy at delivery.

In the review by Landy and Keith loss of one twin could be expected in 40.5% after early identification of two sacs and in only 7.3% if two fetuses were observed, however these percentages were based on only 37 and 41 twin conceptions respectively [2]. In addition patients with SC pregnancies undergo early ultrasonography only because of vaginal bleeding or other high-risk conditions at various gestational ages, while early sonography is routinely performed in ART pregnancies around weeks 6–7.

In summary, the frequency of vanishing twins in ART pregnancies lingers between 6–15%, but the evidence on the rate in SC pregnancies is absent. In many European countries nuchal translucency scans are now being implemented in the national prenatal screening programmes and offered to all pregnant women. Thus a more precise assessment of the frequency of vanishing twins in SC pregnancies will be available in the future.

## Obstetric complications

In 1970 Hewitt and Stewart suggested that the abortion risk for one member of a twin pregnancy is greater than the risks for both members and that the surviving twin is often mistaken for a singleton. In those authors' opinion, misinterpreting the surviving twin as a singleton incorrectly skews data regarding both twinning frequencies and spontaneous abortion statistics [34]. Three decades later this is still relevant, as hidden vanishing twins skew the obstetric outcome of IVF singletons. A possible etiology behind this adverse outcome following spontaneous loss of a co-twin could be inflammatory and catabolic processes secondary to the presence of demised fetal tissue.

Worldwide more than 2 million babies have been delivered after ART and excepting higher childbearing age, the main cause of increasing twin rates is ART as a consequence of the dual- or multiple-embryo transfer policy. Twins carry an increased risk of both short- and long-term adverse outcomes compared with singletons also in ART [30], but the consequences of vanishing twins for the outcome in ART singletons have only been pinpointed during recent years.

The first papers indicating an association between the number of transferred embryos and pregnancy outcome showed that the higher the initial number of gestational sacs the higher the obstetric risks irrespective of the final birth number [25,26,32]. Dickey *et al.* found that after spontaneous reduction with two initial gestational sacs (N = 147), the average length of gestation for singleton births was shortened by 3 days

**Table 25.2** Frequency of pre-term birth (<37 gestational weeks) and very pre-term birth (<32 gestational weeks) in assisted reproductive technology (ART) singleton survivors after either one or two gestational sacs/fetuses had been present at ultrasonography in early pregnancy.

| Percentage with delivery at: | | <37 gestational weeks | | | <32 gestational weeks | | |
|---|---|---|---|---|---|---|---|
| | Survivors | Initial no. of fetuses/sacs | | | Initial no. of fetuses/sacs | | |
| Two gestational sacs | N | Two | One | P-value | Two | One | P-value |
| [32] | 1213 | 18.0% | 13.7% | S | 6.3% | 3.3% | S |
| [26] | 147 | 11.4% | 8.4% | S | 4.5% | 1.4% | S |
| Two fetuses | | | | | | | |
| [30] | 642 | 13.2% | 9.0% | <0.001 | 3.8% | 1.3% | <0.001 |
| [29] | 62 | 19.3% | 16.7% | NS | 4.8% | 2.7% | NS |
| [33] | 46 | 19.6% | 8.7% | 0.067 | 4.3% | 2.2% | 0.47 |
| [35] | 44 | 18.2% | 16.1% | NS | 4.4% | 3.7% | NS |

S, Statistically significant, but no P-value available; NS, Non-significant.

($P$ <0.05) and the mean birth weight was 160 g lower than in singletons with initially one gestational sac ($P$ = 0.002) [26].

Studies on spontaneous reduction in early pregnancy and the frequency of pre-term birth <37 weeks and <32 weeks are summarized in Table 25.2. Apparently all studies with more than 100 survivors show significantly higher frequencies of pre-term and very pre-term birth [26,30,32] and although not statistically significant the smaller studies showed a clear similar trend [29,33,35]. The largest study on spontaneous reduction, an Australian national register-based study with 20 183 singleton pregnancies including 1213 with initially two sacs showed a significant association between the initial number of gestational sacs and risk of prematurity, in particular extremely premature infants, indicating a causal relationship between the numbers of implanted embryos and later outcome in ART singletons [32].

Regarding low birth weight, a very large US population-based controlled cohort study on low birth weight in 18 408 ART singletons found that singletons from pregnancies with initially 2 fetal heartbeats recorded had a frequency of 17.6% with low birth weight (<2500 g) versus 12.6% in singletons with one fetal heartbeat from the start [25].

In a Danish multicenter cohort study on 642 survivors of a vanished co-twin, controlled for maternal age, parity and treatment type (IVF or ICSI), survivors

carried a 2.3-fold increased risk of very pre-term birth (<32 weeks) and a 2.1-fold increased risk of very low birth weight (<1500 g) and a three-fold higher mortality rate [30]. An inverse significant correlation was found between survivors' gestational age at onset of disappearance (early GA <8 weeks, intermediate GA = 8–22 weeks and late GA >22 weeks) and poorer obstetric outcome – the higher gestational age at demise the poorer the outcome regarding both birth weight, pre-term delivery, small-for-gestational age (SGA) and mortality. Even the early and intermediate survivors had significantly poorer outcome than singletons from one gestation with an adjusted risk of child death of 3.3 (95% CI 1.6–7.3) and the early survivors also had significantly lower mean birth weight than singletons from one gestation, indicating that disappearance of a co-twin in the very early pregnancy (<8 weeks) influences the outcome [30].

Results from the same Danish cohort showed a significant inverse correlation between the frequency of babies born SGA and the gestational age at onset of spontaneous reduction and the only independent predictor of SGA in the IVF singleton cohort was vanishing of a co-twin [36].

A recent case–control study on 46 survivors and 92 matched singleton controls confirmed the findings by Schieve and Pinborg on birth weight, as a significantly lower mean ( ± SD) birth weight (2876.3 ± 600.5 g vs 3249.6 ± 624.5 g), a higher frequency of low birth weight (26.1% vs 12.0%) and being small for gestational age (32.6% vs 16.3%) for survivors of the vanishing twin syndrome was found [33].

In summary, ART singletons born after a conception with initially two gestational sacs or fetuses have poorer obstetric outcome than ART singletons born after one initial gestational sac or fetus, even when demise occurs in the very early pregnancy. Evidence of the same vanishing twin effect in SC pregnancies is missing.

## Long-term outcome

Pharoah and Cooke hypothesized that cerebral palsy of unknown etiology could be the result of the vanishing embryo syndrome [37], but the evidence on long-term outcome in survivors of the vanishing twin syndrome is still very limited. Most existing studies on neurological sequelae are based on spontaneously conceived singletons and to death of a co-twin in third trimester. Based on the Western Australian cerebral palsy register, twins in the 1980s born after in-utero death of a co-twin had a prevalence of cerebral palsy of 96.2 per 1000, 15 times higher than for twins where both were live-born (6.4/1000) and 60 times higher than for singletons (1.6/1000) [38]. It has been confirmed since that late intrauterine death of one twin has considerable influence on the risk of cerebral palsy and mortality in the surviving twin [39–40]. Pharoah and Adi found that the liveborn co-twin of a fetus that died in utero was at a 20-fold increased risk of cerebral impairment compared with the general twin risk and Scher et al. found a four-fold increased risk of CP in twin survivors of a stillborn co-twin.

In 2003 Newton et al. conducted a case–control study of vanishing twins as a risk factor for cerebral palsy of unknown etiology. Among mothers of cases, one of 86 had evidence of a vanishing twin on ultrasound, as compared with two of 381 control mothers (OR 2.2, 95% CI 0.2–24.8; $P = 0.5$). Bleeding in early pregnancy may indicate the loss of a co-twin and was reported by 14 case mothers and 46 control mothers (OR 1.6, 95% CI 0.8–3.0; $P = 0.3$). On the basis of their results the authors concluded that the vanishing twin syndrome is unlikely to account for a high proportion of cases of cerebral palsy, but that they had insufficient statistical power to draw firm conclusions [41].

Only two recent studies have looked at cerebral palsy in ART pregnancies after vanishing twins and embryos. In the previously mentioned Danish multicenter study a cross-linkage to the National Patient Register was made to assess the risk of cerebral palsy after loss of a co-twin in either first, second or third trimester [30]. The overall prevalence of cerebral palsy was 8.2 per 1000 in singletons with a disappeared co-twin in the first or second trimester, while 4.2 per 1000 in singletons with only one gestational sac in early pregnancy. Though not statistically significant these results indicate a two-fold increased risk of cerebral palsy (OR 1.9, 95% CI 0.7–5.2) in first and second trimester survivors of a vanished co-twin compared with primary singletons. In addition there was a significant inverse correlation between the gestational age at onset of fetal demise and development of neurological sequelae.

Another Danish population-based cohort study on 9444 IVF/ICSI children revealed a 2.3-fold increased risk of cerebral palsy in children, where the number of children at delivery was smaller than the number of embryos originally transferred compared with pregnancies with equal number of embryos transferred and number of children at birth [27].

Studies on development and neurological function in survivors of a vanished co-twin have appeared only recently. In 2007 Anand and coworkers examined a cohort of 324 children from 229 pregnancies recruited between 1999 and 2001 at the Liverpool Women's Hospital. The authors tested development and neurological function using the Griffiths Mental and Developmental Scales and Optimality score. A neurological examination was performed using an optimality score to exclude those with severe neurodisability. Cerebral impairment was found in two children from the vanishing twin group, two from the twin group and none from the singleton group. When cases with definite vanishing twin were considered there was a significant difference between the vanishing twin and singleton group (relative risk 6.1; 95% CI 1.5–8.3; $P = 0.03$), but their sample size did not allow a very robust conclusion [42]. The sub- and general quotient scores in singletons and surviving co-twins of a vanishing twin did not differ significantly [43].

Pascalis et al. looked at the parent–child relationship in families of 53 singleton births after the vanishing twin syndrome compared with ART parents following a singleton pregnancy with matching for gestational age, maternal age, child's age and child's gender [44].

The authors concluded that despite the perceived motor difficulties and the difficulties in the process of individuation-separation that appear at the beginning of the different educational circumstances, parents of singletons following the "vanishing" twin syndrome perceive their children as "invincible," and thus less vulnerable compared with controls.

In summary, long-term outcome after vanishing twins is still poorly explored, but the present evidence indicates an association between the risk of cerebral palsy and the vanish of a co-twin. The literature on development, neurological function and parent–child relationship is too scarce to draw firm conclusions.

## Conclusions

In recent years large population-based cohort studies have made it evident that IVF singletons have poorer obstetric outcome including perinatal deaths than SC singletons [3–4,45]. The risk of congenital malformations is increased 1.4-fold [5,6] and cerebral palsy increased two- to three-fold [7–9]. More explanations have been proposed for the higher risk in the IVF singleton offspring including the IVF procedures, the subfertility per se and the number of gestational sacs/fetuses in early pregnancy.

The IVF procedures involve ovarian stimulation with its effect on the oocytes, the endometrium, the luteal phase and the pregnancy, and the laboratory procedures with different culture medias and micro-invasive techniques. Studies have shown that children after intrauterine insemination with ovarian stimulation and IVF children have similar neonatal outcome indicating that the ovarian stimulation significantly influences the outcome [46,47]. Further, a recent randomized study found that the proportion of embryos with aneuploidy was lower in mild stimulation cycles than in conventional IVF cycles indicating an effect of the ovarian stimulation on the embryos [48]. However, a large study on more than 32 000 IVF singletons based on the German IVF register revealed no effect of the dose and length of ovarian stimulation; by contrast the duration of infertility and the number of embryos transferred were significant predictors of the singleton offspring [49].

This is not the moment to acquit the IVF procedures of influence on the offspring as more knowledge is warranted comparing children after conventional IVF with appropriate control groups. On the other hand it has been established that a part of the adverse outcome is explained by the unfavorable characteristics of the couples or the infertility per se, i.e. the longer time to pregnancy the higher the risk of prematurity, low birth weight, malformations and neonatal deaths in the offspring [10–14]. The risk of congenital malformations is also related simply to subfertility [15].

As demonstrated in this chapter the vanishing twin phenomenon and the processes of even very-early pregnancy play a significant role for the IVF singleton outcome. In a clinical frame with a double-embryo transfer policy, vanishing twin pregnancies account for about 10% of all singleton births. This high frequency with the associated impaired short- and long-term outcome in ART singletons adds another firm argument for an elective single embryo transfer (eSET) policy in ART.

According to the annual reports from the European IVF Monitoring (EIM) Consortium modest declines in the IVF twin birth rates have been observed, from 25% in 2000 to 21.7% in 2004, with large variations – from 5.6% in Sweden to more than 30% in some Eastern European countries [50]. One of the big challenges in the coming years is to promote the clear trend of declining twin birth rates by the introduction of milder stimulation protocols and transfer of fewer embryos and by encouraging national political and funding initiatives towards eSET. Many couples are still attached to the idea of twins, but patient's attitudes are also changing and once confronted with the actual probabilities of specified perinatal complications associated with a twin pregnancy, couples seem less keen to have them. Thus, the adoption of eSET requires profound counseling, which should include exact twin and vanishing twin risk estimates, eSET pregnancy rates and information on added cycles with cryopreserved embryos. IVF specialists themselves play the most vital role in this counseling process.

## References

1. Landy HJ, Keith L, Keith D. The vanishing twin. *Acta Genet Med Gemellol*, 1982; **31**: 179–94.

2. Landy HJ, Keith L. The vanishing twin: a review. *Hum Reprod Update* 1998; **4**: 177–83.

3. Helmerhorst FM, Perquin DAM, Donker D, Keirse MJNC. Perinatal outcome of singletons and twins after assisted conception: a systematic review of controlled studies. *Br Med J* 2004; **328**: 261–5.

4. Jackson RA, Gibson KA, Wu YW, Croughan MS. Perinatal outcomes in singletons following in vitro fertilization: a meta-analysis. *Obstet Gynecol* 2004; **103**: 551–63.

5. Hansen M, Bower C, Milne E, de Klerk N, Kurinczuk JJ. Assisted reproductive technologies and the risk of birth

defects – a systematic review. *Hum Reprod* 2005; **20**: 328–38.

6. Källén B, Finnström O, Nygren KG, Olausson PO. In vitro fertilization (IVF) in Sweden: risk for congenital malformations after different IVF methods. *Birth Defects Res (Part A)* 2005; **73**: 162–9.

7. Strömberg B, Dahlquist G, Ericson A *et al.* Neurological sequelae in children born after in-vitro fertilisation: a population based study. *Lancet* 2002; **359**: 461–5.

8. Källén B, Finnström O, Nygren KG, Olausson PO. In vitro fertilization in Sweden: child morbidity including cancer risk. *Fertil Steril* 2005; **84**: 605–10.

9. Lidegaard O, Pinborg A, Nyboe Andersen A. Imprinting diseases and IVF. Danish National IVF cohort study. *Hum Reprod* 2005; **20**: 950–4.

10. Henriksen TB, Baird DD, Olsen J et al. Time to pregnancy and preterm delivery. *Obstet Gynecol* 1997; **89**: 594–9.

11. Draper ES, Kurinczuk JJ, Abrams KR, Clarke M. Assessment of separate contributions to perinatal mortality of infertility history and treatment: a case-control analysis. *Lancet* 1999; **353**: 1746–9.

12. Pandian Z, Bhattacharya S, Templeton A. Review of unexplained infertility and obstetric outcome: a 10 year review. *Hum Reprod* 2001; **16**: 2593–7.

13. Basso O, Baird DD. Infertility and preterm delivery, birthweight, and Caesarean section: a study within the Danish National Birth Cohort. *Hum Reprod* 2003; **18**: 2478–84.

14. Basso O, Olsen J. Subfecundity and neonatal mortality: longitudinal study within the Danish National Birth Cohort. *Br Med J* 2005; **330**: 393–4.

15. Zhu JL, Basso O, Obel C, Bille C, Olsen J. Infertility, infertility treatment, and congenital malformations: Danish national birth cohort. *Br Med J* 2006; **333**: 679.

16. Stoeckel W. *Lehrbuch der Geburtschilfe*. Jena: Gustav Fischer, 1945.

17. Finberg HJ, Birnholz JC. Ultrasound observations in multiple gestation with first trimester bleeding: the blighted twin. *Radiology* 1979; **132**: 137–42.

18. Tharapel AT, Elias S, Shulman LP *et al.* Resorbed co-twin as an explanation for discrepant chorionic villus results: Non-mosaic 47, XX,+16 in villi (direct and culture) with normal (46, XX) amniotic fluid and neonatal blood. *Prenat Diagn* 1989; **9**: 467–72.

19. Landy HJ, Weiner S, Corson SL *et al.* The "vanishing twin": ultrasonographic assessment of fetal disappearance in the first trimester. *Am J Obstet Gynecol* 1986; **155**: 14–19.

20. Hofmann G, Gundrun C, Drake L, Bertsche A. Frequency and effect of vaginal bleeding on pregnancy outcome during the first 3 weeks after positive B-hCG test results following IVF-ET. *Fertil Steril* 2000; **74**: 609–10.

21. Pezeshki K, Feldman J, Stein DE, Lobel SM, Grazi RV. Bleeding and spontaneous abortion after therapy for infertility. *Fertil Steril* 2000; **74**: 504–8.

22. Williams MA, Mittendorf R, Lieberman E, Monson RR. Adverse infant outcomes associated with first-trimester vaginal bleeding. *Obstet Gynecol* 1991; **78**: 14–18.

23. Weiss JL, Malone FD, Vidaver J *et al.* Threatened miscarriage: a risk for poor pregnancy outcome, a population based screening study. *Am J Obstet Gynecol* 2004; **190**: 745–50.

24. De sutter P, Bontinck J, Schutysers V *et al.* First-trimester bleeding and pregnancy outcome in singletons after assisted reproduction. *Hum Reprod* 2006; **21**: 1907–11.

25. Schieve LA, Meikle SF, Ferre C *et al.* Low and very low birth weight in infants conceived with use of assisted reproductive technology. *New Engl J Med* 2002; **346** (2002): 731–7.

26. Dickey RP, Taylor SN, Lu PY *et al.* Spontaneous reduction of multiple pregnancy: incidence and effect on outcome. *Am J Obstet Gynecol* 2002; **186**: 77–83.

27. Hvidtjørn D, Grove J, Schendel D *et al.* "Vanishing embryo syndrome" in IVF/ICSI. *Hum Reprod* 2005; **20**: 2550–1.

28. Tummers P, De Sutter P, Dhont M. Risk of spontaneous abortion in singleton and twin pregnancies after IVF/ICSI. *Hum Reprod* 2003; **18**: 1720–3.

29. La Sala GB, Nucera G, Gallinelli A *et al.* Spontaneous embryonic loss following in vitro fertilization: incidence and effect on outcomes. *Am J Obstet Gynecol* 2004; **191**: 741–6.

30. Pinborg A, Lidegaard O, la Cour Freiesleben N, Nyboe Andersen A. Consequences of vanishing twins in IVF/ICSI pregnancies. *Hum Reprod* 2005; **20**: 2821–9.

31. Dickey RP, Sartor BM, Pyrzak R. What is the most relevant standard of success in assisted reproduction? No single outcome measure is satisfactory when evaluating success in assisted reproduction; both twin and singletons births should be counted as successes. *Hum Reprod* 2004; **19**: 783–7.

32. Lancaster PAL. Number of gestational sacs and singleton IVF preterm birth. *Hum Reprod* 2004; **19** (Suppl. 1): Abstr. book: O–245, p. i85.

33. Shebl O, Ebner T, Sommergruber M, Sir A, Tews G. Birth weight is lower for survivors of the vanishing twin syndrome: a case-control study. *Fertil Steril* 2008; **90**: 310–14.

34. Hewitt D, Stewart A. Relevance of twin data to intrauterine selection: special case of childhood cancer. *Acta Genet Med Gemellol* 1970; **19**: 83–6.

35. La Sala GB, Villani MT, Nicoli A *et al.* Effect of the mode of asisted reproductive technology conception on obstetric outcomes for survivors of the vanishing twin syndrome. *Fertil Steril* 2006; **86**: 247–9.

36. Pinborg A, Lidegaard O, la Cour Freiesleben N, Nyboe Andersen A. Vanishing twins: a predictor of small-for-gestational age in IVF singletons. *Hum Reprod* 2007; **22**: 2707–14.

37. Pharoah POD, Cooke RWI. A hypothesis for the aetiology of spastic cerebral palsy – the vanishing twin. *Dev Med Child Neurol* 1997; **39**: 292–6.

38. Petterson B, Nelson KB, Watson L, Stanley F. Twins, triplets, and cerebral palsy in births in Western Australia in the1980s. *Br Med J* 1993; **307**: 1239–43.

39. Pharoah POD, Adi Y. Consequences of in-utero death in a twin pregnancy. *Lancet* 2000; **355**: 1597–602.

40. Scher AI, Petterson B, Blair E *et al.* The risk of mortality or cerebral palsy in twins: a collaborative population-based study. *Pediatr Res* 2002; **52**: 671–81.

41. Newton R, Casabonne D, Johnson A, Pharoah P. A case-control study of vanishing twin as a risk factor for cerebral palsy. *Twin Res* 2003; **6**: 83–4.

42. Anand D, Platt MJ, Pharoah PO. Vanishing twin: a possible cause of cerebral impairment. *Twin Res Hum Genet* 2007; **10**: 202–9.

43. Anand D, Platt MJ, Pharoah PO. Comparative development of surviving co-twins of vanishing twin conceptions, twins and singletons. *Twin Res Hum Genet* 2007; **10**: 210–15.

44. De Pascalis L, Monti F, Agostini F *et al.* Psychological vulnerability of singleton children after the 'vanishing' of a co-twin following assisted reproduction. *Twin Res Hum Genet* 2008; **11**: 93–8.

45. Schieve LA, Ferre C, Peterson HB *et al.* Perinatal outcome among singleton infants conceived through asssisted reproductive technology in the United States. *Obstet Gynecol* 2004; **103**: 1144–53.

46. De Sutter P, Veldeman L, Kok P *et al.* Comparison of outcome of pregnancy after intra-uterine insemination (IUI) and IVF. *Hum Reprod* 2005; **20**: 1642–6.

47. Ombelet W, Martens G, De Sutter P *et al.* Perinatal outcome of 12,021 singleton and 3108 twin births after non-IVF-assisted reproduction: a cohort study. *Hum Reprod* 2006; **21**: 1025–32.

48. Baart EB, Martini E, Eijkemans MJ *et al.* Milder ovarian stimulation for in-vitro fertilization reduces aneuploidy in the human preimplantation embryo: a randomized controlled trial. *Hum Reprod* 2007; **22**: 980–8.

49. Griesinger G, Kolibianakis EM, Diedrich K, Ludwig M. Ovarian stimulation for IVF has no quantitative association with birthweight: a registry study. *Hum Reprod* 2008; **23**: 2549–54.

50. Andersen AN, Goossens V, Ferraretti AP *et al.* Assisted reproductive technology in Europe 2004: results generated from European registers by ESHRE. *Hum Reprod* 2008; **23**: 756–71.

# Chapter 26

# Late pregnancy loss

Roy G. Farquharson

## Definition of late pregnancy loss

Late pregnancy loss (or second-trimester loss) is defined as the loss of a pregnancy between 12 and 23 weeks' gestation inclusive. The true incidence of this complication is difficult to ascertain as no accurate data collection has been published for this event. Nonetheless most clinicians accept the incidence as around 2–3% of pregnancies.

An important consideration is that an underlying cause for late pregnancy loss (LPL) may be present either in isolation in 40%, combined (as dual pathology) in 10% or absent in 50% of cases despite comprehensive investigation. Women who suffer late pregnancy loss represent a heterogeneous group, displaying widely varying presentation and etiology. In addition, the assessment and exclusion of possible dual/triple pathology must always be considered in a woman with repeated second-trimester miscarriage [1].

## Investigation protocol

A standardized approach to the investigation of LPL helps to exclude the possibility of dual pathology and leads to uniformity in treatment analysis when entry to trials is anticipated. In particular there is a growing consensus for all failed pregnancies to have full karyotyping performed, when possible, to exclude the diagnosis of "treatment failure" when an abnormal karyoype is discovered by comparative genomic hybridization (CGH) array or fluorescent in situ hybridization (FISH) spectrum analysis. A typical investigation protocol is given in Figure 26.1.

## Diagnosis

The clinical event history is vitally important in ascertaining a possible cause (Figure 26.2). Maternal thrombophilia may well be associated with intrauterine death in the second trimester while cervical weakness classically presents as silent cervical dilatation with active fetal heart activity. The presence of bacterial vaginosis (BV) can be associated with spontaneous rupture of membranes in the presence of a closed cervix. Cohort analysis of consecutive cases by cause is by no means definitive due to referral bias but gives a reasonable distribution of investigative audit (Figure 26.3).

In clinical practice there is often no clear event sequence that points to a definitive diagnostic cause. In addition many women with repeated late losses show a variety of presentations which should alert the clinician to the possibility of dual pathology as differing causal factors can predominate at different gestations in different pregnancies within the same individual.

## Factors associated with late pregnancy loss

### Antiphospholipid antibody syndrome

Antiphospholipid antibody syndrome (APS) comprises the lupus anticoagulant (LA) and anticardiolipin antibodies (aCL). These are known to bind to negatively charged phospholipids and are regarded as markers of thrombosis [2]. Various theories exist as to how they cause miscarriage: binding to platelet membrane, activating release of thromboxane and subsequent platelet aggregation and thrombosis; binding to endothelial cells, inhibiting prostacyclin production or involvement with other clotting factors. It is likely that APS is a family of autoantibodies. A high index of suspicion is needed in any patient with an unexplained intrauterine death [3], especially if associated with thrombocytopenia and arterial or venous thromboses.

*Early Pregnancy*, ed. Roy G. Farquharson and Mary D. Stephenson. Published by Cambridge University Press.
© Cambridge University Press 2010.

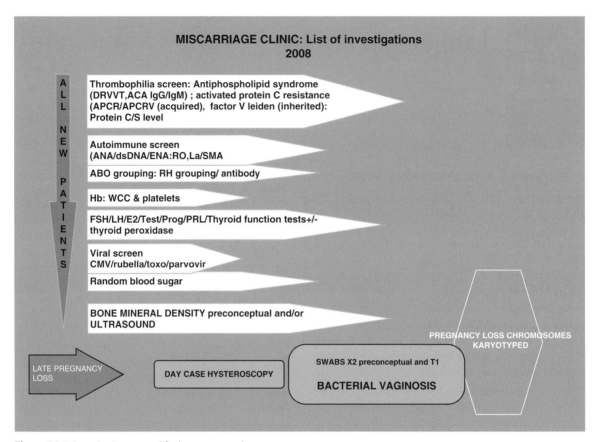

**Figure 26.1** Investigation protocol for late pregnancy loss.

## Event Sequence with Main Cause

| EVENT versus FACTOR | CERVIX | LIQUOR found PV | FETAL HEART ACTION |
|---|---|---|---|
| Cervical Weakness | OPEN | Absent until expulsion of sac | Present |
| Maternal Thrombophilia e.g.APS | Closed | Absent | ABSENT = IUD (Intrauterine death) |
| Bacterial Vaginosis (BV) | Closed | PRESENT | Present ? until sac expulsion |

**Figure 26.2** Clinical history sequence.

Antiphospholipid antibody syndrome is associated with pregnancy loss in any trimester. Early fetal loss commonly occurs in the first trimester [4] while others found that their patients with APS mostly lost pregnancies in the second or early third trimester [5].

Prevalence rates for APS have been recorded in up to 42% of an LPL group [6]. As placental thrombosis has been presumed to be the historical cause, the mainstay of treatment has been the use of anti-coagulants to provide thromboprophylaxis in the form of either low-dose aspirin (LDA) with or without unfractionated/low molecular weight heparin (LMWH). Recent evidence supports the use of LDA alone [7–9] while others support the use of combined LDA/LMWH [10,11].

## Cervical weakness

As stated by the Euro-Team Early Pregnancy Protocol [12], there is no agreed definition of cervical weakness by absolute measurable and reproducible criteria. It is important that before cervical weakness is confirmed, certain diagnostic criteria are applied and other causes excluded, as resultant management is invasive and carries a recurrence risk of an adverse outcome.

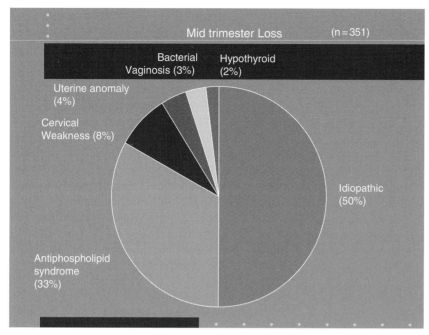

**Figure 26.3** Distribution of cause in 351 consecutive cases of midtrimester loss at Liverpool Women's Hospital.

A consensus definition that is frequently used includes painless dilatation of the cervix followed by ruptured membranes, resulting in second-trimester miscarriage or extreme pre-term delivery. In the non-pregnant state, the passage, without resistance, of a size 9 Hegar dilator through the cervix acts as a surrogate measure. A recent definition for entry into a randomized controlled trial (RCT) includes the initial painless, progressive dilatation of the uterine cervix, where pre-term delivery seems inevitable without interference. The diagnosis is made in the absence of other causes of pre-term delivery such as uterine anomaly, fibroids or infection (vide infra) and where only singleton pregnancies are included [13]. As was written as the premise for another RCT, "the overuse of prophylactic cerclage is a manifestation of our inability to diagnose cervical incompetence with any degree of reliability on the basis of historical criteria alone" [14]. More recently, this message that "prophylactic and reactive interventions remain largely unevaluated or ineffective" has been emphasized [15].

## Bacterial vaginosis

The role of infection in the etiology of miscarriage appears to be in the second trimester rather than the first [16]. Bacterial vaginosis (BV) is known to contribute to late fetal loss [17]. The most sensitive and specific method to diagnose BV is by examining a Gram stain of a vaginal smear for clue cells. Ideally this should be done in the first quarter of the menstrual cycle when levels are highest. A positive diagnosis should be treated with intra-vaginal clindamycin, or alternatively with a combination of oral erythromycin and metronidazole [18]. Antibiotic treatment can eradicate bacterial vaginosis in pregnancy and treatment introduced before 20 weeks' gestation may reduce the risk of pre-term birth [19]. With regard to late pregnancy loss there is RCT evidence of benefit in reducing mid-trimester loss in a BV population [20]. The recent publication of the long-term outcome of the ORACLE II study suggests that the erythromycin in pregnancy should be used with caution in view of an observed increase in cases of cerebral palsy in the offspring of erythromycin users in pregnancy [21].

## Uterine anomaly

The urogenital system develops from a common mesodermal ridge (intermediate mesoderm) along the posterior wall of the abdominal cavity and initially, the excretory ducts of both systems enter a common cavity, the cloaca. Duplication of the uterus results from a lack of fusion of the paramesonephric ducts, in a localized area or throughout the length of the ducts. In its extreme form, the uterus is entirely double (uterus didelphys); in the least severe form, it is only slightly indented in the middle (uterus arcuatus) [22].

In 1931, Smith reported one case of double uterus for every 7040 consecutive obstetric patients in New York from 1899 to 1924 [23]. Having taken an interest in the finding, Smith's detection rate for years 1925 to 1930 increased the reported incidence by five times. Harger *et al.* reported an incidence of 27% of uterine anomalies in their data set of late miscarriage patients [24]. Miscarriage can occur where there is only limited uterine space available, at a point when the semi-uterus is unable to expand further [25] or when implantation occurs into an avascular septum [26]. A recent literature appraisal of congenital uterine anomalies in recurring miscarriage (first and second trimester losses) suggests a high prevalence of 16.7% (95% CI, 14.8–18.6). However this includes the mildest form of arcuate uterus as well as septate uterus so a clear consensus in this area remains elusive [27].

Mode of diagnosis for uterine anomalies has evolved with time. In the past, hysterosalpingography was the mainstay of investigation, but it is painful and is limited by a two-dimensional image. Pelvic ultrasound is highly specific for uterine anomaly and is non-invasive and may be suitable for screening purposes [28]. Magnetic resonance imaging (MRI) has been proposed for the same reason, though is much more expensive [29]. Hysteroscopy is now widely used for directly visualizing septal defects and intrauterine synechiae, which can be combined with laparoscopy to assess fundal dimpling.

# Management

## Cervical cerclage

Treatment of cervical weakness is aimed at strengthening the internal os in order to maintain the pregnancy. Emmett described the first elective reconstruction of the non-pregnant cervix in 1874 [30]. This technique involved a V-shaped incision to remove the scar from a cervix damaged by obstetric trauma. The surfaces were then apposed with silver wire sutures.

In the twentieth century, Shirodkar [31] and McDonald [32] described the two classical techniques of vaginal cervical cerclage. In Shirodkar's technique, the bladder is reflected to enable a suture to be placed

as close to the internal cervical os as possible per vaginum. Bladder reflection is not required for McDonald's described technique.

### Trial results

Although there are no comparative studies, the success rate for both types of vaginal suture is similar. The MRC/RCOG trial on cervical cerclage [33] studied more than 1200 patients and concluded that cerclage is beneficial to patients with three or more pregnancies ending before 37 weeks' gestation (midtrimester losses). Cerclage was also associated with a higher rate of medical intervention, puerperal pyrexia, use of B-sympathomimetics, hospital admissions, induction of labor and cesarean section. More recently, a treatment intervention trial randomly assigned 61 women to either cervical cerclage or no cerclage on presentation with ultrasonographically detected second-trimester pre-term dilatation of the internal os. The study was unable to demonstrate an improved perinatal outcome with cerclage [14]. They proposed a hypothesis that ultrasonographic dilatation of the internal os, prolapse of the membranes into the endocervical canal and shortening of the distal cervix during the second trimester share a final common pathway of multiple pathophysiological processes, such as infection, immunologically mediated inflammatory stimuli and subclinical abruptio placentae.

At a similar time, the preliminary results of the Dutch CIPRACT treatment trial (Cervical Incompetence Prevention Randomized Cerclage Trial) showed no significant differences between the prophylactic cerclage group and the observational group in terms of pre-term delivery rate 34 weeks' gestation and the neonatal survival rate. In this study, patients were initially randomized to cerclage or no cerclage using ultrasound determination of cervical length measurement. If, in the no cerclage arm, the cervical length decreased to <25 mm, the 35 eligible women underwent a second randomization to either cerclage and bed rest or simply bed rest. Interim results indicated that transvaginal ultrasonographic follow-up examination of the cervix can save the majority of women from unnecessary intervention [34]. The final results showed that therapeutic cerclage with bed rest reduces pre-term delivery before 34 weeks' gestation and compound neonatal morbidity but showed no statistically significant difference in neonatal survival between the two groups [13]. By contrast, screening

**Table 26.1** Comparison of vaginal and abdominal procedures for treatment of cervical weakness for late pregnancy loss based on local data from Liverpool Women's Hospital (2001–2008).

|  | Vaginal | Abdominal |
| --- | --- | --- |
| Success rate | 75% | 90% |
| Insertion | 12 weeks' gestation | 10 weeks' gestation or pre-conceptual with less morbidity |
| Morbidity | Minimal | Hemorrhage trauma to bladder/bowel |
| Long term | Removal at 36 weeks | Permanent |
| Delivery | Option of vaginal | Mandatory cesarean section |

for short cervical length (<15 mm, n = 470) in a low risk population (n = 47 123) followed by observation or cervical cerclage failed to reduce pre-term delivery rate before 34 weeks (22% in cerclage versus 26% in observation group, RR = 0.84, 95% CI 0.54–1.31, P = 0.44) [35].

## When vaginal cerclage fails

When cervical cerclage became widely used for the treatment of mid-trimester loss, it became apparent that there was a small sub-group of patients for whom the vaginal approach was inappropriate. This group included those patients in whom the cervix was extremely short or absent secondary to a surgical procedure such as cone biopsy or congenitally deformed as a result of exposure to stilbestrol in-utero. In addition, those patients whose cervices were markedly scarred or lacerated as a consequence of obstetric trauma or as a result of previously failed vaginal cerclage also fell within this group. Local data at Liverpool Women's Hospital (2001–2008) shows that there is a 25% failure rate for elective vaginal cerclage used with mid-trimester loss history associated with cervical weakness (Table 26.1). Mid-trimester loss with previous failed elective cervical vaginal suture comprises the majority of patients requiring abdominal cerclage in our unit.

## Transabdominal cervical cerclage

In developing an abdominal approach, Benson and Durfee [36] uniquely reasoned that "if cervical cerclage during gestation is indicated but the vaginal approach is impossible, why not accomplish constriction from above?"

## Protocol and technique

The first abdominal procedures, as described by Benson and Durfee in 1965 [36], were performed between 14 and 24 weeks' gestation. At this gestation, a midline incision was used to improve access to the cervical region. Dissection involved opening the broad ligament and mobilization of the uterine vessels to identify an avascular space through which to pass a 5 mm Mersilene tape. Several series have been published since 1965 (Table 3) and modifications in timing of the operation, surgical technique, postoperative management and patient selection have been reported to decrease the morbidity (especially hemorrhage) reported with earlier series and secondly, to avoid the necessity for a midline scar.

## Patient selection

Following a second-trimester miscarriage, a detailed history and investigation was undertaken as described above (Figures 26.1 and 26.2). Following analysis and counseling, those patients with diagnosed cervical weakness were offered transabdominal cerclage when they had a failed, elective vaginal cerclage history or where the cervix was so severely damaged that vaginal cerclage was considered impossible. Preconceptual interview required full disclosure and considerable explanation regarding risks of failure, complications of insertion following previous surgery e.g. classical CS delivery, hourglass constriction of cervix and adjacent major vessels, bowel or bladder damage and the need for two major operations. All these factors need to be addressed, ideally by a second counseling interview when consent can be obtained. The patient has by then received all the relevant information before conception and in knowledge that abdominal cerclage should be seen as a last resort.

## The procedure

Laparotomy for insertion of a transabdominal cerclage is performed between 9 and 13 weeks. Fetal viability is confirmed by scan prior to the procedure.

The procedure is performed under general anesthesia. The bladder is emptied and the catheter left in situ during the procedure. In our experience we have found that packing the vagina before laparotomy

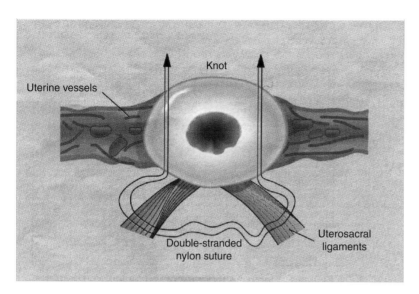

**Figure 26.4** Transabdominal cerclage technique.

can elevate the uterus with improved access to the cervico-isthmic region.

The patient is placed in Trendelenburg position. A low transverse abdominal incision is made and packs used to keep bowel away from the operative field.

The peritoneum of the uterovesical fold is incised transversely in the midline. Often it is not necessary to reflect the bladder inferiorly as the bladder reflection (uterovesical fold) lies at the level of the isthmus. The uterine vessels and isthmus are identified digitally.

Double-stranded 2 gauge nylon suture (Ethicon, UK) is mounted onto a loose 40 mm round-bodied Mayo needle. The isthmus is grasped between the thumb and forefinger to stabilize the uterus. The suture is inserted postero-anteriorly through the window between the substance of the cervix lateral to the canal but medial to the vessels, at the level of the uterine isthmus above the insertion of the utero-sacral ligaments. The needle is remounted and the procedure repeated again postero-anteriorly on the opposite side (Figure 26.4). The knot is tied anteriorly and covered by a loose peritoneal fold and the abdomen closed.

There were no cases of severe hemorrhage requiring blood transfusion in our series although several cases required the knot to be tightly closed to achieve adequate hemostasis in the presence of heavy bleeding [37]. One case of bladder damage and one case of bowel trauma were encountered at operation and treated at the time with good outcome for the patient and pregnancy.

A single dose of intra-operative antibiotics are given. Non-steroidal anti-inflammatory agents (Diclofenac sodium suppositories 100 mg) may be prescribed for pain relief and uterine quiescence over the following 72 hours. Pre-operative thromboprophylaxis was recommened on the first post-operative day using dalteparin 5000 units SC daily and LDA 75 mg PO daily.

Women remained in hospital for 5–7 days and fetal viability was confirmed on scan prior to discharge. Antenatal surveillance included fetal anatomy scan at 20 weeks and serial fetal growth scans. In addition, transvaginal ultrasound of cervical length measurement did not seem to change over trimesters after serial monitoring was commenced at 16 weeks.

Adjuvant treatment was continued for co-existing pathologies, for example LDA with or without LMWH; clindamycin cream for bacterial vaginosis. Prophylactic antenatal steroid treatment was prescribed once only at 24 weeks' gestation where dual pathology was present and the mother consented to the administration. The use of prophylactic bed rest was not used. Pregnancies progressing beyond viability were delivered by cesarean section, and the transabdominal cerclage suture was left in place if the woman wished to consider another pregnancy.

## Results of transabdominal cerclage

Of 40 patients who underwent transabdominal cervical cerclage, 36 have resulted in a successful outcome (defined as a live birth and take-home baby), and four resulted in mid-trimester loss or extreme pre-term

**Table 26.2** Outcome after Transabdominal Cerclage (n = 40).

The presence of dual pathology, such as APS or BV, is associated with increased pre-term delivery before 34 weeks (RR 2.34, 95% CI 1.15–5.58) (BJOG, 2005, 112, 1424–26)

| Dual pathology | <22 | 23–24 | 25–29 | 30–33 | >34 weeks |
|---|---|---|---|---|---|
| Absent (n=22) | 0 | 0 | 0 | 4 | 18 |
| Present (n=18) | 2 | 2 | 3 | 4 | 7 |
| APS (N=11) | 1 | 1 | 1 | 2 | 6 |
| BV (n=7) | 1 | 1 | 2 | 2 | 1 |

delivery and neonatal death. The success rate is 90% (Table 26.2).

Seven pregnancies ended prior to 30 weeks gestation. The recorded failures showed a mixed pattern of presentation. One spontaneously miscarried at 12 weeks' gestation associated with APS. A second had spontaneous rupture of the membranes at 17 weeks associated with BV followed by chorioamnionitis and intrauterine death, requiring hysterotomy followed by severe maternal infection. Three pregnancies were delivered by cesarean section at 23, 24 and 25 weeks following pre-term rupture of the membranes and/or extreme pre-term labor. The infants all died at less than 3 days of age from acute pulmonary hemorrhage and extreme prematurity. Two further deliveries occurred before 30 weeks, progressing to 27 and 29 weeks respectively and both infants subsequently did well. All babies born after 30 weeks did well after delivery.

As 50% of pregnancies progressed to near term, we looked at the presence of other pathologies found on initial screening at the miscarriage clinic (Table 26.2). This demonstrated that 44% (18/40) of delivered patients had pathology in conjunction with the cervical weakness and that the presence of more than one pathology increased the risk of pre-term delivery. In the four patients with two pathologies as well as cervical weakness, 3 delivered prior to 30 weeks and only one of these survived, which emphasizes the importance of coexisting pathology and its detrimental effect. The presence of dual pathology, such as APS or BV, increased the pre-term delivery rate by more than twice (RR 2.34, 95% CI 1.11–5.58).

## The role of transabdominal cerclage

There is little doubt that transabdominal cerclage is an effective surgical technique in reducing fetal loss in a highly selective group of patients with true cervical weakness and/or a past history of failed elective vaginal cerclage [38]. Examination of published series fails to highlight the co-existence of further pathology especially the presence of thrombophilia and clearly demonstrates the lack of standardization and conformity with important pre-conceptual investigations (Table 26.3).

The data from Liverpool suggest that the presence of co-existing pathology increases the risk of pre-term delivery which increases considerably when there are two or more co-existing pathologies. It is important that women are aware of this confounding variable, as the patient will require laparotomy to insert the suture, and abdominal delivery irrespective of gestation.

The presence of co-existing pathology in nearly 50% of patients stresses the need for a full pre-conceptual screen in all patients with cervical weakness to look for dual pathology that can be treated. The commonest co-factor was antiphospholipid syndrome found in 33% of cases. All were treated with LDA with or without LMWH [8,9]. Bacterial vaginosis was treated with oral erythromycin (subsequently suspended following the ORACLE 2 publication in 2008) throughout pregnancy (14 to 32 weeks) combined with a week-long course of Clindamycin cream PV every month. Two cases of uterine anomaly were untreated by surgery and both had a successful outcome.

There is no study comparing insertion of transabdominal cervical cerclage during pregnancy with insertion pre-pregnancy. In the non-pregnant state, more manipulation of the tissues is possible as well as improved access. To counterbalance this advantage, there is the problem of early pregnancy loss before 10 weeks' gestation where spontaneous miscarriage may allow the suture to tear through the substance of the pregnant cervix. In addition fetal loss rates are higher in the presence of the commonest

**Table 26.3** Investigation protocols of recent cerclage studies.

| Author & Year | Number of patients | Pre-conceptual hysteroscopy | Antiphospho-lipid syndrome testing | Bacterial vaginosis or infection tested or treated | TVU of CLM +/- Funneling | |
|---|---|---|---|---|---|---|
| Davis et al. (2000) | 40 TAC | 4 Mullerian anomalies | NO | NO | NO | Failed vaginal cerclage |
| Rust et al. (2000) | 61 RCT of TVC v. TLC | NO | YES | BV & AFV Sample | Inclusion criteria at 16–24/40 | Previous PTD |
| Althuisius et al. (2000) | 67 RCT of TVC v. TLC | No | No | Yes | Inclusion criteria | Previous PTD |
| Gibb et al. (1998) | 50 | No | No | Yes | No | Failed TVC Absent Cx |
| Farquharson et al. (2005) | 40 TAC | Yes | Yes | Yes | Yes | Failed vaginal cerclage |

thrombophilia, antiphospholipid syndrome, where suction evacuation may pose a considerable threat to the integrity of a pre-conceptual abdominal cerclage. An ongoing observational study in Liverpool of consecutive cases undergoing pre-conceptual insertion of transabdominal cerclage has now accumulated over 40 cases with good outcome so far.

Pre-conceptual transabdominal cerclage was performed in two of the first 40 cases. One patient was homozygous for factor V Leiden and at high risk of thrombosis having suffered two previous episodes of venous thromboembolic disease. The second patient had labored at 25 weeks after insertion of her first transabdominal cerclage, and had an emergency classical cesarean section when the suture was removed and subsequent access to the lower segment was poor. Both cases had a successful outcome in subsequent pregnancies.

There are case reports describing insertion and removal of transabdominal cerclage laparoscopically [38,39]; there is at yet no series published using the laparoscopic approach.

Clinical experience with transabdominal cerclage for recurring late pregnancy loss is limited in the UK to a few centers [40–43]. Selection criteria vary between centers and often include patients with pre-term delivery histories and bad outcome as well as classical mid-trimester loss due to true cervical weakness.

There are as yet no randomized trials comparing the use of transabdominal cerclage with the transvaginal approach. A highly selective retrospective study [44] looked at the outcome of a group of patients who had previous failed vaginal cerclage who were assigned either repeat vaginal cerclage or transabdominal cerclage. Assignment to either group was at the discretion of the authors and no randomization occurred. They found that delivery <35 weeks occurred significantly less frequently in the transabdominal group (18% vs 42%) and that pre-term premature rupture of the membranes also occurred less commonly (8% vs 29%). Extrapolation from these data should be viewed with caution as no prospective analysis has been made available and a number of performed cases were excluded from the report.

It is unlikely that an RCT will be feasible; women referred for this procedure often perceive it as their last chance and are unlikely to accept randomization. We are also looking at a small number of patients and the possibility of recruiting sufficient numbers to satisfy a credible power calculation is unlikely.

A recent systematic review [45] stated that transabdominal cervical cerclage may be associated with a lower risk of perinatal death or delivery at less than 24 weeks gestation, but it may also be associated with a higher risk of operative complications. The authors clearly identified a need for a multicenter, randomized controlled trial to address the question.

Although a prospective RCT of elective transabdominal cervical cerclage versus transvaginal cerclage is appealing as a route to evidence-based practice, the numbers of available participants for randomization is small. Added to which many potential recruits are understandably anxious about being randomized to a previous failed treatment arm. There are several pitfalls to a well-designed and robust RCT so the appearance of the multicenter UK trial (MAVRIC) is a welcome addition in attempting to answer a difficult question as to the most appropriate path of treatment intervention where cervical weakness is the major pathology of LPL. An ongoing observational study in Liverpool of consecutive cases undergoing pre-conceptual insertion of TAC has now accumulated over 40 cases with good outcome so far.

The following criteria are examples of important pre-conceptual findings after extensive history taking, event sequence analysis and full investigation protocol compliance.

## Inclusion criteria

(1) A failed elective vaginal cerclage for the treatment of cervical weakness causing mid-trimester loss.
(2) Completion of full investigation protocol for mid-trimester loss.
(3) Viable singleton pregnancy.
(4) Cervical length measurement of more than 20 mm on transvaginal ultrasound.

## Exclusion criteria

(1) Multiple pregnancy.
(2) Untreated co-existing cause of recurring miscarriage.
(3) Violation of pre-conceptual investigation protocol.
(4) Unwillingness to undergo randomization of treatment.

## References

1. Drakeley AJ, Quenby S, Farquharson RG. Mid-trimester loss – appraisal of a screening protocol. *Hum Reprod* 1998; **13**(7): 1975–80.

2. Birdsall MA, Pattison NS. Antiphospholipid antibodies in pregnancy: clinical associations. *Br J Hosp Med* 1993; **50**(5): 251–60.

3. Lubbe WF, Butler WS, Palmer SJ, Liggins GC. Lupus anticoagulant in pregnancy. *Br J Obstet Gynaecol* 1984; **91**: 357–63.

4. Rai RS, Clifford K, Cohen H, Regan L. High prospective fetal loss rate in untreated pregnancies of women with recurrent miscarriages and antiphospholipid antibodies. *Hum Reprod* 1995; **10** (12): 3301–4.

5. Branch DW, Scott JR, Kochenour NK, Hershgold E. Obstetric complications associated with the lupus anticoagulant. *New Engl J Med*. 1985; **313**(21): 1322–6.

6. Unander AM, Norberg R, Hahn L, Arfors L. Anticardiolipin antibodies and complement in ninety-nine women with habitual abortion. *Am J Obstet Gynecol* 1987; **156**(1): 114–19.

7. Pattison NS, Chamley LW, Birdsall MA *et al*. Does aspirin have a role in improving pregnancy outcome for women with the antiphospholipid syndrome? A randomised controlled trial. *Am J Obstet Gynecol* 2000; **183**: 1008–12.

8. Farquharson RG, Quenby SM, Greaves M. Antiphospholipid syndrome in pregnancy: a randomised controlled trial of treatment. *Obstet Gynecol* 2002; **100**: 418–24.

9. Laskin CA, Spitzer KA, Clark CA *et al*. Low molecular weight heparin and aspirin for recurrent pregnancy loss: results from the randomised controlled HepASA Trial. *J Rheumatology* 2009; **36**: 279–87.

10. Kutteh WH. Antiphospholipid antibody – associated recurrent pregnancy loss: treatment with heparin and low dose aspirin is superior to low dose aspirin alone. *Am J Obstet Gynecol* 1996; **174**: 1584–9.

11. Rai R, Cohen H, Dave M, Regan L. Randomised controlled trial of aspirin and aspirin plus heparin in pregnant women with recurrent miscarriage associated with phospholipid antibodies. *Br Med J* 1997; **314**: 253–7.

12. Berry CW, Brambati B, Eskes TKAB *et al*. The Euro-Team Early Pregnancy (ETEP) protocol for recurrent miscarriage. *Hum Reprod* 1995; **10**(6): 1516–20.

13. Althuisius SM, Dekker GA, Hummel P, Bekedam DJ, Gejn HP. Final results of the Cervical Incompetence Prevention Cerclage Trial (CIPRACT): therapeutic cerclage with bed rest versus bed rest alone. *Am J Obstet Gynecol* 2001; **185**: 1106–12.

14. Rust OA, Atlas RO, Jones KJ, Benham BN, Balducci J. A randomized trial of cerclage versus no cerclage among patients with ultrasonographically detected second-trimester preterm dilatation of the internal os. *Am J Obstet Gynecol* 2000; **183**(4): 830–5.

15. Chaniramani M, Shennan AH. Cervical insufficiency: prediction, diagnosis and prevention. *Obstet Gynaecol* 2006; **10**: 99–106.

16. Oakeshott P, Hay P, Hay S *et al*. Association between bacterial vaginosis or chlamydial infection and miscarriage before 16 weeks gestation: prospective community based cohort study. *Br Med J* 2002; **325**: 1334–6.

17. Llahi-Camp JM, Rai R, Ison CR, Regan L, Taylor-Robinson D. Association of bacterial vaginosis with a history of second trimester miscarriage. *Hum Reprod* 1996; **11**(7): 1575–8.

18. Adinkra PE, Lamont RF. Abnormal genital tract flora and pregnancy loss. In RG Farquharson (ed.), *Miscarriage*. Dinton: Mark Allen Publishing Ltd, 2002.

19. McDonald HM, Brocklehurst P, Gordon A. Antibiotics for treating bacterial vaginosis in pregnancy. *Cochrane Database System Rev* 2007; **1**: CD000262.

20. Ugwumadu A, Manyonda I, Reid F, Hay P. Effect of oral clindamycin on late miscarriage and preterm delivery in asymptomatic women with abnormal vaginal flora and bacterial vaginosis: a randomised controlled trial. *Lancet* 2003; **361**: 983–8.

21. Kenyon S, Pike K, Jones DR *et al.* Childhood outcomes after prescription of antibiotics to pregnant women with spontaneous preterm labour: 7-year follow-up of the ORACLE II trial. *Lancet* 2008; **372**(9646): 1319–27.

22. Sadler TW. In TW Sadler (ed.), *Langman's Medical Embryology*. 7th edition. Baltimore: Williams & Wilkins, 1995, pp. 272, 296–7.

23. Smith FR. The significance of incomplete fusion of the Mullerian ducts in pregnancy and parturition, with a report on 35 cases. *Am J Obstet Gynecol* 1931; **22**: 714–28.

24. Harger JH, Archer DF, Marchese SG, Muracca-Clemens M, Garver KL. Etiology of recurrent pregnancy losses and outcome of subsequent pregnancies. *Obstet. Gynaecol* 1983; **62**(5): 574–81.

25. Strassmann EO. Fertility and unification of double uterus. *Fertil Steril* 1966; **17**(2): 165–76.

26. DeCherney AH, Russell JB, Graebe RA, Polan ML. (1986) Resectoscopic management of mullerian fusion defects. *Fertil Steril* 1986; **45**(5): 726–8.

27. Saravelos SH, Cocksedge KA, Li TC. Prevalence and diagnosis of congenital uterine anomalies in women with reproductive failure: a critical appraisal. *Hum Reprod Update* 2008; **14**: 415–29.

28. Jurkovic D, Gruboeck K, Tailor A *et al.* Ultrasound screening for congenital uterine anomalies. *Br J Obstet Gynaecol* 1997; **104**: 1320–1.

29. Kirk EP, Chuong CJ, Coulam CB, Williams TJ. Pregnancy after metroplasty for uterine anomalies. *Fertil Steril* 1993; **59**: 1164–8.

30. Emmett TA. Laceration of the cervix uteri as a frequent and unrecognised cause of disease. *Am J Obstet Gynecol* 1874; **7**: 44–6.

31. Shirodkar VN. A new method of operative treatment for habitual abortion in the second trimester. *Antiseptic* 1955; **52**: 299–300.

32. McDonald IA. Suture of the cervix for inevitable miscarriage. *J Obstet Gynaecol Br Emp* 1957; **64**: 346–50.

33. MRC/RCOG Working Party on Cervical Cerclage Final report of the Medical Research Council/Royal College of Obstetricians and Gynaecologists multicentre randomised trial of cervical cerclage. *Br J Obstet Gynaecol* 1993; **100**: 516–23.

34. Althuisius SM, Dekker GA, van Geijn HP, Bekedam DJ, Hummel P. Cervical Incompetence Prevention Randomized Cerclage Trial (CIPRACT): study design and preliminary results. *Am J Obstet Gynecol* 2000; **183**: 823–9.

35. To MS, Alfirevic Z, Heath VCF *et al.* Cervical cerclage for prevention of preterm delivery in women with short cervix: randomised controlled trial. *Lancet* 2004; **363**: 1849–53.

36. Benson RC, Durfee RB. Transabdominal cervico-uterine cerclage during pregnancy for the treatment of cervical incompetence. *Obstet Gynecol* 1965; **25**: 145–55.

37. Farquharson RG, Topping J, Quenby SM. Transabdominal cerclage: the significance of dual pathology and increased preterm delivery. *BJOG* 2005; **112**: 1424–6.

38. Scibetta JJ, Sanko SR, Phipps WR. Laparoscopic transabdominal cervicoisthmic cerclage. *Fertil Steril* 1997; **69**: 161–3.

38. Novy JJ. Transabdominal cervicoisthmic cerclage. A reappraisal 25 years after its introduction. *Am J Obstet Gynecol* 1991; **164**: 1635–42.

39. Lesser KB, Childers JM, Surwit EA. Transabdominal cerclage a laparoscopic approach. *Obstet Gynaecol* 1998; **91**: 855–6

40. Gibb DMF, Salaria DA. Trans-abdominal cervico-isthmic cerclage in the management of recurrent second trimester miscarriage and pre-term delivery. *Br J Obstet Gynaecol* 1995; **102**: 802–6.

41. Anthony GS, Walker RG, Cameron AD *et al.* Transabdominal cervico-isthmic cerclage in the management of cervical incompetence. *Eur J Obstet Gynaecol Reprod Biol* 1997; **72**: 127–30.

42. Topping J, Farquharson RG. Transabdominal cervical cerclage. *Br J Hosp Med* 1995; **54**: 510–12.

43. Topping J, Farquharson RG. Transabdominal cervical cerclage. In *The Yearbook of Obstetrics and Gynaecology*, Vol. 10. London: RCOG Press, 2002, 254–61.

44. Davis G, Berghella V, Talucci M, Wapner RJ. Patients with a prior failed transvaginal cerclage: a comparison of obstetric outcomes either transabdominal or transvaginal cerclage. *Am J Obstet Gynecol* 2000; **183**: 836–9.

45. Zaveri V, Aghajafari F, Amankwah K, Hannah M. Abdominal versus vaginal cerclage after a failed transvaginal cerclage: a systematic review. *Am J Obstet Gynecol* 2002; **187**: 868–72.

# Index